Hereditary Progressive Dystonia

with
Marked Diurnal Fluctuation

Hereditary Progressive Dystonia

with Marked Diurnal Fluctuation

Edited by Masaya Segawa M.D., Ph.D.

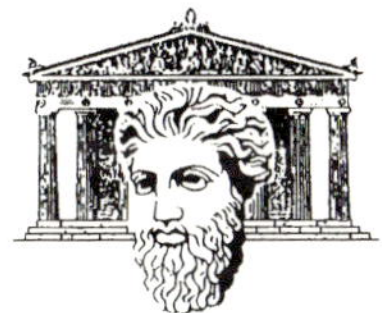

The Parthenon Publishing Group

International Publishers in Medicine, Science & Technology

Casterton Hall, Carnforth,
Lancs, LA6 2LA, UK

One Blue Hill Plaza, Pearl River,
New York 10965, USA

Published in the UK by
The Parthenon Publishing Group Limited
Casterton Hall, Carnforth,
Lancs, LA6 2LA, UK

Published in the USA by
The Parthenon Publishing Group Inc.
One Blue Hill Plaza,
PO Box 1564, Pearl River,
New York 10965, USA

British Library Cataloguing-in-Publication Data
Hereditary progressive dystonia with marked diurnal fluctuation
I. Segawa, M.
616.8

ISBN 1-85070-372-8

Library of Congress Cataloging-in-Publication Data
Hereditary progressive dystonia with marked diurnal fluctuation /
edited by M. Segawa
p. cm
Includes bibliographical references and index.
ISBN 1-85070-372-8
1. Movement disorders in children 2. Dystonia. 3. Parkinsonism.
I. Segawa, M. (Masaya)
[DNLM: 1. Circadian Rhythm. 2. Dystonia–drug therapy.
3. Dystonia–genetics. 4. Parkinson Disease–drug therapy.
6. Parkinson Disease–genetics. WL 359 H5424]
RJ496.M68H47 1992
618.82′74–dc20
DNLM/DLC
for Library of Congress 91-39611
CIP

First published 1993

Phototypesetting by Lasertext Ltd., Manchester
Printed and bound in Great Britain by
Butler & Tanner Ltd., Frome and London

Contents

List of principal contributors ix

Preface xi

Section 1: Clinical characteristics and definition

1 Hereditary progressive dystonia with marked diurnal fluctuation 3
M. Segawa and Y. Nomura

2 Dopa-responsive dystonia: clinical characteristics and definition 21
T.G. Nygaard, B.J. Snow, S. Fahn and D.B. Calne

3 Clinicopathological identification of juvenile parkinsonism in reference to dopa-responsive disorders 37
M. Yokochi

Section 2: Familial parkinsonism dystonia complex: long-term follow-up studies

4 Parkinsonism of early-onset with diurnal fluctuation 51
Y. Yamamura, Y. Hamaguchi, M. Uchida, H. Fujioka and S. Watanabe

5 Idiopathic dystonia-parkinsonism with diurnal fluctuation: a follow-up study and magnetic resonance imaging findings 61
N. Sunohara, K. Ikeda and H. Tomi

Section 3: Intra- and interfamilial variations of hereditary progressive dystonia/dopa-responsive dystonia

6 Intrafamilial and interfamilial variations of symptoms of Japanese hereditary progressive dystonia with marked diurnal fluctuation 73
Y. Nomura and M. Segawa

7 An analysis of North American families with dopa-responsive dystonia 97
T.G. Nygaard

Section 4: Molecular biology

8 Linkage analysis of hereditary progressive dystonia to the tyrosine hydroxylase gene locus 107
S. Tsuji, H. Tanaka, T. Miyatake, E.I. Ginns, Y. Nomura and M. Segawa

Section 5: Tetrahydrobiopterin, dystonia and parkinsonism

9 Neurochemical investigations of dystonia: catecholamine neurotransmitter synthesis 117
P.A. LeWitt

10 Effect of tetrahydrobiopterin and 5-hydroxytryptophan on hereditary progressive dystonia with marked diurnal fluctuation: a suggestion of serotonergic system involvement 125
A. Ishida and G. Takada

11 Tetrahydrobiopterin therapy for juvenile parkinsonism 133
T. Kondo, H. Miwa, Y. Furukawa, Y. Mizuno and H. Narabayashi

Section 6: Clinical neurophysiology of hereditary progressive dystonia, dystonia and parkinsonism

12 Polysomnographical studies on hereditary progressive dystonia with marked diurnal fluctuation 143
M. Segawa and Y. Nomura

13 Deficits in saccadic eye movements in hereditary progressive dystonia with marked diurnal fluctuation 159
O. Hikosaka, H. Fukuda, M. Kato, K. Uetake, Y. Nomura and M. Segawa

Section 7: Neuroimaging: positron-emission tomography scanning

14 Positron–emission tomography scanning in dopa-responsive dystonia, parkinsonism-dystonia and young-onset parkinsonism 181
B.J. Snow, A. Okada, W.R.W. Martin, R.C. Duvoisin and D.B. Calne

Section 8: Role of the subthalamic nucleus in basal ganglia disorders

15 The role of the subthalamic nucleus in parkinsonism: from pathophysiology to novel non-dopaminergic therapeutic approaches 189
J.M. Brotchie, I.J. Mitchell, T.Z. Aziz, M.A. Sambrook and A.R. Crossman

Section 9: General discussion

16 Juvenile parkinsonism with pallidal posture and spastic paraplegia 205
N. Yanagisawa

17 The distinction between early onset idiopathic parkinsonism (juvenile Parkinson disease) and dopa-responsive dystonia (hereditary progressive dystonia, Segawa dystonia) 215
D.B. Calne, T.G. Nygaard and B.J. Snow

18 A case of nigrostriatal dopamine deficiency of juvenile onset 219
H. Narabayashi

Index 227

List of principal contributors

J.M. Brotchie
Experimental Neurology and Myology Gp
Dept. of Cell and Structural Biology
Medical School
University of Manchester
Manchester M13 9PT
UK

D.B. Calne
Dept. of Medicine
University Hospital – UBC Site
2211 Westbrook Mall
Vancouver
BC V6T 1W5
Canada

O. Hikosaka
Segawa Neurological Clinic For Children
2-8 Surugadai Kanda
Chiyoka-ku
Tokyo 101
Japan

A. Ishida
Dept. of Pediatrics
Akita University School of Medicine
1-1-1 Hondo
Akita 010
Japan

T. Kondo
Dept. of Neurology
Juntendo University School of Medicine
2-1-1 Hongo
Bunkyo-ku
Tokyo 113
Japan

P.A. LeWitt
Clinical Neuroscience Program
Sinai Hospital
Detroit
Michigan
USA

H. Narabayashi
Neurological Clinic
5-12-8 Nakameguro
Meguro-ku
Tokyo 153
Japan

Y. Nomura
Segawa Neurological Clinic for Children
2–8 Surugadai Kanda
Chiyoda-ku
Tokyo 101
Japan

T.G. Nygaard
Dept. of Neurology
Columbia-Presbyterian Medical Center
710 West 168th Street
New York
NY 10032
USA

M. Segawa
Segawa Neurological Clinic For Children
2-8 Surugadai Kanda
Chiyoda-ku
Tokyo 101
Japan

B.J. Snow
Dept. of Medicine
University Hospital UBC Site
2211 Westbrook Mall
Vancouver
BC V6T 1W5
Canada

N. Sunohara
Dept. of Neurology
National Center of Neurology and Psychiatry
4-1-1 Ogawa-Higashi-Machi
Kodaira
Tokyo 187
Japan

S. Tsuji
Dept. of Neurology
Brain Research Institute
Niigata University
1 Asahimachi-dori
Niigata 951
Japan

Y. Yamamura
Third Dept. of Internal Medicine
Hiroshima University School of Medicine
Kasumi 1-2-3
Minamiku
Hiroshima 734
Japan

N. Yanagisawa
Dept. of Medicine (Neurology)
Shinshu University School of Medicine
Asahi 3-1-1
Matsumoto 390
Japan

M. Yokochi
Dept. of Neurology
Tokyo Metropolitan Institute for Neurosciences
2-6 Musashidai Fuchu City
Tokyo
Japan

Preface

Hereditary progressive dystonia with marked diurnal fluctuation is a dystonia which has a marked and sustained response to levodopa.

My recognition of this disorder started in February, 1970, when a 5-year, 10-month-old girl was brought to me at the outpatient clinic of the Pediatric Department of Tokyo University Hospital. Her parents complained of her gait disturbance with slowness in movement and clumsiness in skilful hand movements, which had started around 4 years of age and had had a progressive course. These symptoms were said to have improved almost completely in the morning after sleep. The diurnal fluctuation of symptoms manifested as fatigue and eagerness to take a 'nap' in the late afternoon; the latter improved the symptoms, though only mildly. Clinical and surface electromyographical evaluations of the symptoms showed rigid hypertonus, and dysdiadochokinesis, and the gait disturbance was revealed to be due to the disturbance of reciprocal innervation of the agonist and antagonist muscles. It was also shown that the symptoms were aggravated towards the evening, even though she was kept in bed all day. Thus, the diurnal fluctuation appeared to depend on the longevity of the awake period and not the amount of physical activity. Therefore, I considered this to be a disorder of the central nervous system, probably with lesions in the basal ganglia causing parkinsonian symptoms towards the evening, and I supposed the pathogenesis to be disturbances in the dopamine transmission at the basal ganglia. Levodopa was administered to her and soon the marked response supported the above conjectures.

Meanwhile, two more cases were found, one a female cousin of the first case and the other a girl, whose brother and female cousins also had a similar disease. My experience with these cases led me to consider this as a particular inherited disorder. It was easily differentiated from Hunt disease and Hallervorden–Spatz disease. As there was no resting tremor or cogwheel rigidity, even in the aggravated state in the evening, I supposed that this disorder had a different pathophysiology from the classical Parkinson disease. So, in 1971, I reported this as a new disorder with the term 'hereditary basal ganglia disorder with marked diurnal fluctuation'. However, it was not certain whether this childhood-onset disorder developed into Parkinson disease in adulthood, or whether it was different from the familial juvenile Parkinson disease with diurnal fluctuation of symptoms reported in the pre-dopa era in Japan. Actually, at around this time, Dr Yamamura and his colleagues reported familial dopa responsive cases of juvenile Parkinson disease whose symptoms alleviated after sleep.

At the same time, I experienced the fourth case, a 3-year, 7-month-old girl. This patient was an important and very informative case, not only because she was the earliest onset case of our series at 16 months of age, but also because she had two family members who were affected – one her uncle and the other her grandmother. The former case, a 12-year-old boy who had become institutionalized in a home for handicapped children, was actually my first case, whom I had diagnosed, however, as spastic paraplegia. The latter was a 51-year-old woman with a clinical course of 43 years, who showed dystonia as the main symptom, which was apparently different from classical Parkinson disease. After becoming acquainted with this case, we confirmed that the disorder was not Parkinson disease but dystonia, and diagnosed the case as 'hereditary progressive dystonia with marked diurnal fluctuation' (HPD) in 1975, and implicated autosomal dominant inheritance with low penetrance.

The polysomnographical examinations of this disorder, which started from around 1972, were useful in detecting the pathogenesis of HPD and for the pathophysiological differentiation of HPD from other basal ganglia diseases.

After recognition of the report of McGeer and McGeer, I considered the age variation of the dopamine neuron in relation to the pathophysiology of HPD, and suggested HPD as the terminal disorder of the nigrostriatal dopamine neuron. Furthermore, subsequent to our follow-up studies of childhood cases into adulthood, and after examining some affected parents with onset after childhood, I demarcated hereditary progressive dystonia as a disease entity, different from the juvenile parkinsonism (JPA) reported by Dr Yokochi and from the parkinsonism–dystonia complex, although some of these cases had shown diurnal fluctuation of symptoms as reported by Dr Sunohara. However, not all of the dystonia cases who responded to levodopa had the clinical characteristics of HPD; some showed no diurnal fluctuation, some action dystonia and others did not show a complete response to levodopa, or showed unfavourable side-effects.

In 1988 Dr Nygaard and his colleagues collected cases with dystonia responsive to levodopa under the definition of dopa-responsive dystonia (DRD) including all dystonias that responded to levodopa other than HPD.

There has been no autopsy case of HPD and no definite biological markers to differentiate HPD from JPA and the parkinsonism–dystonia complex. It is not clear whether HPD and DRD are the same or whether the former is a disease included in a group of dystonias which respond to levodopa. At this symposium, we discussed the clinical characteristics of these basal ganglia disorders that develop within a certain age-period from childhood to adulthood and the criteria of HPD or DRD. The pathophysiologies of these disorders were also discussed from the standpoints of clinical neurophysiology and neuro-imaging. The putative roles of biopterin in the pathogenesis were also reported. Possible components of the striatum related to the pathophysiology of certain symptoms of movement disorders including dystonia were also discussed. The description of a putative case of juvenile parkinsonism (Yokochi type III) by Yanagisawa was one of the highlights of this symposium, because the pathology of this case is familiar all over the world as having identical features to Parkinson disease. I think that the precise information on the clinical features of this case, and the fact that her brother has identical clinical characteristics will help understanding, not only the pathophysiology of this young onset dopa-responsive basal ganglia disorder but also those of HPD/DRD and juvenile parkinsonism.

From these discussions it has been clarified that hereditary progressive dystonia and dopa-responsive dystonia are different entities from Parkinson disease and juvenile parkinsonism. Some HPDs and DRDs are shown to occur at adult ages while some juvenile parkinsonism cases have clinical onset in childhood. However, the answers to the question of why HPD has dystonia as the main clinical feature throughout the course of the illness (while juvenile parkinsonism develops parkinsonian symptoms as the dominant features in the second decade) and why HPD shows a complete and sustained response to levodopa (while juvenile parkinsonism shows levodopa-induced side-effects soon after its administration even though they start with dystonia in childhood) are left for further study.

Masaya Segawa
Director, Segawa Neurological Clinic for Children
Tokyo

Acknowledgements

The symposium on 'Hereditary Progressive Dystonia with Marked Diurnal Fluctuation' was held in Tokyo, Japan on November 11, 1990 as the Satellite Symposium to the Joint Convention of the 5th International Child Neurology Congress and the 3rd Asian and Oceanian Congress of Child Neurology.

First and foremost I wish to extend my deep gratitude to the participants, both from abroad and in Japan, for their valuable contributions (of time and information) that made this symposium and publication possible. I would also like to express my sincere appreciation to the Foundation for the Advancement of International Sciences, Tokyo, for sponsoring this meeting and publication of the proceedings.

SECTION 1

Clinical characteristics and definition

1

Hereditary progressive dystonia with marked diurnal fluctuation

M. Segawa and Y. Nomura

INTRODUCTION

Hereditary progressive dystonia with marked diurnal fluctuation (HPD) is characterized by aggravation of symptoms towards evening and their alleviation in the morning after sleep, and marked and sustained response to levodopa. Since our first report[1] more than 70 cases have been reported from Japan and other countries, including our personally reported cases. In this paper we review the characteristics of HPD and demarcate this disorder in basal ganglia diseases.

CLINICAL CHARACTERISTICS OF OUR CASES

Our 18 cases include 12 familial cases from six families and six sporadic cases. There is marked sex preference for females (the female-to-male ratio for all our cases is 15:3; for familial cases, 11:1, and sporadic cases, 4:2). This disorder develops insidiously in a normal child without any episodes which cause chronic dopaminergic dysfunction.

Age of onset of the clinical symptoms ranges from 1 to 11 years with an average of 6.03 ± 2.82 years. There is a slight difference between averages of familial (6.12 ± 2.97 years) and sporadic cases (5.85 ± 2.73 years), and between female (6.10 ± 2.91 years) and male cases (5.60 ± 2.78 years). The initial symptoms in most cases are fatigability and gait disturbance due to leg dystonia, with flexion-inversion of one foot (pes equinovarus). However, cases with later onset, at around 10 years of age, may present dystonia in one arm with flexion-pronation of the elbow and palmar-flexion of the wrist and may sometimes be associated with postural tremor of fingers. These symptoms are aggravated or become apparent towards the evening and are markedly alleviated or completely disappear in the morning after sleep.

The symptoms progress gradually, spread to other extremities and, within 5 or 6 years, all limbs become involved. Some cases show an orderly sequence following the shape of letter 'N'[2].

The basic symptom is postural dystonia which becomes apparent when a sitting or standing position is adopted, and is aggravated by voluntary movements or psychological tension. When the patient is standing, the posture appears to be similar to spastic paraplegia with lumbar lordosis, flexion of the hips and hyperextension of the knee joints being marked on the more affected side. In some cases, flexor posture of the trunk, similar to 'pallidal posture', develops when the patient is sitting on the floor or standing with support. However, no cases show action dystonia or axial torsion. Neck muscle involvement is mild with minimal retrocollis; no cases show torticollis.

Neurological examinations reveal rigidity in the affected muscles. In the initial stage, rigidity appears to depend on the postures and movements. In the advanced stage, it is observed constantly, but is not plastic rigidity; thus by repeating stretch reflexes, rigid hypertonus can be occasionally abolished and proves to be hypotonic. The Westphal phenomenon is observed in most cases, particularly in the advanced stage. Postural tremor may become apparent after 10 years of age or later, and in some cases, it appears in the 4th decade of life[2,3]. However, no case shows parkinsonian resting tremor or intention tremor. The pseudo-Babinski posture is observed occasionally, depending on the posture and voluntary movements that require mental tension or skilfulness. Dysdiadochokinesis is observed in all cases, but finger-nose and knee-heel tests are normal in most cases.

The gait is rigid with marked dystonic posture of the extremities, and lumbar lordosis is present. Coordinated movements of the arms are impaired in the affected side in the early stage, but they disappear on both sides in advanced stages. However, no cases show claw-hand and claw-toe posture or petit pas of parkinsonism. No cases show difficulty in crawling. Although in the advanced stage, there is flexor posture in the legs, the pattern of crawling is normal with the swing phase initiated by the legs[4]. Slowness in movement is observed in all cases and later becomes bradykinetic. Pulsion is observed in advanced cases, but it is mild, and none of the cases shows the freezing phenomenon. The face is expressionless and later becomes masklike. In advanced cases, dysarthria may be observed.

The deep tendon reflexes are exaggerated, particularly in the legs. In some, ankle clonus is observed. The pseudo-Babinski reaction, striatal foot, is also detected, but the plantar response is flexor. The tilting reaction is affected, particularly on the side ipsilateral to the more affected limbs. There is no restriction in the ocular movements. The optic fundi are normal, and there is no Kayser-Fleischer ring present. There are no abnormalities in the cerebellum, in the sensory system or in the mental and psychological activities.

The main clinical feature is dystonia which persists throughout the course of the illness. In advanced stages, the symptoms are more marked in the legs, even in cases whose initial symptoms were in the arms. At severely advanced stages, pes equinovarus contracture may develop. The asymmetry, with left-side predominance, is also observed throughout the course of the disease (ratio of left to right, 11 : 7). The diurnal fluctuation becomes less evident with the progression of the disease, when marked generalized dystonia is observed even in the morning.

In a patient (SS) with a clinical course of 43 years without medical treatment, walking became impossible around 15 years of age, eight years after the onset, but from the third decade, the progression of symptoms became less apparent. After the 4th decade, it became almost static with attenuation of the diurnal fluctuation, and postural tremor appeared[2,3,5].

The whole clinical course of dystonia can be observed even in the early stage with the diurnal fluctuation of symptoms. However, the postural tremor does not appear even in the evening at younger ages. In cases with clinical onset after ten years of age the symptoms are milder, or not complete, and the progression is slow. Affected parents also have a milder course than their children.

CASES REPORTED

Up to now, more than 70 cases have been reported in Japan and other countries, under the name of HPD or dopa-responsive dystonia. However, among them there are cases which seem to be different from 'classical' HPD, either in symptoms or in the pattern of response to levodopa (see below). Excluding these, 44 remain as typical or classical cases, 20 from Japan and 24 from other countries. Most of the cases showed initiation of symptoms with dystonia of one leg in the first decade of life (Japanese, 6.2 ± 2.0 years; other countries, 4.7 ± 2.4 years). They showed female predominance (Japanese, 16:4; other countries, 18:6), and side preference to the left in cases where laterality of the symptoms is described (Japanese, 13:5; other countries, 4:2).

Most Japanese cases showed shorter body length than average, which became manifest with the onset of dystonia, but increased to normal range after levodopa[6,7].

INVESTIGATION

Surface EMG reveals nonreciprocal tonic involuntary activity. In aged cases, grouping discharges and tonic stretch reflexes are observed, often with the Westphal phenomenon.

Polysomnography (PSG) revealed particular abnormalities in the phasic component of sleep while the tonic component remained normal[2,6,8]. As the results were uniform among cases and showed no interlaboratory differences[9], these findings are helpful for detecting the pathophysiology of HPD and will be described precisely in another chapter in this monograph.

Examination of voluntary saccade in HPD revealed slow and hypometric anticipatory saccade, similar to Parkinson disease[10]. The results of recent examinations are reported by O. Hikosaka.

Estimation of catecholamine metabolites in CSF revealed low levels of homovanillic acid (HVA)[11–13] and they were lower in the morning than in the afternoon[12,13]. Maekawa and colleagues[14] showed similar results in a sporadic female case with HPD. They also estimated the levels of 3-methoxy-4-hydroxyphenylglycol (MHPG) and 5-hydroxyindolacetic acid (5HIAA) and revealed similar diurnal fluctuations as with HVA, though the level in the morning was below normal in MHPG, while it was within normal range in 5HIAA[14]. The levels of dopamine and dopa in plasma after oral administration of levodopa show a particular time course in correlation with the age of the patients[3].

Brain computerized tomography scan and magnetic resonance imaging were normal in our group. We have made no personal studies on positron emission tomography (PET) scans but according to investigations reported in the literature PET scans revealed decreased absorption of 18-fluorodopa in the left putamen of an 11-year-old dominantly inherited case, but those of a 34-year-old sporadic case were normal[15]. In this monograph Dr Snow and his colleagues present their recent studies showing normal PET scans in HPD.

No abnormalities were observed in the levels of serum ceruloplasmin, copper, copper excretion in urine or serum levels of pyruvate and lactic acid. The routine laboratory examination results were normal.

TREATMENT

In most cases, a dose of 20 mg/kg per day of levodopa without inhibitor alleviates symptoms completely. In a few cases, choreic movements were induced by a rapid increase of dosage or by erroneous administration of a double dose of levodopa, but these symptoms were quickly eliminated by reducing the dose[3]. In triplet patients, early levodopa showed better effects[16]. However, the study of eight patients who had been treated with levodopa for more than 10 years[3] revealed that in HPD, the effects of levodopa persisted without unfavorable side-effects and that the dosage could later be reduced. Patient SS, who was started on levodopa at the age of 51 years, became ambulant within 3 days under treatment with 600 mg levodopa, after a 36-year inambulant period[3]. She is now 70 years of age and is completely normal under a 50–100 mg Sinemet® treatment (Figure 1).

However, in patients who were started on levodopa in childhood, periods of subjective feelings of ineffectiveness developed, and further increases in dosage were necessary[3]. These feelings occurred in the leg in which the first symptoms occurred, but were without objective signs except in one case. This feature occurred from 2 months to 8.6 years (mean 4.2 ± 3.0 years) after the start of levodopa treatment, but this period was age-dependent, and showed development at ages from 11.7 to 14.7 years (mean 12.8 ± 1.2 years). This feature was not observed in those whose levodopa treatments were started after the mid-teens. This feeling of ineffectiveness was alleviated by increasing the dosage of levodopa up to 30 mg/kg per day, and in some cases by additional administration of a decarboxylase inhibitor. Polysomnography (PSG) performed during the period of this feeling of ineffectiveness revealed a decrease in the number of tonic movements in the muscle concerned. However, there were no abnormalities in the other parameters, including the sleep-stage-dependent modulation of gross movements[3].

In HPD, the time course of plasma dopa after administration of levodopa (without decarboxylase inhibitor) showed marked variation according to

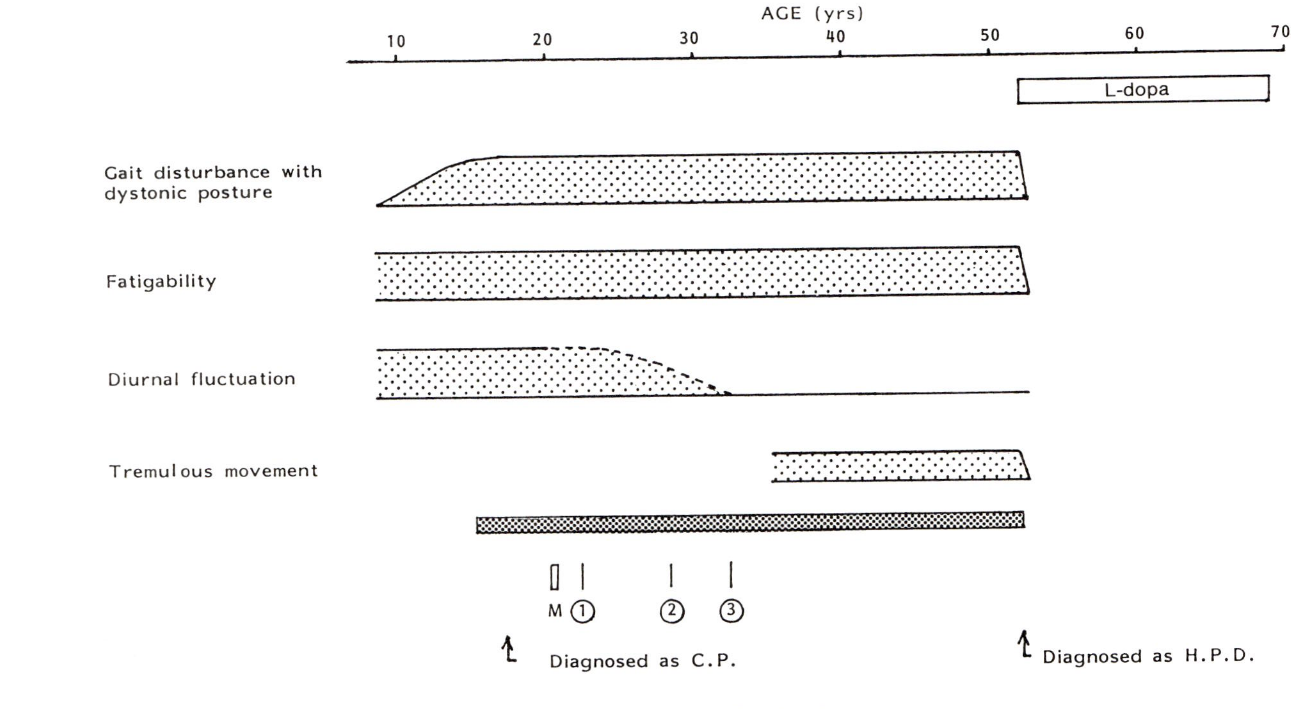

Figure 1 Clinical course of patient SS. Reproduced by kind permission from Segawa, M. (1990). Long-term effects of L-dopa on hereditary progressive dystonia with marked diurnal fluctuation. In Berardelli, R., Benecke, R., Manfredi, M. and Marsden, C.D. (eds.) Motor Disturbances II. (London: Academic Press)

age; that is patients under 12 years of age revealed low levels, while in those over 12 years, the levels increased significantly, even with the same doses of levodopa. Patients with feelings of ineffectiveness showed the pattern of childhood even in adolescence[3].

An anticholinergic drug had a marked and prolonged effect[17,18], but did not afford complete relief, either clinically or polysomnographically, and complete recovery was obtained after replacing it with levodopa[3]. Bromocriptine was also effective but did not afford complete relief[19]. Tetrahydrobiopterin (BH_4) treatment was attempted in HPD patients[20–22], but thus far, levodopa has shown more favorable effects than BH_4, except for one case described by Ishida and colleagues[22].

INHERITANCE

We speculate that HPD comes from autosomal dominant inheritance with low penetrance[6], but recessive inheritance is also suspected[11,12,23]. Thus, no substantial data exist yet for deciding the mode of inheritance. However, cases suggesting recessive inheritance have different clinical features from HPD and may belong to a different category (see below).

DIFFERENTIAL DIAGNOSIS

As for differential diagnosis, movement disorders which develop in childhood with gait disturbance and limb dystonia are taken into consideration. They are Wilson disease, Hallervorden–Spatz disease, hereditary spastic paraplegia and cerebral palsy. HPD is often misdiagnosed as hereditary spastic paraplegia and some patients are initially diagnosed as Duchenne muscular dystrophy, psychological reaction or hysteria. However, the differentiation of HPD from these disorders is rather easy if clinical and laboratory examinations are performed carefully.

On the other hand, differentiation from other types of dystonia and juvenile parkinsonism is important not only for making a precise diagnosis but also for demarcating HPD and considering the pathophysiology of each disorder.

Differentiation from other dystonias

Idiopathic torsion dystonia (ITD) and dystonia with action dystonia vs. HPD

HPD is differentiated from idiopathic torsion dystonia and dystonia with action dystonia by clinical characteristics with lack of axial torsion or action dystonia and the marked and sustained response to levodopa. To clarify the pathophysiological significance of these clinical features, the main characteristic features of clinical and laboratory findings in HPD are correlated with those of symptomatic torsion dystonia and action dystonia (Table 1).

Clinically, cases with torsion dystonia differ from HPD in the pattern of involvement of the sternocleidomastoid (SCM) and muscles of the extremities, that is, the side of the SCM dominantly affected is contralateral to that of the limb muscles in HPD, while it is ipsilateral in cases with axial torsion[24,25]. Brain computerized tomography scans of symptomatic torsion dystonia showed high or low density areas in the putamen, the globus pallidus or the striatum[26]. Studies on neuropathology, or the visual diagnosis of symptomatic torsion dystonia, have revealed the lesion to be in the striatum or the globus pallidus[26]. These findings indicate that the lesion of idiopathic torsion dystonia is in the basal ganglia, the striatum or the globus pallidus. These features were confirmed by PSG[24,25] (see Chapter 12). On the other hand, in cases with Parkinson disease having asymmetrical involvement, the side of the SCM dominantly affected is contralateral to that of the extremities[27]. Thus it is suggested that the lesion of HPD exists in the presynaptic portion of the basal ganglia or in the nigrostriatal dopamine (DA) neurons as in Parkinson disease, and that is not in the basal ganglia, postsynaptic to the nigrostriatal DA neurons as in ITD.

The difference in the locus of the lesion in the nigrostriatal system between ITD and HPD causes the difference in the side of involvement of the SCM to that of the extremities, and shows the symptomatic difference with or without axial torsion. ITD with the lesion in the basal ganglia, consequently, responds poorly to levodopa.

On the other hand, involvement of a neuronal system other than the nigrostriatal system is suspected in the pathophysiology of ITD. In cases with ITD the decrease of 3-methoxy-4-hydroxyphenylglycol in the cerebrospinal fluid has been reported[28] and lesions in the brainstem serotonergic and noradrenergic neurons were demonstrated by PSG[29], and in an autopsied case decreases in noradrenaline and serotonin, as well as dopamine, were detected in the telencephalon, mesencephalon and most areas of the brainstem[30]. Our PSG studies also revealed findings indicating the involvement of noradrenergic and serotonergic neurons of the brainstem as well as the nigrostriatal DA neurons. This evidence implicates the noradrenergic neurons as having a role in the pathophysiology of ITD.

Table 1 Characteristic clinical and laboratory findings of HPD and symptomatic dystonia with action dystonia or axial torsion. (C denotes a clinical finding; PSG, polysomnographic; CT, computerized tomography; MRI, magnetic resonance imaging)

	HPD	*Action dystonia*	*Torsion dystonia*
Postural dystonia (C)	+	+ or −	+
Action dystonia (C)	−	+	+ or −
Axial torsion (C)	−	+ or −	+
Side of sternocleidomastoid dominantly involved and extremities (C, PSG)	Contralateral	Contra- or ipsilateral	Ipsilateral
Response to levodopa (C)	+ + +	+ + or −	− or ±
Synaptic supersensitivity (PSG)	−	+	+ or −
Involvement of the basal ganglia (CT, MRI)	−	− or +	+

In the polysomnographical study of a patient whose symptoms were quite similar to HPD, except for having action retrocollis, a particular abnormality in the pattern of gross movements was observed with a decrease in the rate of occurrence of gross movements in the rapid-eye-movements (REM) stage[25]. This pattern was quite different from that observed in HPD and suggested the existence of a synaptic supersensitivity of the nigrostriatal DA receptors[24]. Similar abnormalities in polysomnography were also observed in other patients with action dystonia and also in patients with oculogyric crisis[24]. Thus the presence of action dystonia or oculogyric crisis suggests the existence of synaptic supersensitivity of the DA receptors, and cases with either symptom imply a pathophysiology different from that of HPD[24,25]. Unsteady or poor response to levodopa, sometimes with aggravation of symptoms, observed in cases with action dystonia or oculogyric crisis is assumed to be due to this modulation of receptors.

Dopa-responsive dystonia vs. HPD

Dopa-responsive dystonias or dystonias that respond to levodopa are a heterogeneous group including various disorders with different clinical features from HPD. That is, there are patients without diurnal fluctuation of symptoms[31,32] (Deonna[23], cases 10, 11, 14–18; Gordon[33], case 1; Rondot and Ziegler[34], cases 1–3); cases without the description of the fluctuation[36–9], cases that seemed to have focal or segmental dystonia[40]; cases with action dystonia, such as action retrocollis or oculogyric crisis[31,32,34,38]; cases that developed the on-and-off phenomenon after levodopa[34,41,42]; cases in whom the effects of levodopa were incomplete or did not last for long (Hirasawa and colleagues[41], case 1; Fink and colleagues[43], cases 3 and 4), and one case in whom a high dose of levodopa was necessary[44]. Case 1 of Hirasawa and colleagues[41] might have been suffering from juvenile parkinsonism, because the features of response to levodopa had the characteristics of juvenile parkinsonism reported by Yokochi[45], and also this patient's elder sister was diagnosed as having type 1 of Yokochi's series[45]. Cases 3 and 4 of Fink's report[43] might have had biopterin deficiency because of the incomplete response to levodopa and the steady progressive course.

When considering the differential diagnosis between dopa-responsive dystonia and HPD the most debatable symptom is diurnal fluctuation. Not all cases of dopa-responsive dystonia have diurnal fluctuation of symptoms[23,46,47]. Among those without diurnal fluctuation or without the description of this symptom, some might nevertheless have HPD because family members have typical HPD (Deonna[23], cases 10, 11), or because they have other characteristics of HPD[21,36,37]. However, others might be different because of an incomplete response to levodopa, with or without unfavorable side-effects[33,34,39,48–51], having action dystonia[31,32,34], resting tremor[35], oculogyric crisis[31,32,38] or an early bulbar involvement (Deonna[23], cases 14–18). Among cases with diurnal fluctuation, those with oculogyric crisis[34] (Nygaard and colleagues[46], case 1), torticollis[52] or on-and-off phenomenon[42] (also Hirasawa and colleagues[41], case 1) could be different from HPD.

Dystonia caused by biopterin deficiency differs from HPD, with relatively poor response to levodopa, and necessitates adding biopterin. Clinically these cases show symmetrical involvement with lack of interlimb coordination. However, the case reported by Ishida[22], with the characteristic features of HPD, suggests involvement of the serotonergic system other than dopamine and indicates the role of biopterin in HPD as the common co-factor.

Dopa-responsive dystonias with different features from HPD tend to affect siblings suggesting recessive inheritance, while those having identical or almost the same features as HPD have transgeneration patients.

Juvenile parkinsonism vs. HPD

Among cases reported as juvenile Parkinson disease or parkinsonism (JPA) or Parkinson-dystonia complex, some patients developed symptoms before the age of 10 years[35] or had diurnal fluctuation of symptoms[53,54]. However, they differ from HPD with parkinsonism resting tremor[35], movement-related fatigability[54] and the progressive course with decrease in responsiveness to levodopa[53]. (see T. Muroga *et al.* (1988). *Shinkei–Naika–Chiryo*, **5**, 339)

Yokochi[45] and Narabayashi and colleagues[55] classified JPA into two types: one having clinical symptoms similar to classical idiopathic Parkinson disease, and the other with dystonia as the main symptom throughout the course of the illness. Recently, Quinn and colleagues[56] documented the same results. The present author has termed the former group tremor-type JPA and the latter dystonic-type JPA, and demonstrated their difference from HPD[2,5,8] (see Table 2).

Comparing with Yokochi's studies[45], tremor-type JPA is easily differentiated from HPD by the age of onset (29.7 ± 6.9 years), parkinsonian resting tremor, and readier development of the up-and-down phenomenon and dyskinesia after levodopa. This type of JPA shows no sex preference, marked pulsion with freezing and difficulty in crawling with total flexor posture[4]. Dystonic-type JPA (group III of Yokochi[45]) has the age of onset as 11.9 ± 4.3 years, slightly but significantly older than that of HPD; differs from HPD in male predominance (female-to-male ratio is 1:7), and has a tendency towards the up-and-down phenomenon and dyskinesia after levodopa.

There are families in which HPD coexists with torsion dystonia with poor response to levodopa[57], parkinsonism with onset in the fourth decade of life[58], or Yokochi's group III, or dystonic-type, JPA[59]. The latter might be JPA because it suggests recessive inheritance. Nomoto and colleagues[58] describe patients with parkinsonism, grand-aunts of a patient with HPD, who showed mild dystonia and postural tremor which responded markedly to relatively low doses of levodopa, and were thought to be cases of late-onset HPD with mild or abortive symptoms. Since late-onset cases of HPD are always mild and abortive, the Sterk and Kellermann patients[57] are quite exceptional, suggesting the probability of a combination of different pathophysiologies in one family.

Table 2 Clinical characteristics of HPD and JPA

Characteristic	*HPD* ($n = 18$)	*Dystonic-type JPA* ($n = 8$)	*Tremor-type JPA* ($n = 32$)
Age of onset (years)	6.03 ± 2.82	11.88 ± 4.26	29.65 ± 6.90
Sex (F : M)	15 : 3	1 : 7	14 : 18
Familial occurrence	12/18 (67%)	4/8 (50%)	13/32 (41%)
Initial signs	gait disturbance, fatigability, flexion-inversion of foot	gait disturbance, dystonic posture of foot	tremor, gait disturbance
Clinical symptoms			
dystonia	+ +	+ +	+
tremor	+ later, postural, 8–10 Hz	− or ±, postural > resting	+ +, resting > postural
pyramidal signs	−	+	±
asymmetry	+	+	+
diurnal fluctuation	+ +	− or +	−
progression	slow, later static	slow	slow
Effects of levodopa	excellent	excellent	excellent, not marked
Levodopa-induced dyskinesia	−	+	+ (levodopa-responsive case)

PATHOPHYSIOLOGY AND POSSIBLE PATHOLOGY

As there have been no autopsy cases, the pathophysiology of HPD must be speculative, using characteristic features observed in clinical and laboratory examinations, which are illustrated in Table 3.

The dramatic and sustained response to levodopa without unfavorable side-effects implies that HPD is a functional disorder in which the lesions are restricted to the nigrostriatal DA neurons. Early-onset extrapyramidal disorders appear as dystonia. The onset of dystonia in the first decade of life generally shows as leg dystonia[60]. This means that the clinical characteristics of HPD are correlated with the age of onset in the first decade. So the pathophysiology of HPD should be considered with reference to the importance of this particular age for the DA neurons, that is, the age variation of the dopamine system.

The tyrosine hydroxylase (TH) of the human striatum, has high activity levels in infancy and decreases its levels with age[61]. The decrement is marked in childhood, moderate in adolescence and therafter attenuated to reach the base levels around the middle of the third decade. On the other hand, TH in the substantia nigra shows no significant age variation, but the number of cells decreases with age, especially after 25 years of age[62].

The age of onset of HPD corresponds to the period of marked age variation of the TH activity of the striatum[61,62], that is, the terminal of the nigrostriatal DA neurons. The clinical course of HPD, that is, a marked progression in childhood with later attenuation in the third decade of life and becoming almost static after the fourth decade exactly follows the age-related decline curve of striatal TH activity.

TH activity in the rat striatum showed a circadian oscillation of increment in the daytime (resting period) and decrement in the night (active period), but TH of the substantia nigra showed no circadian oscillation[61]. In polysomnographic studies, the nocturnal variation of symptoms, with alleviation towards morning of the pattern of rolling over, was detected[63]. Thus the marked diurnal fluctuation (aggravation) as well as the nocturnal fluctuation (alleviation) of symptoms in HPD are thought to reflect the circadian oscillation of the striatal TH activity observed in the rat brain[61].

It is suggested then that the main lesion of HPD is at the terminal of the

Table 3 Clinical and laboratory findings which indicate the pathophysiology of HPD

Age of onset in the first decade
Diurnal fluctuation
Progression in the first two decades
Postural dystonia without axial torsion or action dystonia
Crawling preserved
Marked sustained response to levodopa
No levodopa-responsive side-effects
Side preference
Female predominance
Abnormal voluntary saccade
Particular PSG findings restricted to phasic components

nigrostriatal DA neurons with a decrease in TH activities[2,8]. A similar pathophysiology is suspected in dystonic-type JPA, while in the tremor-type JPA, the main lesion may be in the substantia nigra[2,8] since its age of onset corresponds to the period of cell loss in the structure[61]. Two autopsied cases, one dystonic- and the other tremor-type JPA[64], support this suggestion[2].

The nigrostriatal DA neurons manifest their activities via the basal ganglia. It is therefore necessary to consider the components in the basal ganglia, and particularly their involvement in developing the characteristic symptoms of HPD.

The basal ganglia modulate locomotion via the pedunculo-pontine-nuclei (PPN) with two efferents: one from the substantia nigra pars reticulata (SNr) and the other from the medial segment of the globus pallidus (MGP)[65]. For the development of levodopa-induced dyskinesia, an indirect projection of the striatum, that is, putamen–lateral segment of the globus pallidus (LGP)–subthalamic nucleus (STN)–MGP, which is connected to the thalamic nuclei, is thought to play an important role[66]. The involvement of the ventral lateral nuclei of the thalamus in levodopa-induced dyskinesia has also been demonstrated by the effects of stereotaxic thalamotomy[67]. For voluntary saccadic movement, the caudate nucleus (CN)–SNr–superior colliculus pathway is involved[68] and the same pathway seems to play a role for modulation of REMs during the REM stage[5,24,69]. Gross movements during sleep are thought to be modulated by the pallidofugal thalamic pathway from the MGP and twitch movements by the striatofugal descending pathway, probably via the SNr[24].

Correlation of clinical and laboratory findings of HPD to this evidence implicates the pathophysiology of the neural connection in the basal ganglia related to the affected nigrostriatal DA neurons.

Abnormalities of the voluntary saccade observed in electro-oculography and those of tonic movements and REMs in polysomnography suggest the involvement of the projection of the striatum to the SNr. The abnormal modulation of gross movements in polysomnography implies the involvement of the intra-basal ganglia pathway which is connected to the pallidofugal thalamic pathway from the MGP to the thalamus. But this involvement might be mild as the abnormalities of gross movements are mild and show no remission, once improved after levodopa[3]. On the other hand, the indirect striatal projection might not be involved because levodopa-induced dyskinesia is not observed in HPD. Of the pathways modulating locomotion the MGP–PPN pathway might at least be spared for the normal preservation of locomotive movements. These intrastriatal structures *per se* have to be preserved and postsynaptic supersensitivity might not exist at DA receptors of the striatum. The former is suggested by the lack of axial torsion, marked and sustained responsiveness to levodopa clinically, and the preservation of dopa-acetylcholine interaction observed in polysomnographic examination. The latter is suggested clinically by the absence of action dystonia or of oculogyric crisis, and sustained favorable response to levodopa, and polysomnographically by the absence of a particular modulation of gross movements suggesting synaptic supersensitivity[24,25].

The importance of the direct pathway in the pathophysiology of dystonia has been shown in the neuropathological examination of rigid-type Huntington disease[70]. Estimation of a 2-deoxyglucose autoradiograph in the nucleus of the basal ganglia in the 1-methyl-4-phenyl-1,2,3,6-tetrahydropyridine (MPTP) monkeys revealed 'hot spots' in the lateral segments of the globus pallidus, the specific nuclei of the thalamus and the PPN[66,71]. In cases with levodopa-induced dyskinesia, hot spots were observed in the STN but not in the thalamus or PPN, while in cases with levodopa-induced dystonia, no hot spots were observed in these nuclei[71]. These data cast doubt on the roles of the indirect pathway and the input and output pathways to the MGP in dystonia. It suggests a difference in pathophysiology between dystonia and parkinsonism or Parkinson disease: the former involves the direct pathway mainly to the SNr and the latter both direct and indirect pathways. Sparing of the PPN in the former condition might be related to the preservation of the locomotive activity in dystonia.

Side preference might be a reflection of physiologic asymmetry in the activity of the basal ganglia observed in human autopsies[72]. The abnormal direction of REMs with leftward preference[2,69] also implies that the asymmetry of symptoms depends on the functional asymmetry of the nigrostriatal DA neurons.

Results of polysomnography in HPD fail to show the involvement of the noradrenergic and serotonergic neurons of the brainstem. On the other hand clinicopharmacological evidence[22] and cerebrospinal fluid data[14] suggest the involvement of monoamine neurons other than dopamine.

Female predominance of HPD, in contrast to male predominance in dystonic-type JPA, may prove to be pathognomonic, when the reverse sex preferences observed in disorders with exaggerated DA transmission are compared (that is, male predominance of Gilles de la Tourette syndrome with onset in childhood, and female predominance of Sydenham chorea with onset in adolescence). This evidence, with the age-related alteration in the time course of plasma dopa after oral levodopa, suggests the alteration in modulation of the striatal DA activity between the first and second decades of life.

The mode of inheritance of HPD is suggested as being dominant with low penetrance. This implies that the enzyme deficiency or the degeneration process is unlikely to be the pathogenesis. The gene study of the locus of tyrosine hydroxylase showed negative results.

HPD is a particular disorder different from JPA or Parkinson disease. Among levodopa-responsive dystonias, this disease is defined as an early-onset postural dystonia with diurnal fluctuation of symptoms, and might be demarcated as a dominantly inherited type. As for the pathophysiology, the main lesion is the reduction of the activity of the terminals of the nigrostriatal DA neurons connected to the striatofugal pathway projecting to the SNr. The terminal connected to the indirect striatal projection might not be affected and that connected to the direct striatal projection to the MGP seems to be affected only slightly. The receptors of the nigrostriatal DA neurons might be preserved normally without developing synaptic supersensitivity. Clarification of the pathophysiology requires further evidence from neuropathological and neurohistochemical studies.

REFERENCES

1. Segawa, M., Ohmi, K., Itoh, S., Aoyama, M. and Hayakawa, H. (1972). Childhood basal ganglia disease with remarkable response to L-dopa, 'hereditary basal ganglia disease with marked diurnal fluctuation'. *Chiryo (Tokyo)*, **24**, 667–72
2. Segawa, M., Nomura, Y. and Kase, M. (1986). Diurnally fluctuating hereditary progressive dystonia. In Vinken, P.J., Bruyn, G.W. and Klawans, H.L. (eds.) *Handbook of Clinical Neurology*, Vol. 5 (49), pp. 529–39. (Amsterdam: Elsevier Science)
3. Segawa, M., Nomura, Y., Yamashita, S., Kase, M., Nishiyama, N., Yukishita, S., Ohta, H., Nagata, K. and Hosaka, A. (1990). Long term effects of L-dopa on hereditary progressive dystonia with marked diurnal fluctuation. In Berardelli, A., Benecke, R.M., Manfredi, M. and Marsden, C.D. (eds.) *Motor Disturbances II*, pp. 305–18. (London: Academic Press)
4. Segawa, M. and Nomura, Y. (1991). Pathophysiology of human locomotion: studies on pathological cases. In Shimamura, M., Grillner, S. and Edgerton, R. (eds.) *Neurobiological Basis of Human Locomotion*, pp. 317–28. (Tokyo: Japan Scientific Societies Press)
5. Segawa, M., Nomura, Y. and Kase, M. (1986). Hereditary progressive dystonia with marked diurnal fluctuation: clinicopathophysiological identification in reference to juvenile Parkinson's disease. In Yahr, M.D. and Bergman, K.J. (eds.) *Advances in Neurology*, Vol. 45, pp. 227–34. (New York: Raven Press)
6. Segawa, M., Hosaka, A., Miyagawa, F., Nomura, Y. and Imai, H. (1976). Hereditary progressive dystonia with marked diurnal fluctuation. In Eldridge, R. and Fahn, S. (eds.) *Advances in Neurology*, Vol. 14, pp. 215–33. (New York: Raven Press)
7. Shimizu, N., Hara, M., Yoshihara, S., Tateno, A. and Aoki, T. (1986). Familial (mother–son) cases with hereditary progressive dystonia with marked diurnal fluctuation. *Shonika Rinsho*, **39**, 1442–6
8. Segawa, M. (1981). Hereditary progressive dystonia (HPD) with marked diurnal fluctuation. *Adv. Neurol. Sci.*, (Tokyo), **25**, 73–81
9. Hakamada, S., Watanabe, K., Hara, K. and Miyazaki, S. (1982). A case of 'hereditary progressive dystonia with marked diurnal fluctuation'. *No-To-Hattatsu*, (Tokyo), **14**, 44–8
10. Nomura, Y., Segawa, M., Soda, M. and Hikosaka, O. (1987). Voluntary saccadic eye movements in basal ganglia disorders. In *Highlights in Neuro-Ophthalmology*, (*Proceedings of the Sixth Meeting of the International Neuro-Ophthalmology Society, Hakone, Japan*, 1986), pp. 139–45. (Amsterdam: Aeolus Press)
11. Ouvrier, R.A. (1978). Progressive dystonia with marked diurnal fluctuation. *Ann. Neurol.*, **4**, 412–7
12. Kumamoto, I., Nomoto, M., Yoshidome, M., Osame, M. and Igata, A. (1984). Five cases of dystonia with marked diurnal fluctuation and special reference to homovanillic acid in CSF. *Clin. Neurol.*, (Tokyo), **24**, 697–702
13. Shimoyamada, Y., Yoshikawa, A., Kashii, H., Kihira, S. and Koike, M. (1986). Hereditary progressive dystonia – an observation of the catecholamine metabolism during L-dopa therapy in a 9-year-old girl. *No-to-Hattatsu*, (*Tokyo*), **18**, 505–9
14. Maekawa, N., Hashimoto, T., Sasaki, M., Oishi, T. and Tsuji, S. (1988). A study on catecholamine metabolites in CSF in a patient with progressive dystonia with marked diurnal fluctuation, *Clin. Neurol.*, (Tokyo), **28**, 1206–8
15. Lang, A.E., Garnett, E.S. Firnau, G., Nahmias, C. and Talalla, A. (1988). Positron tomography in dystonia. In Fahn, S., Marsden, C.D. and Calne, D.B. (eds.) *Advances in Neurology*, Vol. 50, pp. 249–53. (New York: Raven Press)
16. Tachi, N., Sasaki, K. and Shinoda, M. (1987). Four cases including identical triplets of progressive dystonia with marked fluctuation. *J. Jpn. Pediatr. Soc.*, **91**, 1403–6
17. Kase, M. (1978). Pitfalls in neurological disorders. *Jpn. Med. J.*, **2850**, 3–11
18. Nomura, Y., Kase, M., Igawa, C., Ogiso, M. and Segawa, M. (1984). A female case of hereditary progressive dystonia with marked diurnal fluctuation with favorable response to anticholinergic drugs for 25 years. *Clin. Neurol.*, (Tokyo), **22**, 723
19. Nomura, K., Negoro, T., Tagesu, E., Aso, K., Furune, S., Takahashi, I., Yamamoto, N. and Watanabe, K. (1987). Bromocriptine therapy in a case of hereditary progressive dystonia with marked diurnal fluctuation. *Brain Dev.*, **9**, 199

20. LeWitt, P.A., Miller, L.P., Newman, R.P., Lovenberg, W., Eldridge, R. and Chase, T.N. (1976). Pteridine cofactor in dystonia: pathogenic and therapeutic considerations. *Neurology*, **33**, (Suppl. 2), 161
21. LeWitt, P.A., Newman, R.P., Miller, L.P., Lovenberg, W. and Eldridge, R. (1983). Treatment of dystonia with tetrahydrobiopterin. *N. Engl. J. Med.*, **308**, 157–8
22. Ishida, A., Takada, G., Kobayashi, Y., Higashi, O., Toyoshima, I. and Takai, K. (1988). Involvement of serotonergic neuron in hereditary progressive dystonia – Clinical effects of tetrohydrobiopterin and 5-hydroxytryptophan. *No-T-Hattatsu*, (Tokyo), **20**, 195–9
23. Deonna, T. (1986). Dopa-sensitive progressive dystonia of childhood with fluctuations of symptoms – Segawa's syndrome and possible variants. *Neuropediatrics*, **17**, 75–80
24. Segawa, M., Nomura, Y., Hikosaka, O., Soda, M., Usui, S. and Kase, M. (1987). Roles of the basal ganglia and related structures in symptoms of dystonia. In Carpenter, M.B. and Jayaraman, A. (eds.) *Basal Ganglia II, Structure and Function*, pp. 489–504. (New York: Plenum Press)
25. Segawa, M., Nomura, Y., Tanaka, S., Hakamada, S., Nagata, E., Soda, M. and Kase, M. (1988). Hereditary progressive dystonia with marked diurnal fluctuation: consideration on its pathophysiology based on the characteristics of clinical and polysomnographical findings. In Fahn, S., Marsden, C.D. and Calne, D.B. (eds.) *Advances in Neurology*, Vol. 50, pp. 367–76. (New York: Raven Press)
26. Rothwell, J.C. and Obeso, J.A. (1988). The anatomical and physiological basis of torsion dystonia. In Marsden, C.D. and Fahn, S. (eds.) *Movement Disorders, Neurology* 2, pp. 367–376. (London: Butterworth)
27. Duvoison, R.C. (1976). Parkinsonism: Animal analogues of the human disorders. In Yahr, M.D. (ed.) *The Basal Ganglia*, pp. 293–303. (New York: Raven Press)
28. Wolfson, L.T., Sharpless, N.S., Thal, L.J., Waltz, J.M. and Shapiro, K. (1983). Decreased ventricular fluid norepinephrine metabolite in childhood onset dystonia. *Neurology (NY)*, **33**, 369–72
29. Jankel, W.R., Allen, R.P., Neidermeyer, E. and Kalsher, M.J. (1983). Polysomnographic findings in dystonia musculorum deformans. *Sleep*, **6**, 281–5
30. Horneykiewicz, O., Stephen, J., Becker, L.E., Farley, I. and Shannak, K. (1986). Brain neurotransmitters in dystonia musculorum deformans. *N. Engl. J. Med.*, **315**, 347–53
31. Rajput, A.J. (1973). Levodopa in dystonia musculorum deformans. *Lancet*, **24**, 432
32. Montanini, R., Basso, P.F. and Gasco, P. (1979). Tranttamento con Levodopa di un caso di spasmo di torsione con atetosi. *Minerva Medica*, **70**, 1551–2
33. Gordon, N. (1982). Fluctuating dystonia and allied syndromes. *Neuropediatrics*, **13**, 152–4
34. Rondot, P. and Ziegler, M. (1983). Dystonia – L-dopa responsive or juvenile parkinsonism? *J. Neural Transmission*, (Suppl.) **19**, 273–81
35. Allen, N. and Knopp, W. (1976). Hereditary parkinsonism-dystonia with sustained control by L-dopa and anticholinergic medication. In Eldridge, R. and Fahn, S. (eds.) *Advances in Neurology*, Vol. 14, pp. 201–13. (New York: Raven Press)
36. Winkelmann, W. (1975). L-dopa – Langzeitbehandlung einer Torsionsdystonie. *J. Neurol.*, **208**, 319–23
37. Maekawa, K., Kitani, N. and Satake, Y. (1972). A case with dystonia responded to L-dopa. *No-T-Hattatsu*, (Tokyo), **4**, 8–15
38. Kaneko, Y., Kumashiro, H., Yashima, Y. and Kowada, M. (1978). Dystonic movement disorders and their treatment – report of three cases. *Fukushima J. Med. Sci.*, **25**, 3–4
39. Garz, B.P. (1982). Dystonia musculorum deformans: implications of therapeutic response to levodopa and carbamazepine. *Arch. Neurol.*, **39**, 376–7
40. Deonna, T. and Ferreia, A. (1985). Idiopathic fluctuating dystonia: a case of foot dystonia and writer's cramp responsive to L-dopa. *Dev. Med. Child. Neurol.*, **27**, 819–21
41. Hirasawa, K., Ochiai, Y. and Fukuyama, Y. (1984). Two cases with hereditary progressive dystonia. *J. Jpn. Pediatr. Soc.*, **88**, 708–13
42. Horiguchi, A., Inami, K., Nagao, H. and Sano, N. (1985). A case with dystonia musculorum deformans responded to L-dopa with drug holiday therapy. *Psychiat. Neurol. Pediatr. Jpn.*, **25**, 67–71
43. Fink, J.K., Barton, N., Cohen, W., Lovenberg, W., Burns, R.S. and Hallett, M. (1988). Dystonia with marked diurnal variation associated with biopterin deficiency. *Neurology*, **38**, 707–11

44. Aggarwal, R., Bagga, A. and Kolra, V. (1984). Progressive dystonia with marked diurnal variation. *Indian J. Paediatr.*, **51**, 747–9
45. Yokochi, M. (1979). Juvenile Parkinson's disease – Part I. Clinical aspects. *Adv. Neurol. Sci.*, (Tokyo), **23**, 1060–73
46. Nygaard, T.G. and Duvoison, R.C. (1986). Hereditary dystonia-parkinsonism syndrome and juvenile onset. *Neurology*, **36**, 1424–8
47. Nygaard, T.G., Marsden, C.D. and Duvoisin, R.C. (1988). Dopa-responsive dystonia. In Fahn, S., Marsden, C.D. and Calne, D.B. (eds.) *Advances in Neurology*, Vol. 50, pp. 377–84. (New York: Raven Press)
48. Still, C.N. and Herberg, K. (1976). Long-term levodopa therapy for torsion dystonia. *South Med. J.*, **69**, 564–6
49. Muenter, M.D., Gomez, M.R., Gordon, H. and Sharpless, N.S. (1982). L-dopa responsive dystonia musculorum deformans with on-off effects. *Neurology*, **32**, (Part 2), A112
50. Gautier, J.C. and Awada, A. (1983). Dystonia musculorum deformans. Effet favorable de la bromocriptine. *Revue Neurologique* (Paris), **139**, 449–50
51. Richards, C.L., Bedard, P.J., Fortin, G. and Malouin, F. (1983). Quantitative evaluation of the effects of L-dopa in torsion dystonia: a case report. *Neurology*, **33**, 1083–7
52. de Yebens, J.G., Moskowitz, C., Fahn, S. and Saint-Hilarie, M.H. (1988). Long-term treatment with levodopa in a family with autosomal dominant torsion dystonia. In Fahn, S., Marsden, C.D. and Calne, D.B. (eds.) *Advances in Neurology*, Vol. 50, pp. 101–11. (New York: Raven Press)
53. Yamamura, Y., Sobue, I., Ando, K., Iida, M., Yanagi, T. and Kono, C. (1973). Paralysis agitans of early onset with marked diurnal fluctuation of symptoms. *Neurology*, **23**, 239–44
54. Sunohara, N., Mano, Y., Ando, K. and Satoyoshi, E. (1985). Idiopathic dystonia: parkinsonism with marked diurnal fluctuation of symptoms. *Ann. Neurol.*, **17**, 39–45
55. Narabayashi, H., Yokochi, M., Iizuka, R. and Nagatsu, T. (1986). Juvenile parkinsonism. In Vinken, P.J., Bruyn, G.W. and Kawans, H.L. (eds.) *Handbook of Clinical Neurology*, Vol. 5 (49), pp. 153–65. (Amsterdam: Elsevier Science)
56. Quinn, N., Critchley, P. and Marsden, C.D. (1987). Young onset Parkinson's disease. *Movement Disorders*, **2**, 73–91
57. Sterk, E. and Kellerman, K. (1984). Unterschiedliche Expressivitat des Segawa Syndrome in einer Familie. Presented at the 10*th Annual Meeting of the 'Gesellschaft fur Neuropadiatrie'*, October, Giessen, Germany
58. Nomoto, M., Kumamoto, K., Sano, Y., Nakajima, H., Osame, M. and Igata, A. (1983). A family of benign juvenile parkinson disease with a child having severe dopa-responsive fluctuating dystonia. *Clin. Neurol.*, (Tokyo), **24**, 1388
59. Ujike, H., Nakashima, M., Kuroda, S. and Otsuki, S. (1989). Two siblings of juvenile Parkinson's disease dystonic type (Yokochi type 3) and hereditary progressive dystonia with marked diurnal fluctuation (Segawa). *Clin. neurol.*, (Tokyo), **29**, 890–4
60. Marsden, C.D. and Harrison, M.H.G. (1974). Idiopathic torsion dystonia (dystonia musculorum deformans): a review of 42 patients. *Brain*, **97**, 793–810
61. McGeer, E.G. and McGeer, P.L. (1973). Some characteristics of brain tyrosine hydroxylase. In Mandel, J. (ed.) *New Concepts in Neurotransmitter Regulation*, pp. 53–68. (New York, London: Plenum Press)
62. McGeer, P.L., McGeer, E.G. and Suzuki, J.S. (1977). Aging and extrapyramidal function. *Arch. Neurol.*, **34**, 33–5
63. Segawa, M. (1982). Catecholamine metabolism in neurological diseases in childhood. In Wise, G., Blaw, M.E. and Procopis, P.G. (eds.) *Topics in Child Neurology*, Vol. 2, pp. 135–50. (New York: Spectrum Publications Inc.)
64. Yokochi, M., Narabayashi, H., Iizuka, R. and Nagatsu, T. (1984). Juvenile parkinsonism – some clinical, pharmacological and neuropathological aspects. In Hassler, R.G. and Christ, J.F. (eds.) *Advances in Neurology*, Vol. 40, pp. 407–13. (New York: Raven Press)
65. Garcia-Rill, E. (1986). The basal ganglia and the locomotor regions. *Brain. Res. Rev.*, **11**, 47–63
66. Crossman, A.R. (1990). A hypothesis on the pathophysiological mechanisms that underlie levodopa dopamine against induced dyskinesia in Parkinson's disease. Implications for future strategies in treatment. *Movement Disorders*, **5**, 100–8

67. Narabayashi, H., Yokochi, F. and Nakajima, Y. (1984). Levodopa-induced dyskinesia and thalamotomy. *J. Neurol. Neurosurg. Psychiatr.*, **47**, 831–9
68. Hikosaka, O. and Sakamoto, M. (1986). Cell activity in monkey caudate nucleus preceding saccadic eye movements. *Exp. Brain Res.*, **63**, 659–62
69. Segawa, M. and Nomura, Y. (1991). Rapid eye movements during REM stage are modulated by nigrostriatal dopamine (NS-DA) neurons? In Bernardi, G., Carpenter, M.B. and Di Chiara, G. (eds.) *Basal Ganglia III*, in press
70. Albin, R.L., Reiner, A., Anderson, K.D., Penney, J.B. and Young, A.B. (1990). Striatal and nigral neuron subpopulations in rigid Huntington's disease: implications for the functional anatomy of chorea and rigidity-akinesia. *Ann. Neurol.*, **27**, 357–67
71. Crossman, A.R. (1990). Animal models of movement disorders. Presented at the *First International Congress on Movement Disorders*, April, Washington, D.C.
72. Glick, S.A., Ross, D.A. and Hough, L.B. (1982). Lateral assymetry of neurotransmitters in human brain. *Brain Res.*, **234**, 53–63

2

Dopa-responsive dystonia: clinical characteristics and definition

T.G. Nygaard, B.J. Snow, S. Fahn and D.B. Calne

INTRODUCTION

In this chapter we delineate our definition of dopa-responsive dystonia (DRD) and its relationship to hereditary progressive dystonia with marked diurnal fluctuation (HPD). We subdivide cases of DRD based on their geographic origin (North America, Japan, and Other), and compare the demographic and clinical features of these cases for any evidence which supports a continued distinction between HPD and DRD. We review clinical and neurochemical data in DRD, and delineate features which we feel distinguish DRD from two other disorders which may present in childhood: idiopathic torsion dystonia (ITD), and childhood-onset parkinsonism (CPD).

HISTORICAL BACKGROUND AND NOSOLOGY

The term 'dystonia' was introduced by Oppenheim[1] in 1911 to describe a clinical condition with coexistent hypertonia and hypotonia. This condition caused rapid, sometimes rhythmic, jerking movements; twisted postures associated with these movements; bizarre gait with axial flexion and twisting, and progressed to sustained fixed postural deformities. We utilize the definition proposed by the Scientific Advisory Board of the Dystonia Medical Research Foundation, hereafter: Dystonia is a syndrome of sustained muscle contractions, frequently causing twisting and repetitive movements, or abnormal postures[2].

The classification of dystonia based on etiology has two major categories, idiopathic (primary) and symptomatic (secondary). Idiopathic dystonia (ITD) represents dystonia which occurs without known etiology or other neurologic deficit[2]. Further analysis of ITD resulted in the appreciation of 'variant forms', distinct from classical ITD[3]. These variant forms include: diurnal dystonia, dopa-responsive dystonia (DRD), paradoxical dystonia, and 'myoclonic' dystonia. Our present focus is the overlapping sets of patients with DRD[4] and diurnal dystonia[5].

Beck[6] made the first apparent clinical description of DRD in 1947, with her report of a girl and her paternal uncle affected with dystonia. A fine rest tremor was present in addition to the dystonic movements. Corner subsequently reported the diurnal nature of this girl's symptoms and a dramatic response to trihexyphenidyl[7]. Proof of dopa-responsiveness in this girl and her affected brother came in 1976 following their treatment with levodopa.

The introduction of levodopa for treatment of Parkinson disease in 1967[8] spurred therapeutic trials in many neurological conditions. Although there was limited success in patients with dystonia[9–12], at least one of these early patients had a dramatic levodopa rsponse[12]. In 1971, Castaigne and colleagues[13] reported two brothers with a 'progressive extrapyramidal disorder', and Segawa and colleagues[14] reported two cousins with 'hereditary basal ganglia disease with marked diurnal fluctuation', who experienced a remarkable response to levodopa therapy. The impact of these observations on Western neurologists may have been blunted by Irving Cooper[15], who cautioned that levodopa rendered patients less responsive to thalamotomy; a major treatment modality for dystonia at the time. Eldridge and co-workers[16] echoed this caution, but noted that about 5% of patients with dystonia reported their greatest therapeutic benefit from levodopa. There were several subsequent reports of levodopa-responsive dystonia[17–23].

In 1975, at the First International Symposium on Torsion Dystonia, there was more complete characterization of this disorder. Allen and Knopp[24] reported a family with a disorder characterized by onset of dystonia in childhood with later development of parkinsonian features. These patients were responsive to levodopa and trihexyphenidyl in low doses. These authors failed to note, however, the prominent diurnal variation of symptoms, and significant exacerbation of symptoms with menstruation experienced by their proband. Segawa and colleagues[5] presented additional levodopa-responsive patients. They stressed the progressive nature of the dystonia and the diurnal fluctuation of symptoms. They also described features of parkinsonism, including 'cogwheel-like rigidity' and rest tremor in the older patients, 'frozen gait', 'pulsion', and 'mask-like face'. These authors concluded that, 'some cases reported as juvenile parkinsonism may be the same disorder'.

Appreciation of the parkinsonian features in DRD has led to increased awareness of the potential clinical overlap between DRD and childhood-onset parkinsonism[25–7]. The concept of 'juvenile Parkinson disease', as a specific entity with onset before age 40, is a topic of much debate. Willage, in 1911[28], analyzed reported cases of parkinsonism with onset before age 30 and concluded that age 20 (or possibly 18) should be the lower age limit accepted for the onset of Parkinson disease. Quinn and colleagues[29] also concluded from their series that parkinsonism beginning before age 21 represents a separate clinical entity. Review of neuropathological data may support this notion as no case with 'typical Lewy body pathology' has been reported with an onset earlier than age 19[30]. The clinical profile of Professor Narabayashi's patient and a refined analysis of her neuropathology are discussed elsewhere in this volume (see Chapter 18). The consensus on this case appears to be that it represented CPD. A division of the first two decades of life into childhood (0–12 years) and adolescence (13–20 years)

Table 1 Nosological designations of included cases used in prior reports

Dystonia musculorum deformans[6]
Hereditary progressive dystonia with marked diurnal variation[5]
Hereditary parkinsonism-dystonia[24]
Fluctuating dystonia[61,72]
Dopa-sensitive progressive dystonia of childhood[69]
Segawa's sydrome[69]
Hereditary dystonia-parkinsonism syndrome of juvenile onset[34]
Dystonia with marked diurnal variation associated with biopterin deficiency[36]
Autosomal dominant torsion dystonia[35]

seems relevant as the classic cases of DRD represent a childhood-onset cohort.

The nosological designations used for some reports of DRD appear in Table 1. The designation 'dopa-responsive dystonia' evolved from an appreciation that the key features linking all cases are dystonia and its dopa-responsiveness[4]. Diurnal fluctuations do not occur in about a quarter of cases and have not been present in all members within several affected families. Although elements of parkinsonism (rigidity, bradykinesia, postural instability, and, rarely, rest tremor) commonly occur in DRD, the designation 'dopa-responsive dystonia' attempts to minimize confusion with other disorders causing 'childhood-onset parkinsonism' (CPD)[30].

It is significant to note that the appreciation or consideration of DRD in many of these patients came through awareness of this disorder from Dr Segawa's untiring efforts over the past two decades. It is, thus, fitting that this symposium to delineate our state of knowledge of DRD is being hosted by Dr Segawa.

CLINICAL MATERIAL

Our minimal inclusion criteria for consideration of a case as DRD include: childhood onset of dystonia or gait disorder, complete or near-complete responsiveness of symptoms to low doses of levodopa (generally less than 300 mg/day, in combination with a dopa-decarboxylase inhibitor), and maintenance of a smooth clinical response duration of levodopa treatment for which data is available. We have arbitrarily divided these 156 cases to reflect North American, Japanese, or Other (predominantly European) origin (Tables 2 and 3). Each of these divisions will be reviewed in other chapters. We have personally examined 70 of these patients. We have limited the cases to those in which there has been proven benefit from levodopa therapy. We excluded other affected family members who remain untreated or are treated only with other agents (i.e. anticholinergics or carbamazepine).

North American cases

We include 55 cases, the majority of whom have a European ethnic background[4,18,21,24,27,31–41]. We have examined 41 of these patients. The

Table 2 Demographics of previously reported or examined cases of DRD

	Geographic origin			
	North America	*Japan*	*Europe and Other*	*Totals*
Total	55	35	66	156
Female:male	44:11	30:5	44:22	118:38
Sporadic	16	17	34	67
Hereditary cases	39 (18 families)	18 (9 families)	32 (18 families)	88 (45 families)
Mean age (years) at onset (range)	5.8 (1.2–12)	5.9 (1.2–10)	5.7 (1.2–12)	5.8 (1.2–12)

Table 3 Laboratory analyses in previously reported cases of DRD

	CSF		
Geographic Origin	*Homovanillic acid*	*Biopterin*	*Fluorodopa PET scans*
North America	reduced	reduced	normal
Japan	reduced	reduced	normal
Europe and other	reduced	not studied	normal

smaller number of 'sporadic' probands in this group may reflect the thorough analysis of families in this cohort (see Chapter 7).

Japanese cases

We were aware of reports including 35 Japanese cases[5,14,17,42–55]. (a larger set of 55 Japanese cases is detailed by Dr Nomura in Chapter 6). We included one patient reported by Dr Segawa whom he would not consider as having HPD on the basis of action retrocollis[52]. We have been fortunate to examine nine of these patients.

Other cases

We include 66 cases who are predominantly European in origin[4,6,13,20,22,23,27,56–79]. We have examined 20 of these patients.

CLINICAL OBSERVATIONS IN DRD

The typical clinical features of DRD include: onset with dystonia in childhood, usually affecting gait; the concurrent or later development of signs of parkinsonism in most affected individuals; and a dramatic therapeutic response to levodopa[4]. Signs and symptoms in DRD often worsen later in the day ('diurnal fluctuation') or increase following exertion.

In general, early motor development is normal. However, several cases had an unexplained delay in attainment of early motor milestones that preceded overt dystonic manifestations in later infancy or childhood[24,41]. Following onset of dystonia in one or both legs or a gait disorder, there is increasing disability in the legs and appearance of postural instability. A small number of cases have had onset with arm dystonia[38,54], torticollis[38], retrocollis[27], 'poor co-ordination'[54] or slowness in dressing[5], before manifesting leg involvement. Clinical features suggestive of spasticity (hyperreflexia and ankle clonus with intermittent extensor plantar responses) occur in a significant proportion of patients. Symptomatic arm involvement ultimately occurs in most patients. Over one-half develop axial manifestations (increased lumbar lordosis, scoliosis, or torticollis) before treatment. Progression to generalized dystonia occurred in most patients. The rate of progression was difficult to determine with certainty, but generalization occurred within a year in several patients. Two women had rapid progression following non-encephalitic illnesses soon after symptom onset. A small number of patients have experienced only exercise-induced dystonia that resolved following 1–2 hours rest (without sleep). Increased awareness of DRD has resulted in earlier treatment and shorter periods of deficit.

The degree of disability tends to correlate inversely with age at onset, being more severe in early-onset cases. However, a few patients with onset of toe walking and postural instability at age 4–5 years, had symptoms that remained restricted to occasional leg 'cramps' with equinovarus posturing through their teens and early adulthood. Later onset cases tended to have more restricted disability, but developed symptomatic worsening from parkinsonism in late adult life. Rest tremor appeared in a few of the more severely affected patients after several years of disease.

Diurnal fluctuations occurred in 77% of cases. These varied widely in degree from some patients being 'normal' in the morning to others who were obviously affected but less severely than later in the day. In our experience, patients still have obvious signs during periods when they report being asymptomatic. A few patients did not develop fluctuations until several years into their clinical course. In several patients there was an attenuation in the degree of variation with disease progression. Importantly, in at least six families there were affected members with and without fluctuations[27,38,77]. In one family, the father and brother of a girl with diurnal fluctuations experienced only exercise-induced exacerbations of dystonia[71]. Rest, without sleep, was sufficient to cause a significant reduction in the dystonia in several personally examined cases.

Levodopa has been effective in all cases. This responsiveness has been present in patients who were symptomatic for as long as 58 years before treatment[27]. Doses required vary from as little as 50 mg (with a peripheral dopa-decarboxylase inhibitor) on alternate days, to 2000 mg levodopa (without inhibitor). The longest duration of treatment with continued stable response is 23 years[27].

The failure of 'patient 2' of Muller and colleagues[77] to initially respond to levodopa at 500 mg levodopa/day may have been due to peripheral metabolism of the drug, as this boy later became 'almost normal' on 125 mg levodopa with carbidopa and 2–4 mg trihexyphenidyl a day. We are not aware of any instance in which one family member responded to levodopa and another fully affected member did not respond.

In contrast to the response of the diffuse dystonic elements in DRD, the response in long-standing focal dystonias may not always be good. In one large DRD family, a man (IV-96 in pedigree[38]) with spastic dysphonia as his only finding, had no benefit when levodopa was tried at 300 mg/day (with decarboxylase inhibitor) for several months after 37 years of symptoms. His position as a 'gene carrier' is evident as his daughter is now considered definitely affected with DRD[39]. A sporadic rise with pronounced writer's cramp in addition to leg symptoms and imbalance was the response of these latter symptoms to low dose levodopa while the writer's cramp was unaffected by levodopa up to 1000 mg/day (with decarboxylase inhibitor), first tried 20 years after its symptomatic onset. There is, however, another case in which writer's cramp responded after being symptomatic for 9 years[68]. This suggests that long-standing task-specific focal dystonic elements in DRD may not always be responsive. Early treatment would seem desirable in such cases to preserve dopa-responsiveness or prevent emergence of these symptoms.

Chorea appeared in a number of patients early in their treatment. This has responded to dose adjustment and has not proved to be a problem in chronic treatment. Dose requirements have remained stable in patients using levodopa with a peripheral dopa-decarboxylase inhibitor and have diminished in some cases. Anticholinergics, carbamazepine, and bromocriptine have had variable effects as prior treatment in many of these patients[27].

LABORATORY STUDIES

Cerebrospinal fluid (CSF) monoamine metabolites

Cerebrospinal fluid levels of homovanillic acid (HVA) have been reduced in most patients studied[4,24,41,43,48–51,53–5,57,66,69,79,80] and have been comparable in all three cohorts. Diurnal determinations revealed afternoon increases[36,51] and decreases[36,54] in HVA. The serotonin metabolite, 5-hydroxyindoleacetic acid has been variable with normal[4,36,43,48,49,51,54,62,80], elevated[36,51,57] and reduced[4,24,36,57,66,81] values reported.

Biopterin pathway metabolites

Cerebrospinal fluid biopterin (a tyrosine hydroxylase cofactor) has been markedly reduced in all patients studied[27,33,36,50]. Neopterin, a biopterin metabolite, has also been reduced[33,36,50,80,81]. These studies have been undertaken in both American and Japanese patients.

Positron emission tomography (PET) scanning

At least ten patients with DRD have had fluorodopa PET[37,82,83]. The consensus is emerging that fluorodopa PET scanning is normal or near normal in DRD in contrast to CPD. A critical analysis of the PET data is presented by Snow and colleagues (see Chapter 14).

RESULTS

As shown in Tables 2 and 3, there are no obvious differences evident in the clinical features, age at onset, sex distribution, heredity, CSF profiles, or PET findings comparing these populations. This conclusion may not be surprising in comparing the North American and Other (mainly European) cohorts since they possess a similar ethnic background. However, the similarity of the Japanese patients to all others is an important finding.

DISCUSSION

The fundamental clinical features of DRD are: dystonia, a dramatic clinical response to small doses of levodopa, and long-term stability of this response. Diurnal fluctuations are frequent but may vary from patient to patient within a family or with the stage of the disease. Features of parkinsonism (rigidity, bradykinesia, postural instability, and, rarely, rest tremor) are commonly appreciated in DRD, and have been present in each case we have had the opportunity to examine without treatment.

A few cases reported as DRD may not conform to this general definition. One case labeled by Agrawal and co-workers[84] as 'progressive dystonia with marked diurnal variation' developed her dopa-responsive condition following tuberculous meningitis. This girl remained severely affected in the evening despite treatment and should clearly be considered to have a symptomatic disorder.

Case 3 of Costeff and colleagues[72] developed 'wearing-off' and more obvious parkinsonism suggesting that her diagnosis is CPD (Costeff, personal communication, 1989). In addition, we have follow-up information on two other cases, previously considered by us as possible DRD, that suggest we misapplied this label. Case 2 reported by Kaneko and colleagues[85] developed generalized dystonia and had a less satisfactory response to levodopa on chronic treatment (Kaneko, personal communication, 1986). Another patient with isolated torticollis, onset at age 16, had resolution of this following institution of levodopa. The reappearance of the torticollis after a few years despite continued therapy (Rajput, personal communication, 1991) suggests this case may represent a case of idiopathic torticollis with a spontaneous remission[86].

Distinction of DRD from idiopathic torsion dystonia (ITD) and childhood-onset parkinsonism (CPD)

Table 4 outlines the major clinical points differentiating DRD from childhood-onset ITD and childhood-onset parkinsonism. The major diagnostic alternative in most of these patients was ITD.

Table 4 Differential aspects of dopa-responsive dystonia, childhood-onset idiopathic torsion dystonia, and childhood-onset parkinsonism

	DRD	*Childhood-onset ITD*	*CPD*
Age at onset	infancy to 12 years	less common before 6 years	rarely before 8 years
Initial signs	foot dystonia, gait disorder	arm or leg dystonia	foot dystonia, rigidity, bradykinesia, and rest tremor
Foot dystonia	usually at onset, all eventually	onset in 40%, 65% eventually	frequently
Arm dystonia	rarely onset, 75% eventually	onset in 45%, 86% eventually	rarely
Axial dystonia	rarely onset, 50% eventually	onset in 15%, 65% eventually	rarely
Bradykinesia	present in nearly all, may be mild early	not present	mild to moderate, early
Rigidity	may be prominent with 'activation'	not a feature	present at rest or with activation
Rest tremor	rarely, late in course	no	may be initial or early sign
Hyperreflexia	common, usually parallels rigidity	no	sometimes, associated with rigidity
Striatal toe	common	may be present if leg involved	may occur
Levodopa response	marked with low doses	may have mild non-specific effect	yes, with small to moderate doses
Anticholinergic response	may be marked	may be marked	yes, early
Long-term levodopa response	continued smooth response with chronic treatment		may need increasing doses with time. Wearing-off and peak-dose dyskinesias generally occur within 5 years of treatment

Clinical elements suggesting a corticospinal deficit (Achilles shortening, brisk reflexes with varying degrees of ankle clonus, and extensor plantar responses) occurred in a number of cases and gave cause for consideration of spastic paraplegia or diplegic cerebral palsy[18,36,41,73–75]. Magnetoelectrical stimulation of the motor cortex failed to reveal any disturbance of corticospinal activity in DRD[77].

In ITD, muscle tone may vary from moment to moment in an affected limb, but rigidity is not a feature. ITD begins in the legs in about 70% of cases, with onset before age 10 years[87,88]. Among leg-onset cases, almost all develop generalized dystonia. Severe disability with wheelchair dependency or severe gait disturbance occurred in many childhood-onset cases, particularly those with leg-onset. Although DRD begins in the leg with greater regularity than ITD, the rate of progression, and the severity of disability in untreated cases does not distinguish between these conditions.

Age at onset has been suggested as a criterion to separate DRD from ITD and 'juvenile parkinsonism'[45,52], but we find there is broad overlap. Figure 1 shows the number of cases of DRD, ITD, and parkinsonism with onset before 21 years which have been seen at the Columbia– Presbyterian Medical Center in the past 20 years. The relative frequencies of these diagnoses are similar to those at the London Dystonia Research Centre[4,29]. The Japanese experience appears to differ in that classic ITD is relatively uncommon in Japan.

The absence of neck involvement has also been suggested as discriminating DRD from other forms of dystonia. We found neck involvement in more than one-third of DRD patients and this should not exclude consideration of DRD. The dramatic response to levodopa in DRD readily establishes the distinction between DRD and ITD.

Comparing site of onset and rate of progression of disability in CPD and DRD is more difficult because of the rarity of the former condition. In the 'juvenile parkinsonism' cases described by Narabayashi[25] and in several other reports[25,29,30,89–92] there were no patients with onset before age six. Foot dystonia, rigidity, slowness, and variable-to-absent tremor are frequent presenting features of CPD, and diurnal fluctuation of symptoms has been apparent in several patients. In CPD, severe disability developed over the first 10 years. Parkinsonism tended to predominate over the dystonic elements during early progression, and the progression of disability in later childhood-onset cases was greater in CPD. The increasing levodopa dose requirements, fluctuations in response, and drug-induced dyskinesias which tend to develop within 5 years of treatment stand in contrast to the stability of treatment response in DRD.

These latter observations, however, only provide for a retrospective diagnosis to be made. In a few cases with CPD that we personally examined, the early clinical presentation was indistinguishable from DRD and the appropriate diagnosis only became obvious after several years of follow-up[27].

CSF monoamine metabolite and PET may offer a means of discriminating between these diagnoses (Table 5). None of the indices in these studies are consistently abnormal in ITD. CSF homovanillic acid and biopterin and its metabolites are reduced in both DRD and CPD, although the degree of reduction seems to be more severe in DRD. PET scanning offers a clear distinction between these conditions with normal studies in DRD and reduced fluorodopa uptake and retention in CPD.

CONCLUSIONS

DRD is a clinical designation which may be applied to a group of children possessing a rather characteristic set of clinical features. The essential elements of this diagnosis are dystonia and its dopa-responsiveness. Within the differential diagnosis of a single case are ITD and CPD. Clinically, the distinction from ITD is clarified by demonstration of a dramatic levodopa benefit in DRD. The distinction of DRD from CPD may be more difficult because their clinical presentations may be similar and the initial response

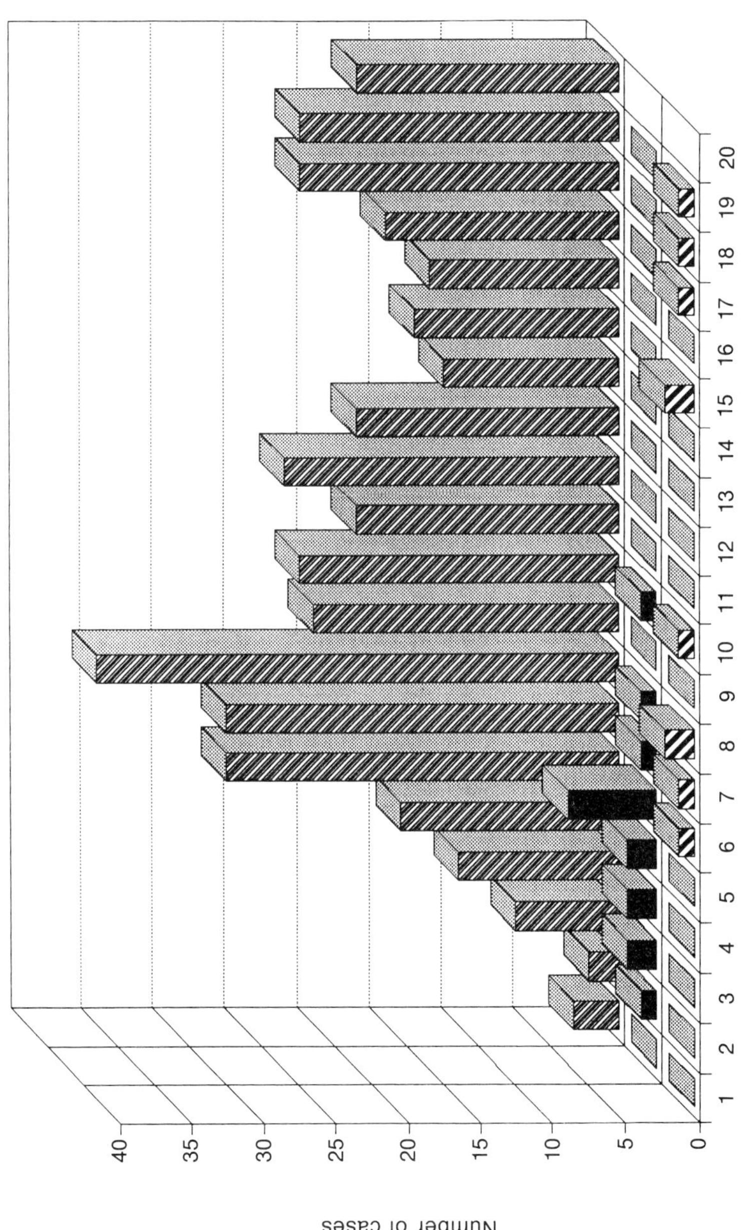

Figure 1 The number of cases of dopa-responsive dystonia (middle row), idiopathic dystonia (back row) and parkinsonism (front row) with onset before 21 years, seen at the Columbia–Presbyterian Medical Center over a period of 20 years (1971–1991)

Table 5 Metabolic studies in dopa-responsive (DRD), and idiopathic (ITD) dystonia and childhood-onset parkinsonism (CPD)

	DRD	*ITD*	*CPD*
CSF homovanillic acid	reduced	normal	reduced
CSF biopterin	markedly reduced	normal	mildly to moderately reduced
Fluorodopa PET scanning	normal	normal	reduced uptake and retention

to levodopa may be dramatic in both disorders. A demonstration of a stable long-term treatment may be necessary in isolated cases before allowing a correct categorization. Although additional clinical elements such as age at onset, and frequency of diurnal fluctuations may reveal differences when comparing groups of patients with each diagnosis, the overlap of these criteria between groups makes them unsuitable to distinguish the diagnosis in an individual case.

In our analysis of the clinical and laboratory data available in DRD and HPD, and after personal examination of patients with these diagnoses, we could not find sufficient evidence to justify their separation. The final resolution of this issue may need to await the identification of the disease gene.

ACKNOWLEDGEMENTS

This work was supported in part by the Dystonia Medical Research Foundation, the Parkinson's Disease Foundation, and NIH Grant HD00914-01 (Dr Nygaard)

REFERENCES

1. Oppenheim, H. (1911). Uber eine eigenartige Krampfkrankheit des kindlichen und jugendlichen Alters (Dysbasia lordotica progressiva, Dystonia musculorum deformans). *Neurologie Centralblatt*, **30**, 1090–107
2. Fahn, S., Marsden, C.D. and Calne, D.B. (1987). Classification and investigation of dystonia. In Marsden, C.D. and Fahn, S. (eds.) *Movement Disorders*, **2**, 332–58. (London: Butterworths)
3. Fahn, S. (1989). Clinical variants of idiopathic torsion dystonia. *J. Neurol. Neurosurg. Psychiatr.*, (Suppl.), 96–100
4. Nygaard, T.G., Marsden, C.D. and Duvoisin, R.C. (1988). Dopa-responsive dystonia. In Fahn, S., Marsden, C.D. and Calne, D.B. (eds.) *Advances in Neurology*, *Vol.* 50, pp. 377–84. (New York: Raven Press)
5. Segawa, M., Hosaka, A., Miyagawa, F., Nomura, Y. and Imai, H. (1976). Hereditary progressive dystonia with marked diurnal fluctuation. In Eldridge, R. and Fahn, S. (eds.) *Advances in Neurology*, *Vol.* 14, pp. 215–23. (New York: Raven Press)
6. Beck, D. (1947). Dystonia musculorum deformans with another case in the same family. *Proc. R. Soc. Med.*, **40**, 551
7. Corner, B.D. (1952). Dystonia musculorum deformans in siblings: treated with Artane (trihexyphenidyl). *Proc. R. Soc. Med.*, **45**, 451–2
8. Cotzias, G.C., VanWoert, M.H. and Schiffer, L.M. (1967). Aromatic amino acids and modification of parkinsonism. *N. Engl. J. Med.*, **276**, 374–9
9. Coleman, M.P. and Barnet, A. (1969). L-dopa reversal of muscular spasm, vomiting and

insomnia in a patient with an atypical form of familial dystonia. *Trans. Am. Neurol. Assoc.*, **94**, 91–5
10. Mandell, S. (1970). The treatment of dystonia with L-dopa and haloperidol. *Neurology*, **20** (Suppl. 2), 103–6
11. Barrett, R.E., Yahr, M.D. and Duvoisin, R.C. (1970). Torsion dystonia and spasmodic torticollis. Results of treatment with L-dopa. *Neurology*, **20** (Suppl. 2), 107–13
12. Chase, T.N. (1970). Biochemical and pharmacologic studies of dystonia. *Neurology*, **20** (Suppl. 2), 122–30
13. Castaigne, P., Rondot, P., Ribadeau Dumas, J.L. and Said, J. (1971). Affection extrapyramidale evoluant chez deux jeunes freres: Effets remarquables du traitement par la L-dopa. *Rev. Neurol.*, **124**, 162–6
14. Segawa, M., Ohmi, K., Itoh, S., Aoyama, M. and Hayakawa, H. (1971). Childhood basal ganglia disease with remarkable response to L-dopa, 'hereditary progressive basal ganglia disease with marked diurnal variation'. *Shinryo*, **24**, 667–72
15. Cooper, I.S. (1972). Levodopa-induced dystonia. *Lancet*, **2**, 1317–8
16. Eldridge, R., Kanter, W. and Koerber, T. (1973). Letter: Levodopa in dystonia. *Lancet*, **2**, 1027–8
17. Maekawa, K. and Kitani, N. (1972). Remarkable effect of L-dopa idiopathic dystonia: a case report. *No To Hattatsu*, **4**, 274–81
18. Hongladarom, T. (1973). Levodopa in dystonia musculorum deformans. *Lancet*, **1**, 1114
19. Mayman, C.I. and Cullen, R. (1973). Salutary effect of L-dopa on dystonia musculorum deformans. *Neurology*, **23**, 392 (Abstr.)
20. Melnichuk, P.V. and Sosnovskaia, L.S. (1973). Lechenie deformiruiushchei myshechnoi dystonii u detei preparatom L-dopa. *Zh. nevropatol. Psikhiatr.*, **73**, 1495–8
21. Rajput, A.H. (1973). Levodopa in dystonia musculorum deformans. *Lancet*, **1**, 432
22. Schenck, E. and Kurschke, U. (1975). Familiare progressive Dystonie mit Tagesschwankungen. Fallbeschreibung. Erfolgreibung Behandlung mit L-dopa. *Klin. Wochenschr.*, **53**, 779–80
23. Winkelmann, W. (1975). L-dopa Langzeitbehandlung einer Torsiondystonie. *J. Neurol.*, **208**, 319–23
24. Allen, N. and Knopp, W. (1976). Hereditary parkinsonism-dystonia with sustained control by L-dopa and anticholinergic medication. In Eldridge, R. and Fahn, S. (eds.) *Advances in Neurology*, *Vol.* 14, pp. 201–13. (New York: Raven Press)
25. Narabayashi, H., Yokochi, M., Iizuka, R. and Nagatsu, T. (1986). Juvenile parkinsonism. In Vinken, P.J., Bruyn, G.W. and Klawans, H.L. (eds.) *Handbook of Clinical Neurology*, *Vol.* 49, pp. 153–65. (Amsterdam: Elsevier Science)
26. Segawa, M., Nomura, Y. and Kase, M. (1987). Hereditary progressive dystonia with marked diurnal fluctuation: clinicopathophysiological identification in reference to juvenile Parkinson's disease. In Yahr, M.D. and Bergmann, K.J. (eds.) *Advances in Neurology*, *Vol.* 45, pp. 227–34. (New York: Raven Press)
27. Nygaard, T.G., Marsden, C.D. and Fahn, S. (1991). Dopa-responsive dystonia – long-term treatment response and prognosis. *Neurology*, **41**, 174–81
28. Willage, H. (1911). Uber paralysis agitans in jugendlichem. *Alter. Z. Ges. Neurol. Psychiatr.*, **4**, 520–87
29. Quinn, N., Critchley, P. and Marsden, C.D. (1987). Young-onset Parkinson's disease. *Movement Disorders*, **2**, 73–91
30. Gershanik, O.S. and Nygaard, T.G. (1990). Parkinson's disease beginning before age 40. In Streifler, M.B., Korczyn, A.D., Melamed, E. and Youdim, M.B.H. (eds.) *Advances in Neurology*, *Vol.* 53, pp. 251–8. (New York: Raven Press)
31. Garg, B.P. (1982). Dystonia musculorum deformans. Implications of therapeutic response to levodopa and carbamazepine. *Arch. Neurol.*, **39**, 376–7
32. Richards, C.L., Bedard, P.J., Fortin, G. and Malouin, F. (1983). Quantitative evaluation of the effects of L-dopa in torsion dystonia: a case report. *Neurology*, **33**, 1083–7
33. LeWitt, P.A., Miller, L.P., Levine, R.A., Lovenberg, W., Newman, R.P., Papavasiliou, A., Rayes, A., Eldridge, R. and Burns, R.S. (1986). Tetrahydrobiopterin in dystonia: identification of abnormal metabolism and therapeutic trials. *Neurology*, **36**, 760–4
34. Nygaard, T.G. and Duvoisin, R.C. (1986). Hereditary dystonia–parkinsonism syndrome of juvenile onset. *Neurology*, **36**, 1424–8

35. de Yebenes, J.G., Moskowitz, C., Fahn, S. and Saint Hilaire, M.H. (1988). Long-term treatment with levodopa in a family with autosomal dominant torsion dystonia. In Fahn, S., Marsden, C.D. and Calne, D.B. (eds.) *Advances in Neurology, Vol.* 50, pp. 101–11. (New York: Raven Press)
36. Fink, J.K., Barton, N., Cohen, W., Lovenberg, W., Burns, R.S. and Hallett, M. (1988). Dystonia with marked diurnal variation associated with biopterin deficiency. *Neurology*, **38**, 707–11
37. Lang, A.E., Garnett, E.S., Firnau, G., Nahmias, C. and Talalla, A. (1988). Positron tomography in dystonia. In Fahn, S., Marsden, C.D. and Calne, D.B. (eds.) *Advances in Neurology, Vol.* 50, pp. 249–53. (New York: Raven Press)
38. Nygaard, T.G., Trugman, J.M., de Yebenes, J.G. and Fahn, S. (1990). Dopa-responsive dystonia: the spectrum of clinical manifestations in a large North American family. *Neurology*, **40**, 66–9
39. Kwiatkowski, D.J., Nygaard, T.G., Schuback, D.E., Perman, S., Trugman, J.M., Bressman, S.B., Burke, R.E., Brin, M.F., Ozelius, L., Breakefield, X.O., Fahn, S. and Kramer, P.L. (1991). Identification of a highly polymorphic microsatellite VNTR within the argininosuccinate synthetase locus – exclusion of the dystonia gene on 9q32-34 as the cause of dopa-responsive dystonia in a large kindred. *Am. J. Hum. Genet.*, **48**, 121–8
40. Geller, M., Kaplan, B. and Christoff, N. (1974). Dystonic symptoms in children: treatment with carbamazepine. *J. Am. Med. Assoc.*, **229**, 1755–7
41. Nygaard, T.G., Waran, S. and Chutorian, A.M. (1989). Unexplained cerebral palsy: dopa-responsive dystonia? *Ann. Neurol.*, **26**, (Abstr.), 485–6
42. Segawa, M. (1981). Hereditary progressive dystonia (HPD) with marked diurnal fluctuation. *Adv. Neurol. Sci.*, **25**, 73–81
43. Hakamada, S., Watanabe, K., Hara, K. and Miyazaki, S. (1982). A case of 'hereditary progressive dystonia with marked diurnal fluctuation'. *Brain and Development*, **14**, 44–8
44. Kumamoto, I., Nomoto, M., Yoshidome, M., Osame, M. and Igata, A. (1984). Five cases of dystonia with marked diurnal fluctuation and special reference to homovanillic acid in CSF. *Rinsho Shinkeigaku*, **24**, 697–702
45. Nomoto, M., Kumamoto, K., Sano, Y., Nakajima, H., Osame, M. and Igata, A. (1984). A family with benign juvenile Parkinson disease with a child having severe dopa-responsive fluctuating dystonia. *Rinsho Shinkeigaku*, **24**, (Abstr.), 1388
46. Komatsu, K., Takada, G., Kobayashi, Y., Onodera, H., Ishida, A. and Higashi, O. (1986). Two cases of hereditary progressive dystonia with marked diurnal fluctuation. *Brain And Development*, **8**, (Abstr.), 189
47. Segawa, M., Nomura, Y. and Kase, M. (1986). Diurnally fluctuating hereditary progressive dystonia. In Vinken, P.J., Bruyn, G.W. and Klawans, H.L. (eds.) *Handbook of Clinical Neurology*, Vol. 5(49), *Extrapyramidal Disorders*, pp. 529–39. (Amsterdam: Elsevier Science)
48. Shimoyamada, Y., Yoshikawa, A., Kashii, H., Kihira, S. and Koike, M. (1986). Hereditary progressive dystonia – an observation of the catecholamine metabolism during L-dopa therapy in a 9-year-old girl. *No To Hattatsu*, **18**, 505–9
49. Nomura, K., Yamamoto, N., Takahashi, I., Furune, S., Aso, K., Negoro, T. and Watanabe, K. (1987). Bromocriptine and L-dopa therapy: comparison in a case of hereditary progressive dystonia with marked diurnal fluctuations. *No To Hattatsu*, **19**, 244–8
50. Ishida, A., Takada, G., Kobayashi, Y., Toyoshima, I. and Takai, K. (1988). Effect of tetrahydrobiopterin and 5-hydroxytryptophan on hereditary progressive dystonia with marked diurnal fluctuation: a suggestion of the serotonergic system involvement. *Tohoku. J. Exp. Med.*, **154**, 233–9
51. Maekawa, N., Hashimoto, T., Sasaki, M., Oishi, T. and Tsuji, S. (1988). A study on catecholamine metabolites in CSF in a patient with progressive dystonia with marked diurnal fluctuation. *Rinsho Shinkeigaku*, **28**, 1206–8
52. Segawa, M., Nomura, Y., Tanaka, S., Hakamada, S., Nagata, E., Soda, M. and Kase, M. (1988). Hereditary progressive dystonia with marked diurnal fluctuation – consideration on its pathophysiology based on the characteristics of clinical and polysomnographical findings. In Fahn, S., Marsden, C.D. and Calne, D.B. (eds.) *Advances in Neurology*, Vol. 50, pp. 367–76. (New York: Raven Press)
53. Oki, J., Sasaki, N., Kusunoki, Y. and Cho, K. (1989). Response to haloperidol and analysis

of growth curve in hereditary progressive dystonia with marked diurnal fluctuation. *No To Hattatsu*, **21**, 569–73

54. Iwami, O., Kawamura, J., Hashimoto, S., Suenaga, T. and Nakamura, M. (1990). Hereditary progressive dystonia with marked diurnal fluctuation – a report of two siblings, one of them showing age-dependent changes of symptoms. *Rinsho Shinkeigaku*, **30**, 961–5
55. Watanabe, K., Ebi, T., Morishima, T., Tsuchiya, I., Sahashi, I. and Mitsuma, T. (1990). Four cases in two families of hereditary progressive dystonia with circadian rhythm. *Nippon Naika Gakkai Zasshi*, **79**, 102–3
56. Haidvogel, M. and Stogmann, W. (1978). Progressive Dystonie mit Tagesschwankungen (Segawa-Syndrom): Behandlung mit niedrigen Dosen von L-dopa und Benserazid. In Groh, C. and Rosenmayr, W. (eds.) *Jahrestagung der Gesellschaft fur Neuropadiatrie, Wein* 1978, pp. 171–8. (Vienna)
57. Ouvrier, R.A. (1978). Progressive dystonia with marked diurnal fluctuation. *Ann. Neurol.*, **4**, 412–17
58. Montanini, R., Basso, P.F. and Gasco, P. (1979). Trattamento con levodopa di un caso di spasmo di torsione con athetosi. *Min. Med.*, **70**, 1551–3
59. Bugiani, O. and Gatti, R. (1980). L-dopa in children with progressive neurological disorders. *Ann. Neurol.*, **7**, 93
60. Balottin, U., Lanzi, G. and Zambrino, C.A. (1981). Illustrazione di un caso di dystonia musculorum deformans tratto con L-dopa. *Riv. Neurobiol.*, **27**, 584–90
61. Gordon, N. (1982). Fluctuating dystonia and allied syndromes. *Neuropediatrics*, **13**, 152–4
62. Rolando, S. and Cremonte, M. (1982). Dystonia progressive con marcata fluttuazone mattine-sera. *Instituto Gaslini (Genova)*, **14**, 176–9
63. Martinius, J. and Neuhauser, G. (1983). Segawa-syndrome. Torsionsdystonie mit Begin im Kindesalter und deutlicher Fluktuation der Symptomatik im Tagesverlauf. Kasuistischer Beitrag. *Padiat. Prax.*, **28**, 45–9
64. Chan Lui, W.Y. and Low, L.C. (1984). Progressive dystonia with marked diurnal fluctuation in a Chinese family. *Aust. Paediatr. J.*, **20**, 143–6
65. Chan Lui, W.Y. and Low, L.C. (1984). A patient with myasthenia gravis and progressive dystonia with marked diurnal fluctuation. *Dev. Med. Child. Neurol.*, **26**, 665–8
66. Willemse, J., van Nieuwenhuizen, O., Gooskens, R.H. and Westenberg, H.G. (1984). Treatment of non-fluctuating progressive dystonia: a neuropharmacological approach. *Neuropediatrics*, **15**, 208–10
67. Bertelsmann, F.W. and Smit, L.M.E. (1985). Progressive dystonia with marked diurnal fluctuation, report of a case. *Clin. Neurol. Neurosurg.*, **87**, 123–6
68. Deonna, T. and Ferreira, A. (1985). Idiopathic fluctuating dystonia: a case of foot dystonia and writer's cramp responsive to L-dopa. *Dev. Med. Child Neurol.*, **27**, 819–21
69. Deonna, T. (1986). Dopa-sensitive progressive dystonia of childhood with fluctuations of symptoms – Segawa's syndrome and possible variants. Results of a collaborative study of the European Federation of Child Neurology Societies (EFCNS). *Neuropediatrics*, **17**, 81–5
70. Torelli, D., Lamontanara, G., Bracciolini, M. and Ciaravolo, G.A. (1986). Hereditary progressive dystonia with marked diurnal fluctuation in a family with pigmentary retinopathy. *Acta Neurol. (Napoli)*, **8**, 626–32
71. Vogel, H.P. (1986). Zum Problem der L-dop-sensiblen Dystonie. *Akt. Neurol.*, **13**, 102–5
72. Costeff, H., Gadoth, N., Mendelson, L., Harel, S. and Lavie, P. (1987). Fluctuating dystonia responsive to levodopa. *Arch. Dis. Child.*, **62**, 801–4
73. Arens, L.J., Silber, M.H. and Leary, M. (1989). Progressive dystonia with diurnal fluctuation. [Letter], *J. Child Neurol.*, **4**, 227–8
74. Boyd, K. and Patterson, V. (1989). Dopa responsive dystonia: a treatable condition misdiagnosed as cerebral palsy. *Br. Med. J.*, **298**, 1019–20
75. de Jong, A.P., Haan, E.A., Manson, J.I., Wise, G.A., Ouvrier, R.A. and Wadman, S.K. (1989). Kinetic study of catecholamine metabolism in hereditary progressive dystonia. *Neuropediatrics*, **20**, 3–11
76. Hwu, W.L., Wang, P.J. and Shen, Y.Z. (1989). Hereditary progressive dystonia with marked diurnal fluctuation: report of a case. *Acta Paediatr. Sin.*, **30**, 46–51
77. Muller, K., Homberg, V. and Lenard, H.G. (1989). Motor control in childhood-onset dopa-responsive dystonia (Segawa syndrome). *Neuropediatrics*, **20**, 185–91

78. Nygaard, T.G., Gardner-Medwin, D. and Marsden, C.D. (1989). Dopa-responsive dystonia: the spectrum of clinical manifestations in a family. In Crossman, A.R. and Sambrook, M.A. (eds.) *Neural Mechanisms in Disorders of Movement*, pp. 367–70. (London: John Libbey)
79. Gorke, W. and Bartholome, K. (1990). Biochemical and neurophysiological investigations in two forms of Segawa's disease. *Neuropediatrics*, **21**, 3–8
80. LeWitt, P.A., Newman, R.P., Miller, L.P., Lovenberg, W. and Eldridge, R. (1983). Treatment of dystonia with tetrahydrobiopterin (Letter). *N. Engl. J. Med.*, **308**, 157–8
81. Fink, J.K., Ravin, P., Argoff, C.E., Levine, R.A., Brady, R.O., Hallett, M. and Barton, N.W. (1989). Tetrahydrobiopterin administration in biopterin-deficient progressive dystonia with diurnal variation. *Neurology*, **39**, 1393–5
82. Martin, W.R., Stoessl, A.J., Palmer, M., Adam, M.J., Ruth, T.J., Grierson, J.R., Pate, B.D. and Calne, D.B. (1988). PET scanning in dystonia. In Fahn, S., Marsden, C.D. and Calne, D.B. (eds.) *Advances in Neurology*, *Vol.* 50, pp. 223–9. (New York: Raven Press)
83. Sawle, G.V., Leenders, K.L., Brooks, D.J., Harwood, G., Lees, A. J., Frackowiak, R.S.J. and Marsden, C.D. (1991). Dopa-responsive dystonia: [^{18}F]dopa positron emission tomography. *Ann. Neurol.*, **30**, 24–30
84. Agrawal, R., Bagga, A. and Kaira, V. (1984). Progressive dystonia with marked diurnal variation. *Indian J. Pediatr.*, **51**, 747–9
85. Kaneko, Y., Kumashiro, H., Yashima, Y. and Kowada, M. (1978). Dystonic movement disorders and their treatment. *Fukushima J. Med. Sci.*, **25**, 109–20
86. Friedman, A. and Fahn, S. (1986). Spontaneous remissions in spasmodic dystonia. *Neurology*, **36**, 398–400
87. Marsden, C.D. and Harrison, M.G.H. (1974). Idiopathic torsion dystonia (dystonia musculorum deformans). A review of forty-two patients. *Brain*, **97**, 793–810
88. Burke, R.E., Brin, M.F., Fahn, S., Bressman, S.B. and Moskowitz, C. (1986). Analysis of the clinical course of non-Jewish, autosomal dominant torsion dystonia. *Movement Disorders*, **1**, 163–78
89. Martin, W.E., Resch, J.A. and Baker, A.B. (1971). Juvenile parkinsonism. *Arch. Neurol.*, **25**, 494–500
90. Horowitz, G. and Greenberg, J. (1975). Pallido-pyramidal syndrome treated with levodopa. *J. Neurol. Neurosurg. Psychiatr.*, **38**, 238–40
91. Naidu, S., Wolfson, L.I. and Sharpless, N.S. (1978). Juvenile parkinsonism: a patient with possible primary striatal dysfunction. *Ann. Neurol.*, **3**, 453–5
92. Clough, C.G., Mendoza, M. and Yahr, M.D. (1981). A case of sporadic juvenile Parkinson's disease. *Arch. Neurol.*, **38**, 730–1

3

Clinicopathological identification of juvenile parkinsonism in reference to dopa-responsive disorders

M. Yokochi

INTRODUCTION

Levodopa treatment during the last twenty years has greatly influenced the study of extrapyramidal disease. Clinical experience has contributed to the nosological categorization of extrapyramidal diseases. Namely, it has shown which of the disorders of the extrapyramidal system correspond to levodopa-responsive disease, that is, a dopamine-deficiency state in the brain. As a result, a group of diseases with the main symptom of dystonia was also classed with parkinsonism. This has made for a complex, but very interesting, discussion.

Regular doses of levodopa have no obvious effect on patients with no pathological abnormality in the brain. Supplementation of dopamine content to target structures with pathological lesions results in certain clinical manifestations. In general, the administration of levodopa affects patients with extrapyramidal symptoms. For instance, it might aggravate the degree of certain involuntary movements such as chorea. On the other hand, as a clinically positive effect, it alleviates the severity of the symptoms in cases where parkinsonism predominates or in some cases where dystonia predominates. In other words, the deficiency of dopamine in the brain might be responsible for two clinically different groups of symptoms of parkinsonism and dystonia. However, parkinsonism and dystonia have been symptomatologically recognized to exhibit clear differences. The fact is that, at the present time, the two sets of symptoms must be recognized as existing on a spectrum of conditions responding to levodopa.

It is important to study the correlation between 'hereditary progressive dystonia' (HPD), with onset in childhood, and 'juvenile parkinsonism' (JP) with onset in adolescence or after, and to determine on a nosological or pathological basis whether these two syndromes are related to or are separate from Parkinson disease (PD) with onset after middle age. HPD and JP eliminate the factors related to aging from the symptomatological, physiological, biochemical and pathological perspectives for study of the dopamine deficiency syndromes. This paper focuses in particular on the clinicopathological characteristics of JP and on the relationship between JP and the two diseases which manifest before and after its onset age, that is, HPD and PD, on the bases of the results of our study and recent publications.

DEFINITION FOR DIAGNOSIS OF JUVENILE PARKINSONISM

The 40 cases of JP discussed by this author in the first publications[1,2] in 1979 have been followed for the last 15 years. The fundamental diagnostic definition for selecting the index cases has not changed. It followed a simple guideline: an illness with onset below the age of forty, showing major symptoms of parkinsonism and whose symptoms improved significantly with levodopa treatment. The most important condition is definite improvement of the disability by levodopa administration, compensating for a deficiency of dopamine. The degree of efficacy should be dramatic or at least demonstrate a marked improvement. This condition is important for differentiating JP from other extrapyramidal diseases.

EPIDEMIOLOGICAL CHARACTER OF JUVENILE PARKINSONISM

JP with an onset age of below 40 years accounts for around ten percent of all Parkinson disease. The onset-age-specific distribution of Parkinson disease is shown in Figure 1 from hospital statistics[3,4] and prevalences of JP are listed in Table 1 from other publications[1,4–8]. The majority of authors adopted an onset age of 40 years or below. As shown in Figure 1(c), however, Gershanik and Leist[4] opted for an onset age of 35 years or below for JP, on the basis of it being two standard deviations from the mean onset age of all Parkinson disease cases. This appears to be a valid method to determine the range of the onset age and to collect the purer index cases of JP. The onset-age-specific distribution in Figure 1 indicates that the age of onset in Japan (Figures 1(a) (b)) is, on average, 10 years younger than that in Argentina, according to the results obtained by Gershanik and Leist[4] (Figure 1(c)), as well as that in Europe and the USA. On the basis of these findings, the author had pointed out the possibility of a much higher prevalence of JP in Japan[9]. However, as shown in Table 1, similar prevalences of JP are observed in Japan and other countries.

PD is not considered to have a high dependence on genetic factors since the concordance between monozygotic twins appears to be low[10], and because the disease is considered to have a multifactorial origin contributed to by environmental factors[11]. Nonetheless, cases of JP have high familial incidence rates. Table 2 shows that the familial incidence rates related to onset age for the combined survey in Japan are higher for the younger proband. The frequencies of familial history for onset ages under 40 years and those of 40 years or more were 36.7% vs. 4.8%, respectively. Among our follow-up cases, 15 out of 35 families had familial incidence, a high

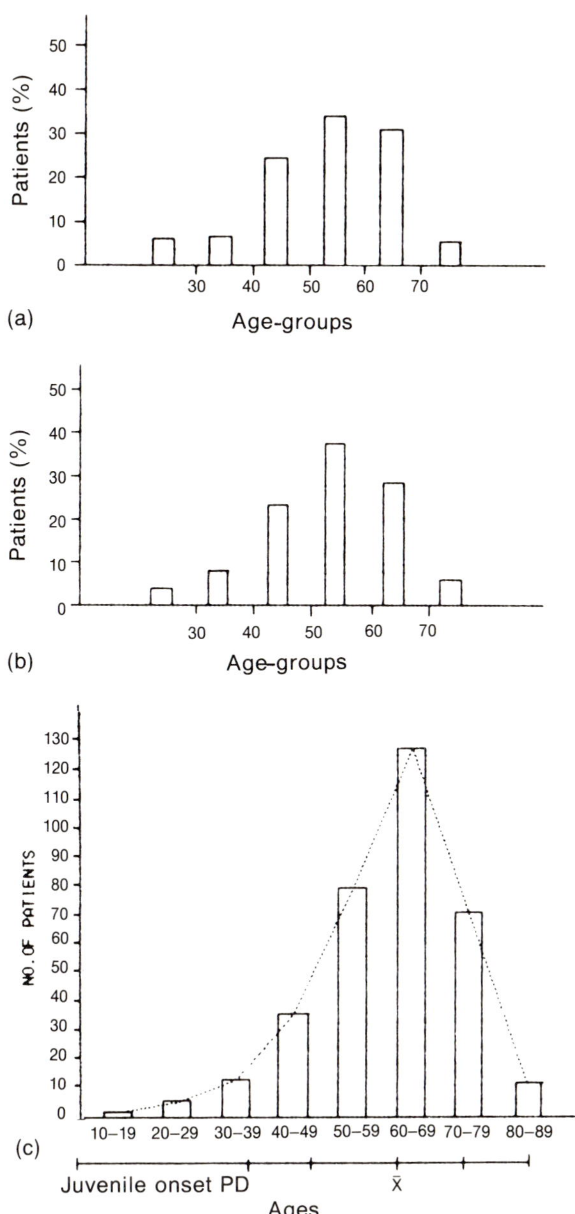

Figure 1 (a) The frequency distribution ($n = 424$) of age of onset in 10-year periods, in Parkinson disease patients from combined survey in seven general hospitals in Japan[3]. (b) The frequency distribution (n = 170) of age of onset in Parkinson disease patients from the survey in the outpatient clinic of the Department of Neurology, Juntendo University Hospital[3]. (c) Distribution of Parkinson disease patients is shown according to age of onset of the disease within 10-year periods; $\bar{X}$, mean age at onset (61.3 years); SD, standard deviation (11.8 years). Juvenile onset Parkinson disease is calculated as the 5-year period falling below SD + 2 (−2SD from $\bar{X}$) (reproduced from Gershanik and Leist[4])

Table 1 Prevalence of juvenile parkinsonism. All these JP cases had an age of onset < 40 years, except for Gershanik and Leist's (≤ 35)

Authors	*Frequency (%) of cases of juvenile parkinsonism*	*Total cases*
Hoehn and Yahr[5]	10.1	672
Yokochi[1]	10.6	170*
	11.5	424†
Barbeau and Pourcher[6]	9.4	–
Gershanik and Leist[4]	3.8	336
Rajput *et al.*[7]	4.8	505
Lima *et al.*[8]	9.2	228

*, Cases in outpatient clinic of Juntendo University; †, cases from combined survey of general hospitals in Japan.

Table 2 The frequency (%) of familial history by age of onset in Parkinson disease patients from a combined survey in seven general hospitals in Japan[1]

Age at onset (years)	*Frequency* (%)		
≤ 29	47.8	36.7 (≤ 29, ≤ 39)	8.5 (all)
≤ 39	29.6		
40 ≤	5.2	4.8 (40 ≤ to 70 ≤)	
50 ≤	6.7		
60 ≤	3.2		
70 ≤	0		

incidence rate of approximately 43%. Table 3 shows that recent reports[4,6,8,12–14] of JP also present much higher familial incidence than average familial incidence for all PD. Genetic factors in JP are considered quite important according to the above data. The transmission traits of familial cases involved with JP seem to demonstrate neither autosomal recessive nor dominant traits. Large families with autosomal dominant PD have been reported. Nukata and colleagues[15] presented a family with 36 affected members over five generations. In this family, the age of onset varied from 38 to 69, but the younger generations had a younger age of onset.

Table 3 Frequency of family history

Authors	*Frequency (%)*	*Positive members/parameters*
Yokochi *et al.*[12]	42.9	15/35 families
Barbeau and Pourcher[6]	45.9	62/135 cases
Gershanik and Leist[4]	23.1	3/13 cases‡
Lima *et al.*[8]	9.5	2/21 cases
Quinn *et al.*[13]	25.0	15/60 cases
	(100)*	(4/4 cases)*
	(19.6)†	(11/56 cases)†
Ludin and Ludin[14]	21.7	5/23 cases

*, Only the cases for onset age below 20 years; †, only the cases for onset age 25–39 years; ‡, only the cases for onset age below 35 years

Golbe and colleagues[16] reported two large families with 41 affected members in four generations. It is pointed out that the illness had an earlier onset at a mean age of 46.5 years. These results are interesting from the standpoint of understanding JP.

SYMPTOMATOLOGICAL CHARACTERISTICS OF JUVENILE PARKINSONISM

Although we have already described the details of symptoms of JP in previous publications[9,17], these characteristics are briefly enumerated as follows:

(1) There is much higher familial incidence;

(2) Progression is much slower and the prognosis seems benign;

(3) Difficulty of gait or drawing is often the first sign, rather than tremor;

(4) Half the cases are of a rigid and bradykinetic type without tremor. If tremor exists, it is seen in posture or in action, but not at rest;

(5) In the case of a much younger onset, inverted, Spitzfuss and dystonic features are often exhibited;

(6) Autonomic symptoms are seldom displayed;

(7) Dramatic or marked responses to levodopa are obtained;

(8) Cumulative levodopa therapy often has the following adverse effects: the wearing-off phenomenon occurs soon after treatment and severe induced dyskinesia appears in the extremities.

It should be emphasized that the characteristics mentioned above are not absolutely necessary conditions for the diagnosis of JP. If only these characteristics (especially the third, fourth and fifth) are predominant, the diagnosis of JP should be abandoned. For instance, two of 40 cases among our follow-up patients were misdiagnosed as JP. These patients (belonging to group III of the follow-up patients mentioned later) had complications of peculiar symptoms with the limitation of beneficial response to levodopa treatment soon after the first examination. (One patient is surviving, the other is deceased and the case has been described[18].)

PATHOLOGICAL OBSERVATION OF JUVENILE PARKINSONISM

The previous pathological reports related to JP are limited. Ota and Miyoshi[19] reported three sibling cases of a juvenile type of paralysis agitans. The autopsy findings of one of them, whose illness started at the age of 20 years and had a duration of 27 years, were described and shown to be very similar to those of classical paralysis agitans (the Lewy body was not mentioned). For a long time, this was the sole autopsy report of JP.

The patients focused on in this paper are different from those described by Hunt[20] in 1917, which have been used as textbook cases of juvenile parkinsonism.

Recently, Gibb and Lees[21] studied preserved brains and compared 12 cases with onset ages from 23 to 40 years, and 22 cases with onset ages of 70 years and above. Although the juvenile group had a stronger decrease in cells containing melanin, this was assumed to be related to the length of illness, and the report determined that an inherent difference could not be found between the two groups. Sage and colleagues[22] reported male autopsied cases (Figure 2), one with onset at age 25 who died at age 67, and an autosomal dominant inherited patient with onset at age 38 (although disease symptoms may have been present since age 32) who died at age 49. (This is the same case reported by Golbe and colleagues[16].) They concluded that their postmortem findings were typical of Lewy body Parkinson disease. Ikeda and colleagues[23] reported a sporadic case, with onset at age 30, which showed specific neuropathological findings with the diffuse appearance of intracytoplasmic inclusions of the Lewy type in the cerebral cortex, in addition to many Lewy bodies in the pigmented brainstem nuclei. Yoshimura and colleagues[24] reported a sporadic case with onset at the age of 24, which also showed diffuse appearance of Lewy bodies in thc brain. Miyazawa and colleagues[25] reported a sporadic case with onset at age 24 years which lacked Lewy bodies.

We had the opportunity to perform autopsies in seven cases and are

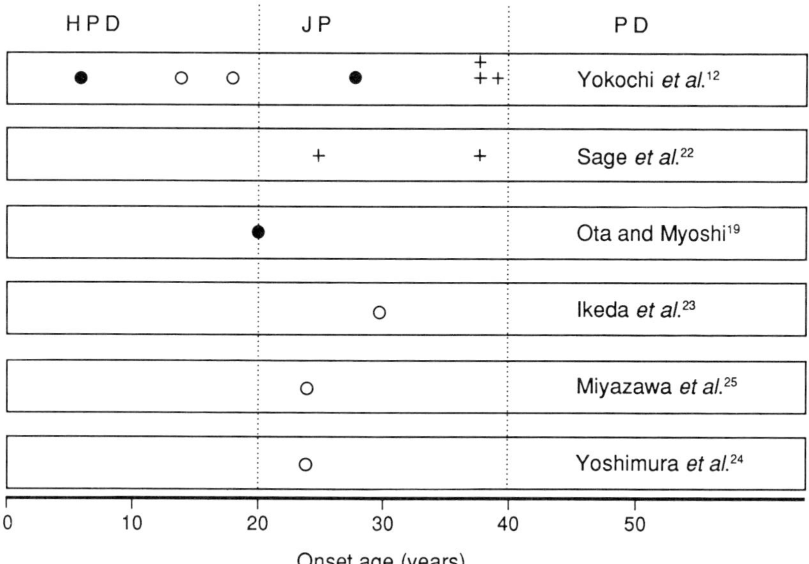

Figure 2 Onset age distribution of autopsied cases of JP, HPD and related cases; + = no contradictory findings compared to PD pathology; ○ = atypical findings with lack of Lewy bodies or with diffuse appearance of numerous Lewy-body additions to brainstem melanin-containing cells; ● = peculiar pathological findings, rather than PD pathology.

presently analyzing them. The distribution of pathological lesions for all cases was consistent with Parkinson disease, but the conditions of the substantia nigra were varied. We are currently performing a study in which the cases are classified into three categories:

(1) Typical Lewy body pathology in cases of onset at ages 38, 38 and 39, with no contradiction with Parkinson disease.

(2) Lewy body absence in cases of onset at ages 14 and 18.

(3) Peculiar substantia nigra pathology in two cases.

Regarding the third category, in one case with onset at age 28 and duration 24 years, gliosis was quite mild and did not match the duration of the illness or the degree of the decrease in cell population. In another patient whose age at onset was 6 years and who died at 39 years of age, the substantia nigra appeared to exhibit hypoplasia or poor neuronal maturation[26].

To this author's knowledge, autopsies of JP are limited to the above cases (Figure 2). The pathological findings are resolved into the following. All cases have no contradiction with Parkinson disease in the distribution of pathology in the brain. This supports the clinical evidence of symptoms, course and response to levodopa. In the patients with onset at ages of about 40, the findings are completely compatible with those of Lewy body Parkinson disease. In the younger-onset cases, the pathological lesions have noticeably peculiar findings. The cases with onset at ages 14, 18 and 24 had a lack of Lewy bodies, and the cases with onset at age 6 exhibited no Lewy bodies in the hypothalamus, the nucleus basalis and dorsal nucleus of the vagus nucleus. Furthermore, in the case with onset at age 25, Lewy bodies were not found in the locus ceruleus, and only a few were found in the nucleus basalis. Thus, in younger onset cases, that is, in the rapid degenerative process, Lewy bodies do not readily appear in the target lesions related to parkinsonism. On the other hand, most cases with widespread Lewy bodies, accompanying dementia and akinetic mutism, showed the involvement of some pathological changes in the striatum or the striatum and pallidum. Such being the case, it can be prudently assumed that they belong to the same disease entity as other cases of JP.

SUBGROUP ESTABLISHMENT

It is difficult to introduce *en bloc* the tenatively collected cases with onset age below 40 for discussion of clinical features. For this reason, authors divide them into several subgroups. This author[1] presented the follow-up patients by dividing them into three groups in consideration of the symptoms and the response to levodopa. Patients in group I exhibited dramatic effects with levodopa, followed by severe adverse effects within the early stage of treatment. Those in group II suffered much milder effects than group I. The patients with complications such as dystonia, inverted posture of the feet and a peculiar gait different from that typical of parkinsonism were designated as group III. This was a classification determined from the symptoms, but all cases in this group unexpectedly experienced onset of the disease at extremely young ages (all cases under 16 years). Subsequently, interest has arisen regarding the differences and similarities between group III and HPD or dopa-responsive dystonia.

Ishikawa and Miyatake[27] proposed classification of the groups as follows: I, the type with autosomal recessive inheritance that shows improvement of symptoms after sleep; II, the type of idiopathic PD; III, hereditary progressive dystonia that shows marked diurnal fluctuations.

Quinn and co-workers[13] developed their theory classifying patients, whose age at onset was less than 40, as under or over 21 years of age at onset. The former is 'juvenile parkinsonism' and the latter is 'young-onset Parkinson disease'. They hypothesized that the former four cases with family history were parkinsonism associated with heredity, and the latter cases occupied the lower end of the skewed deviation of the onset age distribution of Parkinson disease, as long as their clinical characteristics could be shown and no additional factor causing early onset could be confirmed.

Yamamura and colleagues[28] and Sunohara and colleagues[29] reported symptom groups having combined characteristics of both HPD and JP, and suggested that they might be independent types. Other authors[6,8] have advocated classification by a 'group mainly characterized by rigidity and akinesia' and a 'group mainly characterized by tremor'.

Each type of classification has its own basis; however, practically speaking, it is difficult to classify each individual case, and the assignments inevitably become artificial. Actually, classification for the individual case changes according to the course of illness and the result of levodopa treatment.

SIMILARITIES AND DISSIMILARITIES BETWEEN JP AND HPD

Neurological and neuropediatric consultations are clearly distinguished in major hospitals in Japan. Therefore, children are seldom examined by neurologists and adults by neuropediatriststs. Under these circumstances, JP and HPD, described by Segawa and colleagues[30–32] have been individually experienced by different physicians. It is reasonable and beneficial for both neurologists and neuropediatrists to discuss the continuities and similarities between the two diseases. The dissimilarities are listed as follows:

(1) Onset age during childhood in HPD, and at adolescence or after in JP;

(2) HPD has much higher familial incidence than JP. It is inherited in an autosomal dominant fashion;

(3) Symptoms of HPD are mainly characterized by dystonia, and JP by parkinsonism;

(4) Diurnal fluctuation of symptoms is characteristically recognized in HPD, but is not characteristic of JP;

(5) Beneficial response to levodopa therapy of HPD reveals an almost curable condition; and

(6) Adverse effects such as wearing off and dopa-induced dyskinesia by levodopa administration rarely appear in HPD.

As shown above, there are significant clinical differences between HPD and JP; however, no evidence exists for final differential diagnosis according to the borderline cases. In Figure 3, several reported cases with the diagnostic titles given by the authors (see Table 4) themselves are plotted against the ages of onset. It is difficult to draw a distinct line for dividing HPD and its related cases from JP. However, it seems to be possible to reach a consensus for separating HPD and JP at the age of 10–15 years. The onset ages of the cases accompanied with dystonia are earlier in comparison to cases without dystonia.

NOSOLOGICAL INDEPENDENCE OF JP

Although JP is distinguished by some clinical characteristics from PD, no apparent evidence for the diagnosis of JP as a nosological entity is proposed. A common pathogenic basis may put it on a continuum with PD in terms of nosology. For instance, the onset age distribution curve of Parkinson disease does not have peaks but is a normal curve. Quinn and co-workers[13] proposed that the onset age of JP should occupy only the lower end of a skewed distribution of onset age of all Parkinson disease cases. However, the author believes that the two large groups of JP type and PD type, according to the differences of response to levodopa and symptoms, overlap around the age of 40 at onset.

Also, the current tendency is to recognize HPD or dopa-responsive dystonia as a nosological entity. However, as mentioned in the last paragraph, no evidence for distinguishing between the cases of HPD and of JP with mainly much younger onset has been exhibited. HPD and JP specifically respond to the administration of levodopa as much as PD does. This shows that these three diseases are caused by the dysfunction of dopamine systems in the brain. According to the concept of pathogenesis, they belong to such a nosological entity as to exist on the same spectrum and they are consecutively arranged on the axis of onset age.

From a different point of view, in the clinical sense, it is unnatural that HPD, characterized by dystonia, and PD, characterized by parkinsonism, exist as the same symptomatological entity. Moreover, some peculiar pathological conditions in the substantia nigra have been shown in the autopsies of much younger JP cases. Further, there have been no autopsies of definite HPD.

In conclusion, these ambivalent findings support the hypothesis that pathological conditions and symptoms might change their expression according to the age of a harmful exposure, in spite of common disturbance of the catecholaminergic system by a common factor.

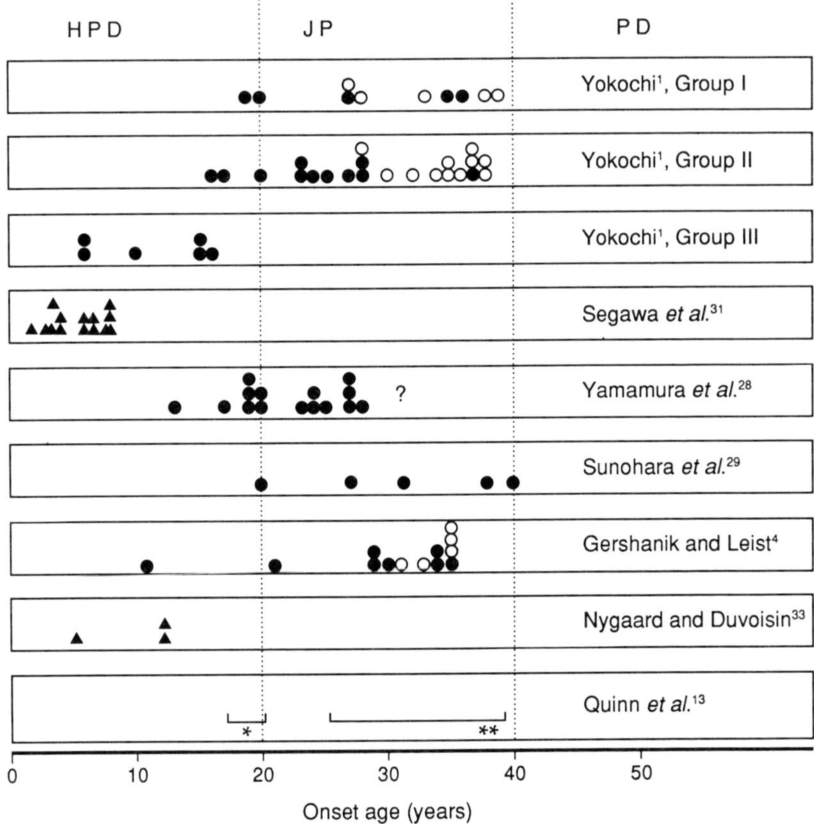

Figure 3 Onset age distribution of JP, HPD and related cases. Quinn *et al.*[13] described only the youngest and eldest cases. ▲ = cases characterized by dystonia ● = cases accompanied by dystonic feature (Yamamura *et al.*, Quinn *et al.* cases not individually mentioned). For the diagnostic classifications given by authors see Table 4.

Table 4 Author's diagnostic titles for cases shown in Figure 3

Reference	*Diagnostic title*
1	juvenile parkinsonism (JP) groups I, II and III
31	hereditary progressive dystonia (HPD) with marked diurnal fluctuation
28	paralysis agitans of early onset with marked diurnal fluctuation
29	idiopathic dystonia-parkinsonism with marked diurnal fluctuation of symptoms
4	juvenile onset Parkinson disease
33	hereditary dystonia-parkinsonism syndrome of juvenile onset
13	(*) juvenile parkinsonism
	(**) young-onset Parkinson disease

REFERENCES

1. Yokochi, M. (1979). Juvenile Parkinson's disease: Part I. Clinical aspects. *Adv. Neurol. Sci.* (Tokyo), **23**, 1048–59
2. Yokochi, M. (1979). Juvenile Parkinson's disease: Part II. Pharmacokinetic study. *Adv. Neurol. Sci.* (Tokyo), **23**, 1060–73
3. Yokochi, M. and Narabayashi, H. (1981). Clinical characteristics of juvenile parkinsonism. In Rose, F.C. and Capildeo, R. (eds.) *Research Progress in Parkinson's Disease*, pp. 35–9. (Pitman Medical Ltd)
4. Gershanik, O.S. and Leist, A. (1986). Juvenile onset Parkinson's disease. In Yahr, M.D. and Bergmann, K.J. (eds.) *Advances in Neurology*, Vol. 45, pp. 213–16. (New York: Raven Press)
5. Hoehn, M.M. and Yahr, M.D. (1967). Parkinsonism: onset, progression, and mortality. *Neurology*, **17**, 427–42
6. Barbeau, A. and Pourcher, E. (1982). New data on genetics of Parkinson's disease. *Can. J. Neurol. Sci.*, **9**, 53–60
7. Rajput, A.H., Uitti, R.J., Stern, W. and Laverty, W. (1986). Early onset Parkinson's disease and childhood environment. In Yahr, M.D. and Bergmann, K.J. (eds.) *Advances in Neurology*, Vol. 45, pp. 295–7. (New York: Raven Press)
8. Lima, B., Neves, G. and Nora, M. (1987). Juvenile parkinsonism: Clinical and metabolic characteristics. *J. Neurol. Neurosurg. Psychiatr.*, **50**, 345–8
9. Narabayashi, H., Yokochi, M., Iizuka, R. and Nagatsu, T. (1986). Juvenile parkinsonism. In Vinken, P.J., Bruyn, G.W. and Klawans, H.L. (eds.) *Handbook of Clinical Neurology*, Vol. 5(49), pp. 153–65. (Amsterdam: Elsevier Science)
10. Ward, C.D., Duvoisin, R.C., Ince, S.E., Nutt, J.D., Eldridge, R. and Calne, D.B. (1983). Parkinson's disease in 65 pairs of twins and in a set of quadruplets. *Neurology*, **33**, 815–24
11. Kondo, K., Kurland, L.T. and Schull, W.J. (1973). Parkinson's disease. Genetic analysis and evidence of a multifactorial etiology. *Mayo Clin. Proc.*, **48**, 465–75
12. Yokochi, M., Mizutani, Y., Narabayashi, H. and Tsuboi, T. (1988). Long term follow-up study in patients with juvenile parkinsonism. Presented at *9th International Symposium on Parkinson's Disease*, Israel, Abstracts, p. 70
13. Quinn, N., Critchley, P. and Marsden, C.D. (1987). Young-onset Parkinson's disease. *Movement Disorders*, **2**, 73–91
14. Ludin, S.M. and Ludin, H.P. (1989). Is Parkinson's disease of early onset a separate disease entity? *J. Neurol.*, **236**, 203–7
15. Nukata, H., Kowa, H., Saitoh, T., Tazaki, Y. and Miura, J. (1978). A big family of paralysis agitans. *Clin. Neurol.* (Tokyo), **18**, 627–33
16. Golbe, L.I., Iorio, G.D., Bonarita, V., Miller, D.C. and Duvoisin, R.C. (1990). A large kindred with autosomal dominant Parkinson's disease. *Ann. Neurol.*, **27**, 276–82
17. Yokochi, M., Narabayashi, H., Iizuka, R. and Nagatsu, T. (1984). Juvenile parkinsonism – some clinical, pharmacological and neuropathological aspects. In Hassler, R.G. and Christ, J.F. (eds.) *Advances in Neurology*, Vol. 40, pp. 407–13. (New York: Raven Press)
18. Funata, N., Maeda, Y., Koike, M., Yano, Y., Kaseda, M., Muro, T., Okeda, R., Iwata, M. and Yokochi, M. (1990). Neuronal intranuclear hyaline inclusion disease: report of a case and review of the literature. *Clin. Neuropathol.*, **9**, 89–96
19. Ota, U. and Miyoshi, S. (1958). Familial paralysis agitans juveniles: a clinical, anatomical and genetic study. *Folia Psychiatr. Neurol. Jpn.*, **12**, 112–21
20. Hunt, J.R. (1917). Progressive atrophy of the globus pallidus. *Brain*, **40**, 58–148
21. Gibb, W.R.G. and Lees, A.J. (1988). A comparison of clinical and pathological features of young- and old-onset Parkinson's disease. *Neurology*, **38**, 1402–6
22. Sage, J.I., Miller, D.C., Golbe, L.I., Walters, A. and Duvoisin, R.C. (1990). Clinically atypical expression of pathologically typical Lewy-body parkinsonism. *Clin. Neuropharmacol.*, **13**, 36–47
23. Ikeda, K., Yoshimura, T., Kato, H. and Namba, M. (1978). Idiopathic parkinsonism with Lewy-type inclusions in cerebral cortex. A case report. *Acta Neuropathol.*, **41**, 165–8
24. Yoshimura, N., Yoshimura, I., Asada, M., Hayashi, S., Fukushima, Y., Sato, T. and Kudo, H. (1988). Juvenile Parkinson's disease with widespread Lewy bodies in the brain. *Acta Neuropathol.*, **77**, 213–18

25. Miyazawa, Y., Abe, N., Ohtoh, T. (1987). An autopsy case of juvenile parkinsonism. *Neurol. Med.* (Tokyo), **26**, 578–83

26. Mizutani, Y., Yokochi, M. and Oyanagi, S. (1991). Juvenile parkinsonism: A case with first clinical manifestation at the age of six years and with neuropathological findings suggesting a new pathogenesis. *Clin. Neuropathol.*, **10**, 91–7

27. Ishikawa, A. and Miyatake, T. (1988). Juvenile parkinsonism. In Miyatake, T. (ed.) *Niigata Symposium Series on Neurology*, No. 5, *Parkinsonism*, pp. 22–49. (Tokyo: Kagaku Hyoronsya)

28. Yamamura, U., Sobue, I., Ando, K., Iida, M., Yanagi, T. and Kono, C. (1973). Paralysis agitans of early onset with marked diurnal fluctuation of symptoms. *Neurology*, **23**, 239–44

29. Sunohara, N., Mano, Y., Ando, K. and Satoyoshi, E. (1985). Idiopathic dystonia-parkinsonism with marked diurnal fluctuation of symptoms. *Ann. Neurol.*, **17**, 39–45

30. Segawa, M., Hosaka, A., Miyagawa, F., Nomura, Y. and Imai, H. (1976). Hereditary progressive dystonia with marked diurnal fluctuation. In Eldridge, R. and Fahn, S. (eds.) *Advances in Neurology*, Vol. 14, pp. 215–33. (New York: Raven Press)

31. Segawa, M., Nomura, Y. and Kase, M. (1986). Hereditary progressive dystonia with marked diurnal fluctuation: clinicopathological identification in reference to juvenile Parkinson's disease. In Yahr, M.D. and Bergmann, K.J. (eds.) *Advances in Neurology*, Vol. 45, pp. 227–34. (New York: Raven Press)

32. Segawa, M., Nomura, Y., Tanaka, S., Hakamada, S., Nagata, E., Soda, M. and Kase, M. (1988). Hereditary progressive dystonia with marked diurnal fluctutation – consideration on its pathophysiology based on the characteristics of clinical and polysomnographical findings. In Fahn, S., Marsden, C.D. and Calne, D.B. (eds.) *Advances in Neurology*, Vol. 50, pp. 367–76. (New York: Raven Press)

33. Nygaard, T.G. and Duvoisin, R.C. (1986). Hereditary dystonia-parkinsonism syndrome of juvenile onset. *Neurology*, **36**, 1424–8

SECTION 2

Familial parkinsonism dystonia complex: long-term follow-up studies

4

Parkinsonism of early-onset with diurnal fluctuation

Y. Yamamura, Y. Hamaguchi, M. Uchida, H. Fujioka and S. Watanabe

INTRODUCTION

Since early-onset paralysis agitans was first described in 1911 its nosological identification has been debated. In 1968 and 1973 we[1,2] reported cases of early-onset parkinsonism, mostly familial, in which parkinsonism and dystonia showed marked diurnal fluctuation. In the intervening years similar cases have been noted in Japan[3–5], and the cumulative experience of investigators has confirmed the excellent effect of levodopa therapy, which is, however, almost invariably complicated by dyskinesia or the 'wearing-off' phenomenon appearing relatively soon after commencement of treatment. The condition investigated in this study, hereafter referred to as parkinsonism of early onset with diurnal fluctuation (PEDF), has some similarities to juvenile parkinsonism type III described by Yokochi and colleagues[6] and, more importantly, to hereditary progressive dystonia with marked diurnal fluctuation (HPD) reported by Segawa and colleagues[7,8]. In this paper we clarify the differences betweeen PEDF and early-onset Parkinson disease and compare PEDF with HPD and related disorders.

MATERIALS AND METHODS

For the purpose of long-term observation of PEDF, previously observed patients were re-examined after 17–23 years. Of 11 patients from four families[2] one patient (F-III) had already died at the time of the previous study and, subsequently, two others died; N-I of cerebral hemorrhage and F-I of cardiac arrest. Therefore, eight patients were examined in the present study. Brain computerized tomography (CT), magnetic resonance imaging (MRI), and single photon emission CT (SPECT) with ^{125}Imipramine were performed in some of the patients.

To differentiate PEDF from early-onset Parkinson disease we collected data for 40 cases of parkinsonism with onset before the age of 40, including cases referred to above, from our cumulative case records. All patients were thoroughly examined to exclude those with any known cause of secondary parkinsonism (Huntington disease, etc.). The 40 cases were divided into two groups according to the presence or absence of diurnal fluctuation, and differences between the two in familial occurrence, sex ratio, age at onset, and neurological manifestations were evaluated.

RESULTS

Long-term follow-up study of previously described PEDF patients

Clinical manifestations of the eight patients from four families for 1973 and 1990 are shown in Table 1. In two families the parents were consanguineously related. All patients were female. On the previous examination marked diurnal fluctuation and alleviation after sleep had been observed. In three patients (Sa-I, O-I, O-II) the initial symptoms of parkinsonism had started during pregnancy or postpartum, and the symptoms were aggravated during menstruation. With the start of the therapy the magnitude of diurnal fluctuation decreased or was masked. Most patients, however, had brief remission of the symptoms after sleep, even 40 years after onset. All eight patients were ambulatory, and were maintained at Hoehn–Yahr stage II to III with the aid of appropriate medication. Levodopa coupled with other antiparkinsonism drugs had been successfully used in five patients (Sa-I, Sa-II, O-I, N-II, N-III), but in two (F-II and F-IV) levodopa had been discontinued because of adverse effects and substituted with other drugs including amantadine, trihexyphenidyl and bromocriptine. In one patient (O-II) a small dose of trihexyphenidyl was potent enough to improve the symptoms. The patients habitually took the drugs in small divided doses several times a day for the purpose of minimizing adverse effects.

In patients with long-standing PEDF, a stooped posture, kyphoscoliosis, pes equinovarus or talipes equinus was manifest. All patients had dysarthria due to striatal pseudobulbar palsy, but deglutition was not disturbed. Hyperactive deep reflexes without pathological reflexes were common to all the patients. Patient F-II had impaired fast eye movement and saccadic movement on smooth pursuit. Cerebellar coordination was intact in all patients. Autonomic disorders were minimal; five patients had constipation, but other autonomic deficits were not elicited on physical examinations. None had progressive mental disorders.

CT and MRI revealed mild to moderate atrophy of the cerebral cortex (especially of the frontal lobe), midbrain and cerebellum, along with enlargement of the third ventricle in four patients (O-I, O-II, F-II, F-IV), (Figures 1 and 2). In the other three patients (Sa-I, N-II and N-III) CT revealed slight frontal atrophy with or without cerebellar vermis atrophy and enlargement of the third ventricle. SPECT revealed decreased perfusion of the basal ganglia regions in four patients (O-I, O-II, F-II and F-IV).

In addition, three patients (Sa-I, Sa-II and O-II) had simple goiter and one patient (N-III) had hyperthyroidism. Two patients (S-I and O-II) had

Table 1 Long-term follow-up study of parkinsonism of early-onset with diurnal fluctuation. Diurnal fluctuation is shown as previous state →present state. Elsewhere, + + + represents marked; + +, moderate; +, mild; ±, slight; —, absent; THP, trihexyphenidyl; DOPS, L-threo-3,4-dihydroxyphenylserine

	Patients							
	SA-I	*SA-II*	*O-I*	*O-II*	*N-II*	*N-III*	*F- II*	*F-IV*
Family history	siblings consanguineous parents		siblings consanguineous parents		siblings		siblings	
Sex	F	F	F	F	F	F	F	F
Age at onset	24	19	28	27	20	20	25	23
Duration of illness (years)	33	29	40	27	48	45	44	24
Diurnal fluctuation	+4→0	+4→0	+3→+1	+4→+1	+3→+1	+2→+1	+2→+2	+3→+2
Hoehn-Yahr stage	III	III	III	III	III	II	III	II
Treatment	levodopa THP bromocriptine	levodopa	levodopa THP amantadine	THP amantadine	levodopa THP	levodopa THP	Amantadine THP bromocriptine	Amantadine THP bromocriptine DOPS
Drug-induced dyskinesia	+ + +	+ + +	±	±	+ +	±	±	±
Postural abnormalities	+ +	+	+ + +	+ + +	+ +	+ +	+ + +	+ + +
Hyper-reflexia	+ +	+ +	+ +	+ +	+ +	+ +	+ +	+ +
Autonomic symptoms	±	—	±	±	—	±	±	—

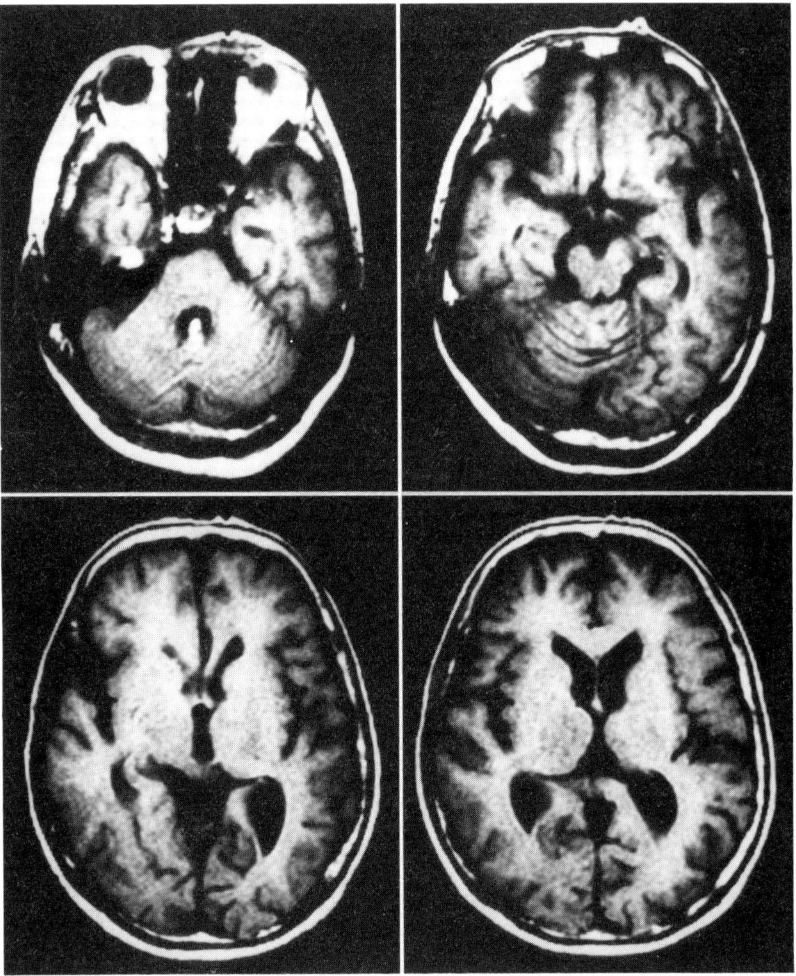

Figure 1 MRI T_1-weighted images of patient O-I (a 68-year-old woman with a 40-year history of parkinsonism) showing atrophy of the midbrain along with cerebral and cerebellar cortical atrophy

glucose intolerance, and four patients (O-I, O-II, N-II and F-II) had hypertension.

Comparative study of early-onset parkinsonism with and without diurnal fluctuation

There were distinct differences between the groups with and without diurnal fluctuation in familial occurrence, sex ratio, and age at onset (Table 2). The

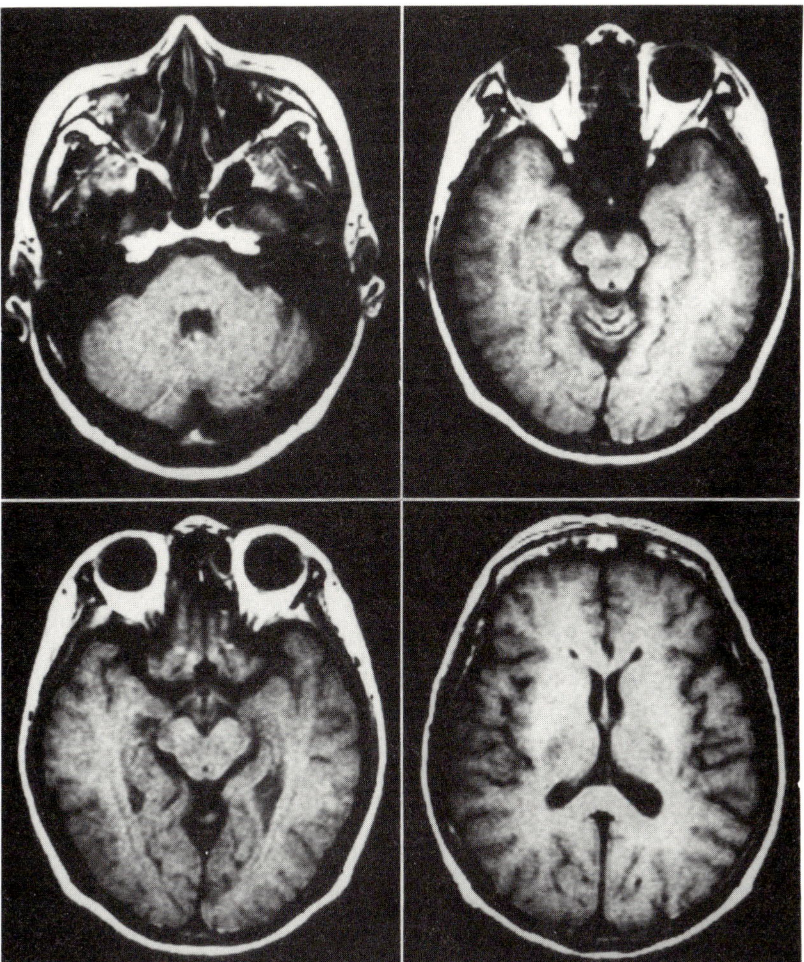

Figure 2 MRI T_1-weighted images of patient O-II (54-year-old woman with 27-year history of parkinsonism) showing less remarkable changes than that of her sister, patient O-I

group with diurnal fluctuation showed higher incidence of familial occurrence, while most of the patients without diurnal fluctuation were the sole family members affected. The male-to-female ratio of patients with diurnal fluctuation was 1:3.3, and of those without was 1:0.4. Mean age at onset of the group with diurnal fluctuation was 22.6 years (range 12–38), which was 11 years younger than that of the group without diurnal fluctuation (33.7 years; range 25–39). The age distribution of the group without diurnal fluctuation was positively skewed and peaked at 40 years of age.

Dystonic posture of the neck, trunk and extremities before starting therapy was present in most patients with diurnal fluctuation, while it was rare and mild in those without diurnal fluctuation. Hyperreflexia was frequent in the

Table 2 Comparison of two groups of early-onset parkinsonism patients, with and without diurnal fluctuation. (Percentages in brackets)

	With diurnal fluctuation ($n = 26$)	*Without diurnal fluctuation* ($n = 14$)
Familial occurrence		
present	19 (73.1)	3 (21.4)
absent	7 (26.9)	11 (78.6)
Sex		
male	6 (23.1)	10 (71.4)
female	20 (76.9)	4 (28.6)
male : female	1 : 3.3	1 : 0.4
Age at onset (years)		
10–19	8 (30.8)	–
20–29	15 (57.7)	3 (21.4)
30–39	3 (11.5)	11 (78.6)
mean	22.6	33.7
Minor dystonia		
present	20 (76.9)	2 (14.3)
absent	6 (23.1)	12 (85.7)
Hyperreflexia		
present	22 (84.6)	3 (21.4)
absent	4 (15.4)	11 (78.6)
Levodopa treatment		
useful	19 (73.1)	14 (100)
discontinued	7 (26.9)	–
dyskinesia	21 (80.8)	6 (42.9)

group with diurnal fluctuation, but it was not as frequent in the other group. No patient had any distinct progressive mental disorders. Levodopa therapy had been effective in both groups. The wearing-off phenomenon and/or drug-induced dyskinesias were seen in most patients with diurnal fluctuation, in seven of whom levodopa therapy was discontinued. In most patients without diurnal fluctuation, levodopa was useful for a long enough period without serious adverse effects.

DISCUSSION

The present study shows that early-onset parkinsonism without diurnal fluctuation is mostly, if not exclusively, Parkinson disease, which is characterized by a wide range of onset ages. On the other hand PEDF shows the following characteristic features:

(1) High incidence of familial occurrence and parental consanguinity, and therefore probably an autosomal recessive trait;

(2) Early onset (mean, 22.6 years);

(3) It is more frequent in females than in males;

(4) Diurnal fluctuation of parkinsonism-dystonia, reduced in range with the development of postural changes;

(5) Frequent hyperreflexia;

(6) Minimal autonomic failures;

(7) No dementia, no serious bulbar signs or cerebellar disorders;

(8) Marked effect of antiparkinsonism drugs, almost invariably complicated by drug-induced dyskinesias and other adverse effects; and

(9) Slow progression of the disease through life.

Idiopathic dystonic parkinsonism, as reported by Sunohara and colleagues[3], and juvenile parkinsonism with marked diurnal fluctuation reported by Yamada and colleagues[4] and Ishikawa and colleagues[5], are almost the same condition as PEDF. Juvenile parkinsonism type III of Yokochi and Narabayashi[6] is differentiated from PEDF by its lack of diurnal fluctuation. Progressive atrophy of globus pallidus[9] is known as a type of juvenile paralysis agitans, but the clinical manifestations in reported cases are different from those of PEDF described here.

HPD reported by Segawa[7,8] is a disease of childhood-onset, predominantly found in females. It is mainly characterized by dystonia rather than parkinsonism. Levodopa-induced dyskinesia is not a significant concern in the treatment of HPD. Dopa-responsive dystonia (DRD)[10] is a childhood- or adolescent-onset disease, where the parkinsonian signs – dramatic response to levodopa, diurnal fluctuation, and autosomal dominant inheritance – are notable. From the clinical perspective, PEDF can be differentiated from HPD and DRD. It is, however, possible that the underlying pathological and biochemical abnormalities of both conditions are similar. Analogously, in Huntington chorea a particular pathological process causes a fluctuating dystonia in the first decade, but is more typically manifested as parkinsonism in older patients[11].

To discriminate PEDF from HPD and related disorders pathological and biochemical data of these conditions are needed. In this context, the autopsy report described by Yokochi and co-workers[12] is important. In a woman with a long-standing history of parkinsonism without diurnal fluctuation the cells of the substantia nigra had decreased amounts of melanin pigment, although the cellular population was normal. CT and MRI examinations in our study, however, indicate that the cerebral cortex and cerebellum as well as brain stem could be involved in PEDF. This pathological change of PEDF is more extensive than expected from its clinical picture.

It seems reasonable to suppose that a diurnal fluctuation of symptoms reflects a specific metabolic, functional defect of the nigrostriatal system rather than structural alteration[1,5]. Increasing postural abnormality with diminution of diurnal fluctuation suggests morphological alteration could ensue in the later stages. One of the putative metabolic abnormalities which would account for the diurnal fluctuation of the dopaminergic system is that of tyrosine hydroxylase, whose striatal activity shows a circadian variation[13]. Another candidate is estrogen. Striatal dopamine activity in experimental animals is both enhanced and blocked by estrogens[14]. Clinical observations which support the implication of female sex hormones in the pathophysiology of Parkinson disease and dopa-induced dyskinesias have been documented[15]. In some cases of PEDF the initiation of disease and temporary worsening of symptoms in relation to pregnancy or menstruation has been noted. A third possibility is a defect of dihydrobiopterin synthesis, reported by Tanaka and colleagues[16]. Fluctuation of symptoms in PEDF and HPD may also be related to impaired synthesis of neurotransmitters due to biopterin deficiency[16].

CONCLUSION

The results of our clinical studies show that PEDF can be differentiated from Parkinson disease of early-onset and is considered to be a distinct clinical entity. Most probably PEDF is closely related to HPD, but biochemical and pathological evidence for this supposition is not available.

REFERENCES

1. Yamamura, Y., Iida, M., Ando, K. and Sobue, I. (1968). A juvenile familial disorder with marked rigidospasticity, bradykinesia and minor dystonia alleviated after sleep. *Clin. Neurol.*, (Tokyo), **5**, 233–43
2. Yamamura, Y., Sobue, I., Ando, K., Iida, M., Yanagi, T. and Kono, C. (1973). Paralysis agitans of early onset with marked diurnal fluctuation of symptoms. *Neurology*, **23**, 239–44
3. Sunohara, N., Mano, Y., Ando, K. and Satoyoshi, E. (1985). Idiopathic dystonia-parkinsonism with marked diurnal fluctuation of symptoms. *Ann. Neurol.*, **17**, 39–45
4. Yamada, T., Koguchi, Y. and Hirayama, K. (1989). Juvenile parkinsonism with marked diurnal fluctuation. *Jpn. J. Psychiatr. Neurol.*, **43**, 205–12
5. Ishikawa, A. and Miyatake, T. (1988). Juvenile parkinsonism. In Miyatake, T. (ed.) *Parkinsonism*, pp. 22–49. (Tokyo: Kagaku-Hyouron-Sha)
6. Yokochi, M. and Narabayashi, H. (1981). Clinical characteristics of juvenile parkinsonism. In Rose, F.C. and Capildeo, R. (eds.) *Research Progress in Parkinson Disease*, pp. 35–9. (Tunbridge Wells, UK: Pitman Medical)
7. Segawa, M., Hosaka, A., Miyagawa, F., Nomura, Y. and Imai, H. (1976). Hereditary progressive dystonia with marked diurnal fluctuation. In Eldridge, R. and Fahn, S. (eds.) *Advances in Neurology*, Vol. 14, pp. 215–33. (New York: Raven Press)
8. Segawa, M., Nomura, Y. and Kase, M. (1987). Hereditary progressive dystonia with marked diurnal fluctuation: clinicopathophysiological identification in reference to juvenile Parkinson disease. In Yahr, M. and Bergmann, K.J. (eds.) *Advances in Neurology*, Vol. 45, pp. 227–34. (New York: Raven Press)
9. Jellinger, K. (1968). Progressive pallidumatrophy. *J. Neurol. Sci.*, **6**, 19–44
10. Nygaard, T.G., Marsden, C.D. and Duvoisin, R.C. (1986). Dopa-responsive dystonia. In Fahn, S., Marsden, C.D. and Calne, D.B. (eds.) *Advances in Neurology*, Vol. 50, pp. 377–84. (New York: Raven Press)
11. Ouvrier, R.A. (1978). Progressive dystonia with marked diurnal fluctuation. *Ann. Neurol.*, **4**, 412–17
12. Yokochi, M., Narabayashi, H., Iizuka, R. and Nagatsu, T. (1984). Juvenile parkinsonism: Some clinical, pharmacological, and neuropathological aspects. In Hassler, R.G. and Christ, J.F. (eds.) *Advances in Neurology*, Vol. 40, pp. 407–13. (New York: Raven Press)
13. McGeer, E.G. and McGeer, P.L. (1973). Some characteristics of brain tyrosine hydroxylase. In Mandel, J. (ed.) *New Concepts in Neurotransmitter Regulation*, pp. 53–68. (New York: Plenum Press)
14. Bedard, P.J., Langelier, P., Dankova, J., Villeneuve, A., Di Paolo, T., Barden, N., Labrie, F.,

Voissier, J.R. and Euvrard, C. (1979). Estrogens, progesterone, and the extrapyramidal system. In Poirier, L.J., Sourkes, T.L. and Bedard, P.J. (eds.) *Advances in Neurology*, Vol. 24, pp. 411–22. (New York: Raven Press)

15. Sandyk, R. (1989). Estrogen and the pathophysiology of Parkinson disease. *Intern. J. Neurosci.*, **45**, 119–22
16. Tanaka, K., Yoneda, M., Nakajima, H., Miyatake, T. and Owada, M. (1987). Dihydrobiopterin synthesis defect: An adult with diurnal fluctuation of symptoms. *Neurology*, **37**, 519–22

5

Idiopathic dystonia-parkinsonism with diurnal fluctuation: a follow-up study and magnetic resonance imaging findings

N. Sunohara, K. Ikeda and H. Tomi

INTRODUCTION

We have previously reported five patients with idiopathic dystonia-parkinsonism in 1985[1]. Before publication of the paper, we had an opportunity to examine two sisters whose clinical manifestations were similar to those in our patients, by courtesy of Dr Kowa, Professor of Kitazato University School of Medicine. Moreover, we had another opportunity to examine Yamamura's first case[2]. From the examinations of these patients, we had confidence that our cases of idiopathic dystonia-parkinsonism were included in a distinct disorder group.

We emphasized the following three points in the papers published in 1982[3] and 1985[1]: the patients had minor dystonia such as dystonia of the foot or legs, or torticollis-like neck dystonia, before administration of antiparkinsonian drugs; secondly, the dystonia was dramatically improved by administration of a small dosage of levodopa, trihexyphenidyl and/or bromocriptine, and thirdly, the dystonia was remarkably increased by exercise, and this contributed to diurnal fluctuation of the symptom.

In this paper, we will report a follow-up study of three of the previously reported patients with idiopathic dystonia-parkinsonism, that is patients 1, 2 and 5 in the paper[1], and we will also report magnetic resonance imaging (MRI) findings from these patients.

FOLLOW-UP STUDY

Patient 1 is a 55-year-old woman. There is no family history of neurological disorders. She had noticed dorsiflexion of the right large toe, tremor of the right hand and generalized bradykinesia at age 27 years. At the age of 30 years, her symptoms, including gait disturbance, bradykinesia and dystonia, became worse after exercise. Trihexyphenidyl (6 mg daily) was given to the patient. The drug effect was remarkable, with abolition of parkinsonian symptoms and dystonia for 15 successive years. At age 45, she was admitted to our hospital because of slight worsening of the symptoms.

Neurological examination at age 45 years showed mild emotional lability, monotonic speech and masked face, with plastic and cogwheel rigidity, bradykinesia and poor postural reaction. These manifestations were mild in the morning, but increased in the evening or after exercise. Resting tremor was seen in the limbs and trunk. This was exaggerated by movements and emotional stress. There was pes equinovarus, extreme dorsiflexion of the large toes (Figure 1(b)) and flexion dystonia of the limbs. These dystonias were also exaggerated after exercise. Figure 1(a) shows a small-stepped gait with no arm movement in the patient. This picture was taken 2 weeks after discontinuation of trihexyphenidyl administration.

The patient was given 6 mg of trihexyphenidyl, 200 mg of levodopa and 21.6 mg of carbidopa. A dramatic effect on all symptoms was obtained. At the present time (55 years), she has slight dorsiflexion of the large toes, and mild fluctuation of symptoms, which may be side-effects of the long-term administration of antiparkinsonian drugs, because these become worse with increase of the dose.

Patient 2 is now 73 years old. She had first noticed tremor and bradykinesia at the age of 38 years. She was treated with trihexyphenidyl, but it was discontinued because of nausea, vomiting and anorexia. At age 40 years, she had severe tremor of all limbs, gait disturbance, and dystonia of the left limbs and neck. At the same time, she had diurnal fluctuation of the symptoms. Her symptoms had remained unchanged without medication for the last 24 years prior to admission.

At age 64 years, when she was admitted to our hospital, she showed monotonic speech, resting tremor of the hand and limbs, plastic rigidity, mild bradykinesia, and poor postural reaction. Dystonias, such as torticollis, flexion dystonia of the left arm, hyperextension of the large toes, and pes equinovarus were seen (Figure 2(a)). These dystonias and parkinsonian symptoms revealed marked diurnal fluctuation as with patient 1.

Levodopa (100 mg) and carbidopa (10.8 mg) were given twice daily. The symptoms, including both parkinsonism and dystonia with diurnal fluctuation, were dramatically improved (Figure 2(b)). At the present time (72 years), she is being treated with the same doses of levodopa and carbidopa. Her neurological examination remains unchanged.

Patient 3 (patient 5 in reference 1) is now 48 years old. He had noticed hand tremor and gait disturbance at the age of 22 years. Subsequently he had tremor of all limbs and bradykinesia. At age 29, he had dystonia of the fingers, and at 32 years, dystonia of the neck and left leg. At the same time, he experienced diurnal fluctuation of the symptoms.

At age 40, he was admitted to our hospital. He showed dystonia of the finger (flexion of the proximal interphalangeal finger joints and extension of the distal interphalangeal joints), neck dystonia (Figure 3), and flexion of the leg, in addition to parkinsonian symptoms including rigidity, resting tremor, bradykinesia, small-stepped gait and poor postural reaction. These manifestations became worse after exercise or in the evening, and diminished after rest or sleep (Figure 3).

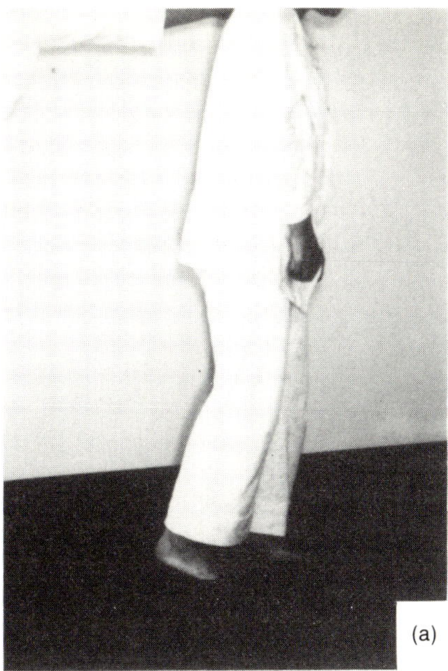

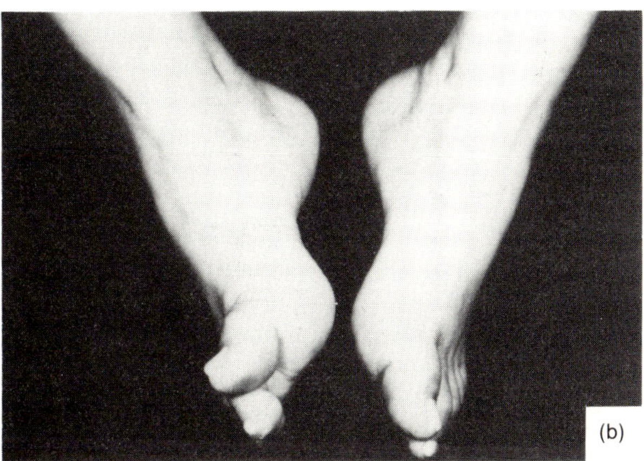

Figure 1 Patient 1: (a) small-stepped gait and poor postural reaction during walking; (b) foot dystonia.

He was given 150 mg of levodopa with 16.3 mg of carbidopa, and 6 mg of trihexyphenidyl, three times daily. His symptoms were markedly improved. At age 48, he still showed a good response with the same dosage of the antiparkinsonian drugs, except for mild diurnal fluctuation of the symptoms. This fluctuation is considered to be due to insufficient dosage of the antiparkinsonian drugs, because increase of the dosage diminished the symptoms, but severe peak-dose dyskinesia appeared.

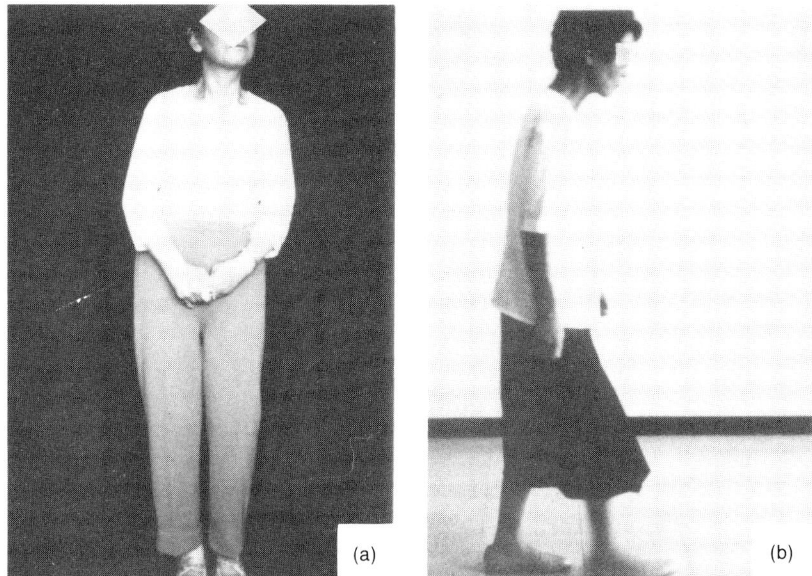

Figure 2 (a) Torticollis and flexion dystonia of the left upper limb which patient 1 is extending with the right hand; (b) neck and limb dystonias disappeared after administration of a small dose of antiparkinsonian drugs.

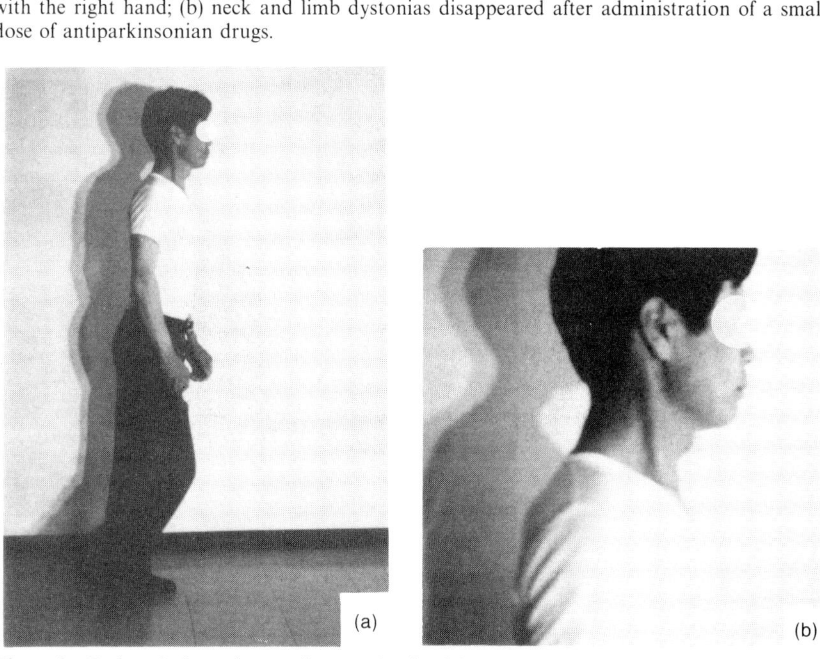

Figure 3 Patient 3 showed a small-stepped gait without arm-swinging (a), and neck dystonia (a), (b).

Table 1 Clinical features of idiopathic dystonia-parkinsonism with marked diurnal fluctuation of symptoms

Early-adult onset
? Autosomal recessive
Parkinsonism and minor dystonia before treatment
Marked diurnal fluctuation of symptoms
Dramatic response to parkinsonism and dystonia with levodopa therapy
Extremely good prognosis

SUMMARY OF THE CLINICAL FEATURES

The disorder is early-adult onset, and it may have an autosomal recessive mode of inheritance. There is minor dystonia in addition to parkinsonism in the pretreatment state, and the symptoms become worse after exercise and diminish in the morning or after rest or sleep. Dramatic improvement is obtained with a small dosage of levodopa. Our follow-up study confirmed that the disorder has an extremely good prognosis (Table 1).

MAGNETIC RESONANCE IMAGING IN IDIOPATHIC DYSTONIA-PARKINSONISM

Materials and methods

MRI was performed on three patients with idiopathic dystonia-parkinsonism (IDP), two patients with juvenile Parkinson disease (JPD), five patients with Parkinson disease (PD), and six normal controls (Table 2). The patients with IDP were patients 1 and 2 mentioned previously, and a new case. The latter was a 67 year old woman. The age of onset had been 27 years. She had torticollis and hyperextension of the large toes in addition to parkinsonism. She was successfully treated with 150 mg of levodopa with 16.2 mg of carbidopa, and 4 mg of trihexyphenidyl.

The patients with JPD showed no dystonia or diurnal fluctuation in the pretreatment state, and response to levodopa was not so dramatic. Their ages were 52 and 54 years old, the duration of the disease being 13 and 15 years, respectively.

The patients with PD had a mean age of 55.2 years (ranging from 49 to 71 years), and the mean duration of the disease was 9.2 years (ranging from 7 to 11 years). The six normal controls had a mean age of 41.8 years (ranging from 30 to 59 years).

Duration of the disease of patients with IDP was much longer than that of other groups. Severity of the disease was evaluated by the Hoehn and Yahr scale. All patients with IDP showed stage II. The patients with JPD or PD, except for one with PD, were classified as stage III or IV.

The magnetic resonance images were obtained using the 2.0 tesla Philips prototype system with spin-echo sequences. T_1-weighted images were obtained using a repetition time of 550 ms and an echo time of 19 ms. T_2-weighted images were obtained using a repetition time of 2100 ms (first and second echoes) and echo times of 29 ms (first echo) and 100 ms (second echo).

Table 2 Width of the pars compacta

Subjects	*Age/sex* (year)	*Age of onset*	*Duration* (years)	*Stage of severity**	*Width*† (mm) *Right*	*Left*
Idiopathic dystonia-parkinsonism (IDP)						
1	55/F	27	38	II	3.0	2.8
2	72/F	38	34	II	2.7	2.6
3	67/F	27	40	II	NA	3.6
Juvenile Parkinson disease (JPD)						
1	52/M	39	13	IV	3.2	2.6
2	45/F	30	15	III	3.2	2.7
Parkinson disease (PD)						
1	52/F	42	10	IV	3.2	3.3
2	53/M	42	11	IV	3.3	3.0
3	51/M	42	9	II	2.9	2.7
4	49/F	42	7	III	2.8	2.6
5	71/F	62	9	III	2.5	2.4
Normal controls						
1	30/M				2.6	2.7
2	35/M				3.6	3.7
3	37/F				2.7	2.8
4	43/M				2.5	2.7
5	47/F				3.1	3.2
6	59/M				3.0	2.8

*: Evaluated by the Hoehn & Yahr's scale; †: width of the pars compacta; NA: not available

An image matrix of 256 × 256 was used. Section thickness was 9 mm for the whole brain, and 5 mm for the midbrain. The scanning plane was axial 0–20 degrees positive to the inferior orbito-meatal line.

T_1- and T_2-weighted images and proton images, obtained from each disorder group and normal controls, were compared with each other. Additionally the width of the pars compacta signal was measured by the method described by Duguid and colleagues[4].

Optical density profiles of the scan, photographed on X-ray film, were obtained using a densitometer. We measured the width of the valley at half-height between the peaks of optical density, representing the red nucleus and crus cerebri–pars reticulata complex (Figure 4).

RESULTS

The T_2-weighted images showed mild, low signals in the postero-lateral portion of the putamen in two patients with IDP, one patient with JPD and three patients with PD, and also one normal subject. However, proton-weighted images showed no abnormality. These findings are considered to be due to the aging process. Very small foci, showing high signals on the T_2-weighted images and low signals on the T_1-weighted images, were observed on the centrum ovale in one patient with IDP and two patients with PD. These suggested lacunae. Stern and colleagues[5] stated that groups

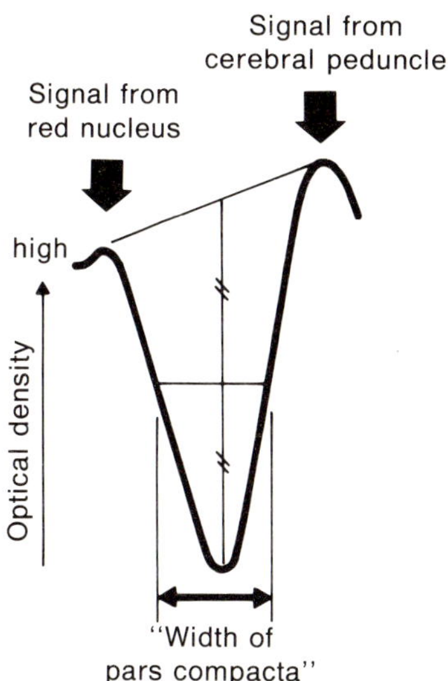

Figure 4 Densitometer profile of the scan to measure width of the pars compacta.

of Parkinson disease and parkinsonian syndrome patients had more of these lesions than controls. Our results disclosed similar findings. Some investigators have reported a distortion of signal in the dorsal lateral aspect of the substantia nigra, or prominent putaminal hypodensity in the T_2-weighted images in PD. However, we did not discover this in any cases. We did not find any specific abnormalities related to the disorders in any groups.

Figure 5 shows axial sections through the basal ganglia and through the red nucleus on T_2-weighted images. The two pictures on the left (5(a)) were taken from patient 1, with IDP, and those on the right (5(b)) from a normal control, aged 59 years. The sections through the basal ganglia show a mild low signal in the postero-lateral portion of the putamen in both patient and normal subject. The MRI of the midbrain shows no abnormality in both patient and normal control. Mukai and colleagues[6] have recently described MRI findings in a 23-year-old woman with hereditary progressive dystonia with diurnal fluctuation. They reported that the MRI revealed no abnormality. Our patients with IDP also showed no specific abnormality. These findings, at least, do not distinguish hereditary progressive dystonia from IDP on MRI examination.

The widths of the pars compacta signal in individual cases and normal controls are shown in Table 2. There was no significant difference between any groups, except that in JPD, there was a prominent difference between the right width and the left. The width in PD was no narrower than those in other groups. We consider that PD patients with a longer duration of disease are needed for analysis. Concerning IDP patients, our study confirmed

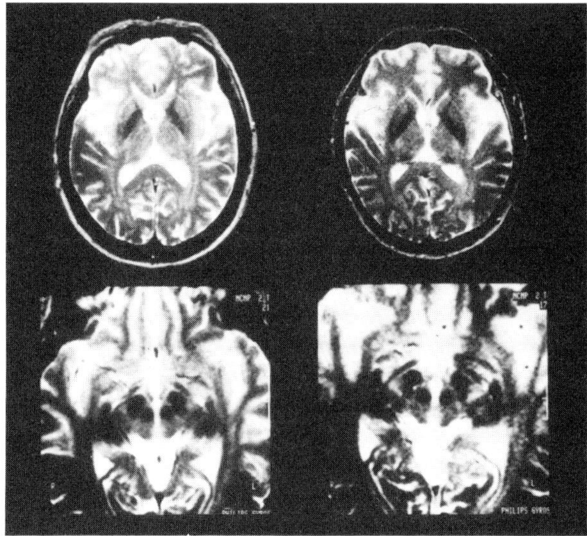

Figure 5 MRI in patient 1 (55 years old) (left) and normal control (59 years old) (right).

that the width of the pars compacta signal revealed no abnormality in spite of the very long duration of disease.

The findings of our MRI study suggested that in IDP, organic lesion of the substantia nigra or other basal ganglia was very mild or there was only functional abnormality.

DISCUSSION

We divided the Japanese patients, who showed both dystonia and parkinsonism with diurnal fluctuation, into two groups, namely early-adult-onset group and childhood-onset group (Table 3).

In 1958, Nasu and his colleagues[7] reported four cases in a family under the title of 'juvenile paralysis agitans'. All the patients had pes equinovarus, and their symptoms revealed marked diurnal fluctuation. Their ages of onset ranged from 19 to 35 years old. They had marked improvement of symptoms with trihexyphenidyl administration. In 1968 and 1973, Yamamura and colleagues[2,8] described 11 cases in three families under the titles 'a juvenile familial disorder with rigido-spasticity, bradykinesia and minor dystonia alleviated after sleep' and 'paralysis agitans of early onset with marked diurnal fluctuation of symptoms'. The patients all showed talipes equinus. Trihexyphenidyl was effective in all patients and one patient showed a dramatic response with levodopa administration. In 1985, we reported five similar cases[1], and in the same year, Ishikawa and colleagues[9] also reported another five cases. In our paper, we directed attention to the presence of minor dystonia, which is improved by levodopa therapy. We, therefore, reported these cases under the title of 'dystonia-parkinsonism'.

Table 3 Dystonia-parkinsonism/parkinsonism-dystonia with marked diurnal fluctuation (Japanese cases)

	Early-adult onset (14–42 years old)	*Childhood onset (1–16 years old)*
1958	'juvenile paralysis agitans'[7]	
1968	'juvenile familial disorder'[2]	
1971		'hereditary progressive extrapyramidal disorder'[10]
1973	'paralysis agitans of early onset'[8]	
(1975)		'hereditary parkinsonism-dystonia'[11]
1979		'juvenile parkinsonism with dystonia'[13]
1982	'juvenile parkinsonism'[3]	'hereditary progressive dystonia;[14]
1984		'dystonia with marked diurnal fluctuation'[15]
1985	'dystonia-parkinsonism'[1] 'juvenile parkinsonism'[9]	

On the other hand, in 1971, Segawa and colleagues[10] described childhood-onset cases of hereditary progressive dystonia with marked diurnal fluctuation of symptoms. In 1975, Allen and Knopp[11] reported childhood-onset cases of hereditary parkinsonism-dystonia. These had gradual onset of dystonia in childhood with later development of parkinsonian features. A marked response to levodopa therapy was obtained. Furthermore, in 1986, Nygaad and his colleague[12] reported similar cases. These cases, of course, were not Japanese. However they are mentioned because we believe that these cases are very relevant to the discussion of the nosological problems of this disorder.

In 1979, Yokochi[13] reported childhood-onset cases of juvenile parkinsonism, manifesting dystonia. He pointed out the similarities between juvenile parkinsonism with dystonia and hereditary progressive dystonia reported by Segawa and colleagues[10].

Whether the disorder of Segawa's cases is the same as that of Yokochi's is now under discussion. When our cases are compared with Segawa's cases, the clinical features of these two groups are very dissimilar: the age of onset is very different between them and, also, the inheritance mode is considered autosomal dominant with incomplete penetrance in Segawa's cases, whereas in ours it is considered autosomal recessive. These findings suggest that these two groups represent different disorders (Table 4).

However, if we could confirm that all patients reported by Segawa and colleagues[10], Yokochi[13], and Allen and colleagues[11] showed different clinical expressions of the same disorder, we would consider that this disorder has a tendency to show more prominent parkinsonism than dystonia as age advances. If so, the early-adult-onset dystonia-parkinsonism might be a mild form of the disorder.

At the present time, however, we have insufficient evidence to indicate that these groups are variable expressions of the same disorder. Therefore, we should keep the early-adult-onset group separate from that of childhood-onset.

Table 4 Dystonia-parkinsonism and parkinsonism-dystonia

	Dystonia/parkinsonism	*Parkinsonism-dystonia*
Onset	early adult	childhood
Heredity	? AR	? AD
Clinical features	parkinsonism > dystonia	parkinsonism < dystonia
Change of clinical features	—	dystonia to parkinsonism
Response to levodopa	dramatic	dramatic
Prognosis	very good	very good

REFERENCES

1. Sunohara, N., Mano, Y., Ando, K. and Satoyoshi, E. (1985). Idiopathic dystonia-parkinsonism with marked diurnal fluctuation of symptoms. *Ann. Neurol.*, **17**, 39–45
2. Yamamura, Y., Iida, M., Ando, K. and Sobue, I. (1968). A juvenile familial disorder with rigido-spasticity, bradykinesia and minor dystonia alleviated after sleep. *Clin. Neurol.*, (Tokyo), **8**, 233–43
3. Sunohara, N., Mano, Y., Toyoshima, E., Ando, K. and Satoyoshi, E. (1982). Juvenile parkinsonism with marked diurnal fluctuation. About new findings. *Clin. Neurol.*, (Tokyo), **22**, 101–10
4. Duguid, J.R., De La Paz, R. and DeGroot, J. (1986). Magnetic resonance imaging of the midbrain in Parkinson's disease. *Ann. Neurol.*, **20**, 744–7
5. Stern, M.B., Braffman, B.H., Skolnick, B.E., Hurtig, H.I. and Grossman, R.I. (1989). Magnetic resonance imaging in Parkinson's disease and parkinsonian syndromes. *Neurology*, **39**, 1524–6
6. Mukai, E., Makino, N. and Fujishiro, K. (1989). Magnetic resonance imaging of parkinsonism. *Clin. Neurol.*, (Tokyo), **29**, 720–5
7. Nasu, H., Aoyama, T. and Morisada, A. (1958). Vier Falle von der juvenilen Paralysis Agitans in einer Sippe. *Psychiatr. Neurol. Jpn.*, (Tokyo), **60**, 178–86
8. Yamamura, Y., Sobue, I., Ando, K., Iida, M., Yanagi, T. and Kono, C. (1973). Paralysis agitans of early onset with marked diurnal fluctuation of symptoms. *Neurology*, **23**, 239–44
9. Ishikawa, A., Atsumi, T. and Miyatake, T. (1985). Efficacy of cigarette smoking in five cases with juvenile parkinsonism. *Neurol. Med.*, (Tokyo), **23**, 562–7
10. Segawa, M., Ohmi, K., Itoh, S., Aoyama, M. and Hayakawa, H. (1971). Childhood basal ganglia disease with remarkable response to L-dopa, 'hereditary basal ganglia disease with marked diurnal fluctuation'. *Shinryo*, (Tokyo), **24**, 667–2
11. Allen, N. and Knopp, W. (1976). Hereditary parkinsonism-dystonia with sustained control by L-dopa and anticholinergic medication. In Eldridge, R. and Fahn, S. (eds.) *Advances in Neurology*, Vol. 14, pp. 201–13. (New York: Raven Press)
12. Nygaard, T.G. and Duvoisin, R.C. (1986). Hereditary dystonia-parkinsonism syndrome of juvenile onset. *Neurology*, **36**, 1424–8
13. Yokochi, M. (1979). Juvenile Parkinson's disease. Part I. Clinical aspect. *Adv. Neurol. Sci.*, (Tokyo), 1060–73
14. Hakamada, S., Watanabe, K., Hara, K. and Miyazaki, S. (1982). A case of 'hereditary progressive dystonia with marked diurnal fluctuation'. *No To Hattatsu*, (Tokyo), **14**, 44–8
15. Kumamoto, I., Nomoto, M., Yoshidome, M., Osame, M. and Igata, A. (1984). Five cases of dystonia with marked diurnal fluctuation and special reference to homovanillic acid in CSF. *Clin. Neurol.*, (Tokyo), **24**, 697–702

SECTION 3

Intra- and interfamilial variations of hereditary progressive dystonia/dopa-responsive dystonia

6

Intrafamilial and interfamilial variations of symptoms of Japanese hereditary progressive dystonia with marked diurnal fluctuation

Y. Nomura and M. Segawa

Hereditary progressive dystonia with marked diurnal fluctuation (HPD) is a clinical entity characterized by postural dystonia which shows marked diurnal fluctuation, childhood onset and complete recovery by levodopa[1,2,3]. On the other hand, as cases accumulated, the similarities and dissimilarities of its clinical features with those of so-called juvenile parkinsonism (JPA)[4,5], dystonia parkinsonism complex,[6,7] and cases recently reported as dopa-responsive dystonia (DRD)[8] have drawn attention and been discussed. It has also been argued that HPD may later turn out to be Parkinson disease.

The crucial question is whether these differently named disorders represent a pathophysiologically and etiologically continuous process with variable clinical manifestations, or whether they are etiologically different disorders with partially similar features.

The purpose of this report is to clarify this question by evaluating the intra- and interfamilial variations of symptoms and signs of Japanese HPD patients, to find the spectrum and variation of the clinical features of HPD and to draw a line of demarcation between the other disorders.

SUBJECTS AND METHODS

Twenty-two personal cases of HPD who have been diagnosed and followed at the Segawa Neurological Clinic for Children (SNCC) and 43 cases reported from other institutions in Japan as HPD or probable HPD were reviewed. Three particular familial cases with different clinical courses from HPD were discussed separately. All the cases were Japanese (Tables 1–6).

Among the 22 SNCC cases, 14 were familial cases from five families and eight were sporadic cases. The reported 43 cases included 32 familial cases from ten families and 11 sporadic cases. These reported familial cases

Table 1 Familial cases at the Segawa Neurological Clinic for Children (SNCC): gait = gait disturbance; l. = left; r. = right; pes eq. = pes equinovarus

	Sex	*Age at report** (years)	*Age at onset* (years, months)	*Symptoms at onset*	*Diurnal fluctuation*	*Tremor*[†]
Family T						
KW: cousin	F	30	6,7	l. hand tremor; slow in dressing/undressing	+	± (8)
RT: proband	F	27	4	r. > l. pes eq.; easy fatigability	+	–
CN: cousin	F	19	4	l. > r. pes eq.	+	–
HN: cousin	F	19	11	bilateral pes eq.	+	–
Family Su						
SSu : grandmother	F	72	8	gait; r. pes eq.	+	+ (30s)
KSu: father's cousin	M	31	2,7	gait; l. pes eq.	+	–
ASu: proband	F	23	1,4	l. > r. pes eq.	+	–
Family Sa						
YSa: mother	F	45	10	r. pes eq.	+	+ (39)
HSa: proband	F	18	6	l. > r. pes eq.	+	–
Family M						
IM: father	M	56	11	r. pes eq.	+	–
SM: proband	F	13	8	gait; l. pes eq.	+	–
Family K						
TS: aunt	F	49	5–6	gait; dragging feet	+	+ (33)
MO: aunt	F	46	7	gait; easy fatigability	+	+ (13–14)
MK: proband	F	8	4,11	l. pes eq.	+	–

*SNCC cases: present age; [†]Age (years) at onset of tremor in parentheses

Table 2 Reported familial cases: Group A; gait = gait disturbance; l. = left; r. = right; pes eq. = pes equinovarus; NM = not mentioned

	Sex	Age at report (years, months)	Age at onset (years, months)	Symptoms at onset	Diurnal fluctuation*	Tremor*
Kumamoto *et al.*, 1984[9]						
Case 3: younger sister	F	16	7	gait; l. pes eq.	+	–
Case 4: elder brother	M	18	7	l. pes eq.	± (15)	–
Tachi *et al.*, 1987[10,11]						
Case 1: elder sister	F	13	4	easy to fall down; l. pes eq.	+	NM
Case 2: } younger sisters, identical triplets	F	11,8	9,1	l. pes eq.	+	NM
Case 3: } younger sisters, identical triplets	F	11,8	9.1	l. pes eq.; l. anklepain	+	NM
Case 4: } younger sisters, identical triplets	F	11,8	9.4	r. pes eq.	+	NM
Ishida *et al.*, 1988[12]						
Case 1: daughter	F	8	4	toe walk; easy to fall down	+	–
Case 2: mother	F	35	34	fatigability of 4 limbs	–	+ (35)
Maeda *et al.*, 1988[13]						
Case 1: elder brother	M	12	6	l. pes eq.	+ (9)	NM
Case 2: younger sister	F	9	7	l. pes eq.; leaning to l.	+	NM
Iwami *et al.*, 1990[14]						
Case 1: } half-sisters	F	50	8	gait; r. pes eq.	+	+ (45)
Case 2: } half-sisters	F	37	8	slow in running; l. dystonic hand	+ (33)	NM
Father (of Cases 1 and 2)	M	(71)†	childhood	stiff 4 limbs	+	NM

*Age (years) at onset in parentheses; †died at 71 years of age

Table 3 Reported familial cases: Group B; gait = gait disturbance; l. = left; r. = right; pes eq. = pes equinovarus; post. = posture; NM = not mentioned

	Sex	*Age at report* (years, months)	*Age at onset* (years)	*Symptoms at onset*	*Diurnal* fluctuation*	*Tremor**
Morone *et al.*, 1983[17]						
Case 1: proband	F	9,5	5–6	l. pes eq.	+ (8)	–
Mother	F	NM	7	toe-in walking	NM	NM
Kumamoto *et al.*, 1984[9]						
Nomoto *et al.*, 1984[15], 1991[16]						
Case 1: proband	F	12	7	l. > r. pes eq.	+	–
Grandmother	F	74	50	gait	–	+
Grandmother's younger sister	F	69	56	tremor (upper limbs)	–	+
Grandmother's younger brother	M	72	57	gait	NM	+
Aunt 1 of grandmother	F	NM	65	forward bending post.; tremor (hand)	NM	+
Aunt 2 of grandmother	F	NM	65	forward bending post.; tremor (hand)	NM	+
Hirasawa *et al.*, 1984[18]						
Case 2: proband	F	8,1	6	leaning to r.	+	+
Grandmother's sibling	NM	NM	NM	gait	NM	NM
Grandmother's sibling	NM	NM	NM	gait	NM	NM
Simizu *et al.*, 1986[19]						
Proband	M	9,4	4	r. pes eq.	+	–
Mother	F	NM	18	gait	NM	–
Ibi *et al.*, 1991[20]						
Sahashi, 1991[21]						
Proband	F	36	early childhood	slow in walking	+	+ ($\leqslant$ 36)
Five cases†	NM	NM	NM	same disorder, details unknown	NM	NM

*Age (years) at onset in parentheses; †in five generations

Table 4 Sporadic cases at the Segawa Neurological Clinic for Children (SNCC); gait = gait disturbance; l. = left; r. = right; pes eq. = pes equinovarus; pron. = pronation

Case	*Sex*	*Age at report** (years)	*Age at onset* (years, months)	*Symptoms at onset*	*Diurnal fluctuation*	*Tremor*†
HN	M	28	6,4	gait; l. pes eq.; easy fatigability	+	+ (10,7)
KN	M	31	8,6	l. elbow pron., then l. pes eq.	+	± (10)
CO	F	26	1	l. > r. pes eq.; lumbar lordosis	+	+ (2,2)
AI	F	21	7,9	l. pes eq.	+	–
MS	F	18	8	r. pes eq.	+	± (10)
YY	F	45	3–4	l. > r. pes eq.	+	–
RK	F	12	8	r. pes eq.	+	–
RM	F	12	6	l. pes eq.	+	–

*SNCC cases: present age; †Age (years, months) at onset of tremor in parentheses

Table 5 Reported sporadic cases: l. = left; r. = right; pes eq. = pes equinovarus; NM = not mentioned

	Sex	*Age at report* (years, months)	*Age at onset* (years, months)	*Symptoms at onset*	*Diurnal fluctuation*	*Tremor**
Hakamada *et al.*, 1982[24]						
One case	F	8	5	l. pes eq.	+	+ (8)
Hiraki *et al.*, 1982[25]						
One case	F	9,2	5	l. arm dystonia	+	NM
Morone *et al.*, 1983[17]						
Case 2	F	7,6	6,2	l. pes eq.	+	+
Kumamoto *et al.*, 1984[9]						
Case 2	F	38	9	easy to fall down	+	NM
Case 5	F	13	9	l. pes. eq.	+	NM
Ishitsu *et al.*, 1986[26]						
One case	M	10,9	7,8	r. pes eq.	+	NM
Shimoyamada *et al.*, 1986[27]						
One case	M	9,6	1,3	bilateral pes eq.	+	–
Nomura *et al.*, 1987[28]						
One case	F	14	6	NM	+	NM
Yamashita *et al.*, 1987[29]						
One case	F	4	2	stiff gait	+	NM
Maekawa *et al.*, 1988[30]						
One case	F	17,5	9	r. pes eq.	+	NM
Nakayama *et al.*, 1988[31]						
One case	M	15	3	r. pes eq.	+	NM

*Age (years) at onset in parentheses

Table 6 Special cases (not hereditary progressive dystonia); gait = gait disturbance; l. = left; r. = right; pes eq. = pes equinovarus; NM = not mentioned; JPA = juvenile parkinsonism

	Sex	*Age at report* (years, months)	*Age at onset* (years, months)	*Symptoms at onset*	*Diurnal fluctuation*	*Tremor**
Hirasawa *et al.*, 1984[18]						
Case 1	F	8,1	5	r. pes eq.	+	+ (resting)
Elder sister†	F	NM	23	JPA	NM	NM
Horiguchi *et al.*, 1985[22]						
One case	F	21	9	r. pes eq.	+	+
Younger sister‡	F	NM	25	gait; l. pes eq.	+	NM
Ujike *et al.*, 1989[23]						
Case 1	M	32	12,5	resting tremor (4–5 Hz); l. pes eq.	–	NM
Case 2: younger brother of Case 1	M	(23)**	8	easy fatigability of legs; l. pes eq.	+	+ (16)

*Age (years) at onset in parentheses; †Y. Hirano, personal communication; ‡Y. Kaji, personal communication; **died at 23 years of age

consisted of 13 cases from five families[9–14], all of whom were diagnosed as HPD (Group A), and 19 cases from five other families[9,15–21] in which probands were reported as HPD but their involved family members were reported with other diagnoses (Group B). All these involved family members of Group B are included in the following analysis because, as will be discussed, they are probably the late-onset cases of HPD.

Three particular cases: Case 1 of Hirasawa and colleagues[18], the case of Horiguchi and colleagues[22] and Case 2 of Ujike and colleagues[23], were diagnosed as HPD at first but were revealed later to have different features, and their affected family members had characteristic features of JPA or movement disorders other than HPD.

In the SNCC cases, in addition to careful evaluations of clinical features which were performed repeatedly, their past histories were cautiously asked and ascertained from photos, if necessary. As for the cases reported from other instititutions, the clinical characteristics described in each article were analyzed prudently, and personal communications were made with the authors or physicians who followed the patients and/or their affected relatives. The natural clinical courses were assessed by evaluation of patients who came to medical attention after long clinical courses since onsets in the first decade.

RESULTS

Mode of inheritance

The details of familial cases evaluated in this study are listed in Tables 1–3. They are divided into two types; one with vertical transmission, or with affected cousins, suggesting dominant inheritance and the other with affected siblings without transgenerational cases.

SNCC familial cases included those with proband and her three cousins (Family T); with proband, her grandmother and a cousin of the father (Family Su); with proband and her mother (Family Sa); with proband and her father (Family M); and with proband and her two paternal aunts (Family K). There were no families with affected siblings among SNCC cases. Consanguinity was present only in one family (Family Su).

Among the reported familial cases, Group A consisted of three families with only sibling occurrence (Cases 3 and 4 of Kumamoto *et al.*[9], Tachi *et al.*[11] and Maeda *et al.*[13]) and two with vertical transmission; one with proband and mother (Ishida *et al.*[12]) and the other with half-sisters and their father (Iwami *et al.*[14]). One of the families with sibling occurrence had four affected siblings including identical triplets (Tachi *et al.*[10,11]).

Group B consisted of two families with child–mother involvement (Morone *et al.*[17], Shimizu *et al.*[19]), two families with affected members in probands' grandparents and their siblings (Case 1 of Kumamoto *et al.*[9], Case 2 of Hirasawa *et al.*[18]) and one family with five members affected in five generations but on whom details were unknown (Ibi *et al.*[20], Sahashi[21]). Thus, all five families revealed transgenerational involvement.

In Group A, consanguinity was not present in four families[11–14] but it was not mentioned in one family[9]. In Group B no consanguinity was seen in two families[9,19] and it was not mentioned in three families[17,18,20].

Thus, 12 families (80%) out of the total 15 were revealed to have transgeneration or cousin cases and suggested dominant inheritance.

Sex ratio

Female:male ratios (Table 7) of familial cases were 12:2 in SNCC cases and 10:3 in Group A. In Group B there were ten females, two males and seven cases whose sex was unknown. As for sporadic cases[9,17,24–31], SNCC cases consisted of six females and two males, and reported cases consisted of nine females and two males. The female:male ratio was 32:7, (i.e. 4.6:1) in familial cases and 15:4 (i.e. 3.8:1) in sporadic cases. There was no statistical difference between them. Thus, Japanese HPD, including both familial and sporadic cases, revealed marked female predominance with a female:male ratio of 47:11 (i.e. 4.3:1).

Age of onset

The age of onset (Tables 8 and 9) of SNCC familial cases ranged from 1 year 4 months to 11 years with a mean of 6.4 ± 2.9 years. The mean age of onset of the eight cases of the proband generation was 5.7 ± 2.7 years and that of the one previous generation was 7.2 ± 3.1 years. The mean age of onset of each family ranged between 4.0 and 8.0 years. The difference between the youngest and the oldest onset cases of Family T with four affected cousins was 7 years. In families Sa, M and K, with transgenerational involvement, the differences of ages of onset between the two generations ranged from several months (Family K) to 4 years (Family Sa), onset being younger in the later generation in each family. Three generations were affected in Family Su and it was also observed that the later generations revealed a younger

Table 7 Sex ratio of hereditary progressive dystonia cases; SNCC = Segawa Neurological Clinic for Children

	Female	*Male*	*No information*	*Total*
Familial				
SNCC	12	2	0	14
Group A*	10	3	0	13
Group B*	10	2	7	19
Total	32	7	7	46
Sporadic				
SNCC	6	2	0	8
Reported*	9	2	0	11
Total	15	4	0	19
Total (all cases)	47	11	7	65

*See text

Table 8 Age of onset of hereditary progressive dystonia cases; SNCC = Segawa Neurological Clinic for Children

	Familial			*Sporadic*		
		Group†				
*Age of onset** (years)	*SNCC*	A	B	SNCC	Reported†	Totals
⩽ 10	13	12	5	8	11	49
10–20	1	–	1	–	–	2
20–30	–	–	–	–	–	0
30–40	–	1	–	–	–	1
40–50	–	–	–	–	–	0
50–60	–	–	3	–	–	3
⩾ 60	–	–	2	–	–	2
Unknown	–	–	8	–	–	8
Total	14	13	19	8	11	65

*Each range given excludes lower limit of age but is inclusive of upper limit; †see text

age of onset and the differences between the 1st and 2nd, and the 2nd and 3rd generations were 5 years 5 months and 1 year 3 months, respectively. This suggests anticipation in families which involved more than two generations, but those differences between generations did not exceed the inter-individual differences observed in Family T, in which all cases belonged to one generation.

In the 13 cases of Group A, the variation of the age of onset was wide, ranging from 4 to 34 years. The oldest onset of 34 years was a mother of a case. The ages at onset of the rest were all in the 1st decade, and ranged between 4 years and 9 years 4 months. The average of the 11 cases who belonged to the probands' generation was 7.1 ± 1.8 years. In two families with vertical transmission, ages at onset of the probands were 4 years[12] and 8 years[14], and difference of age of onset between the two generations were 30 years in the former and no apparent difference in the latter, in which all had onset in the 1st decade. The ages of onset of the three families of sibling occurrence[9,11,13] ranged from 4 years to 9 years 4 months, with an average of 7.3 ± 1.7 years. Intrafamilial differences of the age of onset among these sibling cases ranged from 0 to 5 years 1 month. Two of the triplet cases reported by Tachi and colleagues started at the same time; the other started 3 months later[11].

In the 19 cases of Group B, the ages of onset ranged widely from 4 years to the mid-60s. The ages of onset of probands ranged from 4 to 7 years, with a mean age of 5.6 ± 1.1 years (excluding Ibi's case[20] whose onset was described only as preschool age). The ages at onset of cases of earlier generations were 18 years in the family reported by Shimizu and colleagues[19]; in the 6th to 7th decade in that of Kumamoto and colleagues[9,15,16], and uncertain in the study of families by Morone and co-workers[17], Hirasawa and colleagues[18] and Ibi and colleagues[20]. The family studied by Kumamoto and co-workers had three cases in the two previous generations, whose ages at onset were all in the 50s (i.e. 50, 56 and 57 years), and two cases in three previous generations which both started at 65 years[9,15,16].

Table 9 Mean age of onset (year ± SD) of hereditary progressive dystonia cases; SNCC = Segawa Neurological Clinic for Children

Cases	*Generation(s)*			
	All (n)	*Proband (n)*	*One previous (n)*	*Two previous (n)*
Familial				
SNCC ($n = 14$)	6.4 ± 2.9 (14)	5.7 ± 2.7 (8)	7.2 ± 3.1 (5)	8 (1)
Group A** ($n = 13$)	9.4 ± 7.6 (12)*	7.1 ± 1.8 (11)	34 (1); psa† (1)	
Sibling occurrence	7.3 ± 1.7 (8)	7.3 ± 1.7 (8)		
Vertical transmission	13.5 ± 11.9 (4)*	6.7 ± 1.9 (8)	34 (1); psa† (1)	
Group B**	data incomplete	5.6 ± 1.1 (4)‡	18 (1)	54.3 ± 3.1 (3)
Sporadic				
SNCC	6.1 ± 2.5 (8)			
reported**	5.7 ± 2.7 (11)			

*Excluding a case (father) from the study by Iwami *et al.*[14]; †primary school age; ‡excluding a case (proband) from the study by Ibi *et al.*[20] **see text

In the sporadic cases, the age at onset of SNCC cases ranged from 1 to 8.5 years, with a mean of 6.1 ± 2.5 years, and of the reported cases it ranged from 2 to 9 years, with a mean of 5.7 ± 2.7 years.

Thus, there were no significant differences in the ages at onset among the cases of the proband generations of SNCC familial cases, the probands of Group B, and the sporadic cases, both SNCC and reported. The mean ages at onset of the earlier generations of SNCC familial cases and the probands of Group A, both transgenerationally and sibling occurring cases, were slightly higher than the above groups, but there were no statistically significant differences. In contrast, the ages at onset of cases of earlier generations of Group B were significantly later, but as observed in the family studied by Kumamoto and co-workers,[9,16] the ages at onset within the same generation were similar in each family.

In summary, excluding eight cases whose age of onset was unknown, 49 out of 57 (86.0%) started in the 1st decade, two in the 2nd decade, one in the 4th, three in the 6th and two in the 7th decade of age.

Symptoms at onset

The symptoms of onset (Table 10) were mostly postural dystonia involving the lower extremities usually of one side. Among 14 SNCC familial cases, 11 started with pes equinovarus, six on the left, four on the right and one bilateral, but with asymmetry at 11 years of age. Among the other three cases, one started at 6 years 7 months old with tremulous movement of the left hand which was soon followed by left pes equinovarus, and two began with gait disturbance, the details of which were unknown because they came to us at adult ages. No family showed the intrafamilial concordance of the side of the initial involvement.

Among 13 cases in Group A, 11 showed pes equinovarus as the initial symptom; eight on the left, two on the right and one unilaterally, but side uncertain. One case started with stiffness of four extremities and one adult-onset case started with fatigability of four extremities. In the case of two families[9,13] with sibling occurrence, the side of the initial pes equinovarus showed intrafamilial concordance, the other two families also with sibling occurrence[11,14], including triplet cases, it was discordant and in one family with child–mother involvement[12] the initially affected side was unknown.

Among five probands in Group B, two started with left pes equinovarus, one with right pes equinovarus, one with a leaning of the body toward the right on movement and one who came to medical attention in adulthood was said to have started with slowness in walking in early childhood. The initial symptom of their affected family members in the earlier generations was mostly gait disturbance. One case who started in the second decade with gait disturbance (Shimizu and colleagues[19]) and five cases who had onset after the 6th decade with gait disturbances, hand tremor and forward bending posture (Kumamoto and co-workers[9,15,16]) were initially diagnosed as Parkinson disease.

Among eight SNCC sporadic cases, the initial symptom was pes equino-

Table 10 Initial symptoms of hereditary progressive dystonia; SNCC = Segawa Neurological Clinic for Children

	Familial				*Sporadic*		
			*Group B**				
	SNCC	*Group A**	*Probands*	*Previous generations*	*SNCC*	*Reported**	*Totals*
Pes equinovarus							
right	4	2	1	–	2	3	12
left	6	8	2	–	5	3	24
unilateral side unknown	0	1	0	–	0	0	1
bilateral	1	0	0	–	0	1	2
Total	11	11	3	0	7	7	39
Gait disturbance	2	2†	1	11	0	2	18
Arm dystonia	0	0	0	0	1‡	1	2
Postural abnormality	0	0	1	2**	0	0	3
Hand tremor	1††	0	0	1	0	0	2
No details	0	0	0	0	0	1	1
Total cases	14	13	5	14	8	11	65

*See text; †1 case of stiffness, 1 of fatigability; ‡arm dystonia soon followed by left pes equinovarus; **also associated with hand tremor; ††hand tremor soon followed by left pes equinovarus

varus in seven: five on the left and two on the right and dystonic posture of the left hand and arm, which was soon followed by left pes equinovarus in the remaining one case.

Among eleven reported sporadic cases, seven started with pes equinovarus: three on the left, three on the right and one bilateral; one with dystonic posture of the left arm, one with stiff gait; one with a tendency toward falling, and the details of the initial symptom of the last one was not mentioned[28].

It was suggested that the initial symptoms differed according to the age of onset. Out of 49 cases who had onset under the age of 10 years, 38 (77.6%) started with pes equinovarus, showing left side predominance: 24 on the left (63.2%), 12 on the right (31.6%), one unilaterally side unknown and one bilaterally. In three of these young onset cases, tremor or dystonia of the left arm was the initial sign, but it was transient and was soon replaced by pes equinovarus, the side not necessarily the same. The rest of the cases with onset in the first decade started with gait disturbance, though details were unknown. Thus, most of the cases with onset in childhood had leg dystonia as the initial symptom. In contrast, the main initial symptom of adult onset cases was gait disturbance associated with postural abnormalities or tremor.

Main neurological symptoms

The predominant neurological symptom of the reviewed cases was postural dystonia of the extremities which continued in the foreground throughout the course, most frequently as pes equinovarus. Asymmetry was present in most cases. The predominantly involved side of the present series was left, but this was not consistent and not necessarily concordant within a family. As regards the dystonic posture of the trunk and neck, lumbar lordosis with mild retrocollis upon standing or walking, and forward bending upon sitting or standing with assistance were present in some childhood patients. In older-onset cases in the 6–7th decade the latter was the main feature. Axial torsion or action dystonia was not observed throughout the course.

Basic muscle tone was not a plastic rigidity but a rigidity which became apparent with certain posture and movement. The stretch reflex was mainly hypertonic with rigidity but sometimes, when repeating the stretch reflex, revealed as normotonic or even hypotonic. Case 2 of Ishida and colleagues[12], and the two half-sister cases of Iwami and co-workers[14], when evaluated at adult ages, showed cogwheel rigidity.

The increased deep tendon reflex of lower extremities was observed with unsustained ankle clonus in some patients, but none showed extensor plantar response.

Postural tremor was observed in five of the SNCC familial cases, one in the 1st decade, one in the 2nd decade and three in their 30s. One case showed, also, a tremor at rest (in her 30s) but it was of low amplitude and with a high frequency of 8–10 cycles per second (SNCC case YSa). Two cases in Group A showed tremor; one adult-onset case showed postural tremor, in the mid-30s, as an initial symptom (Case 2 of Ishida and colleagues[12]) and the other case with onset in the first decade developed tremor on action at 11 years of age (Case 1 of Iwami and co-workers[14]). Among the cases in Group B, two with onset in childhood showed tremor, one on posture when examined at 36 years of age (Ibi and colleagues[20]), and the other on action at 7 years (Case 2 of Hirasawa and co-workers[18]). All cases with onset in the 6th and 7th decades (Kumamoto and colleagues[9,16]) showed tremor, the character of which, however, was not described. Four SNCC sporadic cases developed tremor – one in the 1st decade and three at around 10 years of age, but they were all transient, either on posture or action. Of the reported sporadic cases, two[17,24] showed tremor on action in the first decade.

Thus, 14 out of 49 cases with onset in the 1st decade, and all of the six adult-onset cases presented tremor either at the beginning or later in the course; five cases each in the 1st, 2nd, 4th decades and five after their 40s. The character of the tremor observed in the 1st or the 2nd decade was mild, transient and on posture or action. Three adult-onset cases[9,15,16] had tremor as the initial sign. Tremor did not develop if levodopa was started in childhood or in the early stage of the illness. Levodopa completely alleviated the tremor.

Diurnal fluctuation of symptoms

The marked diurnal fluctuation of symptoms was apparent in all SNCC cases and all the reported cases whose ages at onset were in the 1st decade. All of the cases whose onsets occurred in their teens showed diurnal fluctuation, but the grade was less marked. One case whose onset was at 34 years old[12], and cases with onset in the 6th decade[9,15,16] did not show the diurnal fluctuation. Thus, fluctuation of symptoms gradually decreased as the age advanced, but Case 2 of Iwami and colleagues[14] showed marked diurnal fluctuation, even after 33 years of age. Some cases developed fluctuation a few years after the onset of the disorder. The grade of the fluctuation was not consistent either among individual patients or among families; rather, it depended (with a few exceptions) on the age of onset and the age of the patient during the course. Furthermore, fluctuation disappeared after initiation of levodopa treatment.

Clinical course

The mode of progression altered with age, showing apparent progression in the first decade, slowing down in the latter half of the second decade and almost stabilizing thereafter.

The dystonia with onset before 10 years of age spread to all extremities within 5 years and by the mid-teens required assistance in walking from the morning onward. In contrast, dystonia that started after the age of 10 years remained in one leg for almost 10 years showing slow progression. In these cases, aggravation occurred in the 20s or late 30s with general involvement but very mild.

In some cases who had not been treated with levodopa, tremor developed in their mid- and late teens or in their 30s.

SNCC cases showed intrafamilial and inter-individual differences in severity. The cases with older onset tended to follow milder courses, but there were a few patients with early onset with a rather mild course. There were no definite interfamilial differences in severity among SNCC familial cases.

Among five families of Group A, sibling cases of two families (Kumamoto *et al.*[9] and Maeda *et al.*[13]) revealed an almost identical course. The triplet sisters studied by Tachi and colleagues[11] developed symptoms later than their elder sister and their symptoms and clinical courses were milder. Case 1 of Ishida and co-workers was a typical one of HPD, but Case 2, the mother of Case 1, with onset at age 34 years, followed a much milder course[12]. The family studied by Iwami and colleagues[14] showed different features; Case 1 revealed the typical course for HPD at the beginning, spontaneous remission around the early 20s and aggravation in the 40s, whereas Case 2 showed a rather milder course in spite of the age of onset being in the 1st decade, as Case 1. Their father had never received treatment all through his life, but the course was similar to Case 1, with spontaneous remission in his 20s and aggravation around his 40s with diurnal fluctuation. He became bedridden at 53 years old and died at 71 years of age.

The five probands of Group B revealed a typical course of HPD. The case reported by Ibi and colleagues[20,21] had onset at age 6 years, being diagnosed at 36 years of age, and her 30-year clinical course was indentical to that of the SNCC case SSu. The courses of the affected family members of previous generations in both of the families studied by Kumamoto and colleagues[9,15,16] and Shimizu and co-workers[19] were not described in detail, but their symptoms were mild, and recovery was complete after levodopa. The courses of the affected family members of the other three families studied by Morone *et al.*[17], Hirasawa *et al.*[18], and Ibi *et al.*[20], were not described. All sporadic cases showed a typical course.

The effect of treatment

Levodopa demonstrated complete alleviation of symptoms and a sustained effect in all cases; the longest was 22 years (SNCC case RT), without any side-effects such as wearing-off, on–off phenomena or dyskinesia. Its optimal dose was variable among individuals, even within a family, but all required a rather small dose, usually not exceeding 20 mg/kg/day of plain levodopa. A SNCC case (SSu) who had suffered from the disease for more than 40 years without any treatment responded to levodopa completely at 50 years of age and has remained symptom-free for 22 years[2,3,32]. Another SNCC case[33,34] had been under fair control by anticholinergics for more than 25 years, until aggravation took place in her mid-30s. She was switched to levodopa with satisfactory improvement[32].

In the proband case of the family studied by Ishida and co-workers[12], tetrahydrobiopterin (BH_4) had some effect, but it was not as marked as levodopa; the mother's arm dystonia responded fairly well to BH4. 5-Hydroxytryptophan (5-HTP) was also tried on both cases and it lowered the levodopa dose to obtain optimal effect. Ibi and colleagues[20] also tried BH4 on the proband case which alleviated the symptoms fairly well but not completely as observed with the levodopa treatment. Bromocriptine showed a slight effect on one sporadic case[28] but no effect on Case 1 in the study by Iwami and colleagues[14]

Associated diseases

HPD is usually not associated with other disorders. One SNCC family (Family Su) revealed myotonic dystrophy coexisting in the pedigree (Figure 1). Up to now, however, both disorders have not occurred in any case except for one myotonic dystrophy case (IV–10), in whom mild rigidity of extremities was observed at age 37 years.

Among reported sporadic cases, one patient was afflicted with blue sclera and osteogenesis imperfecta[25] and one case was said to have high tone sensory deafness[26].

Case 1 (an elder brother), reported by Maeda and co-workers[13], had low-grade astrocytoma of the cerebellum and had been operated on successfully at 3 years of age, 3 years before the onset of HPD. The course of HPD was not influenced by earlier surgery of the cerebellum.

Particular cases

Among the cases reported as HPD there were three families which should be presented separately, because they had different clinical features from HPD.

The case 1 of Hirasawa *et al.*[18] was originally reported as a sporadic case of HPD. The clinical features of onset did not contradict those of HPD with onset at 5 years of age with unilateral pes equinovarus, but progression of the symptoms was unusual with contractures in the hip and knee joints at 9 years 8 months and presence of resting tremor. The symptoms were progressive, in spite of levodopa treatment and the dose of levodopa had to be increased. The wearing-off, on–off phenomena and dopa-induced dyskinesia developed after a 1-year treatment of levodopa. Various other medications did not seem to be effective. Furthermore, her elder sister developed JPA of Yokochi's Type I at 23 years of age. The symptoms of this later onset sibling were more severe from the onset than the younger-onset proband and required a higher dose of levodopa which soon caused unfavorable side-effects. The authors later concluded that the original case was probably categorized as JPA of Yokochi and not HPD (Y. Hirano, personal communication).

The case of Horiguchi *et al.*[22] was reported as 'dystonia musculorum deformans with diurnal fluctuation of symptoms and levodopa responsiveness' with onset at 9 years of age, and the authors concluded that this patient was a sporadic case of HPD. However, the effectiveness of levodopa

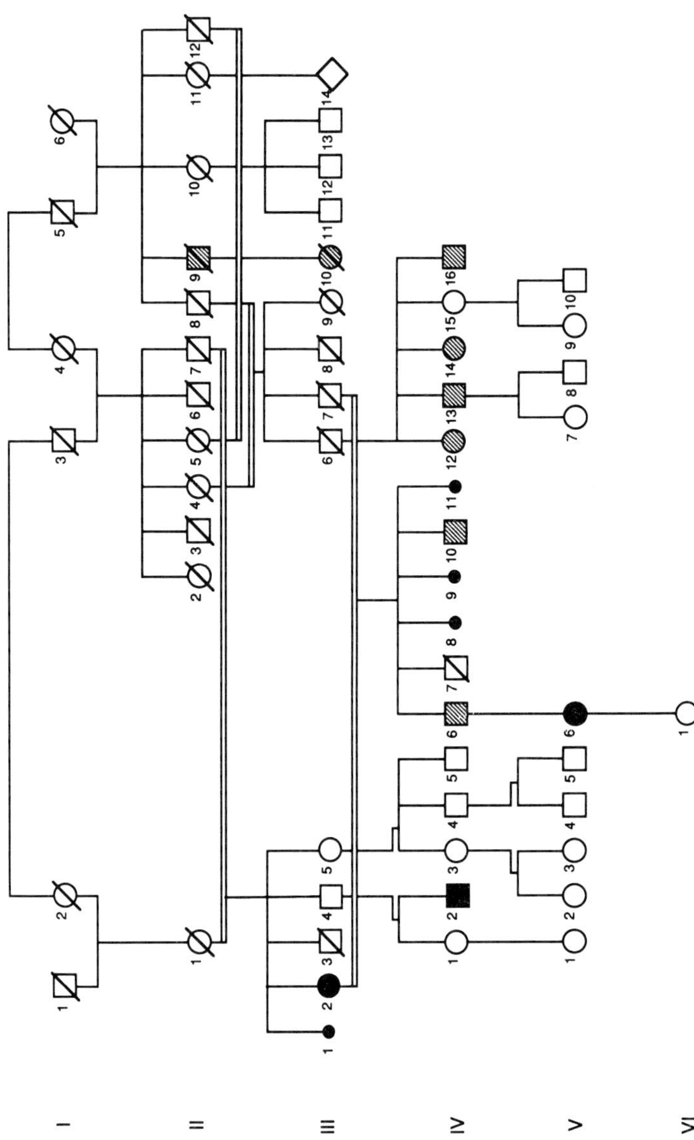

Figure 1 The pedigree of one family (Su) at the Segawa Neurological Clinic for Children, showing co-existence of myotonic dystrophy (hatched symbols) with hereditary progressive dystonia (filled symbols), III–2: SSu, IV–2: KSu, V–6: ASu (see Table 1)

was not as marked as HPD and she soon manifested up-and-down phenomena and dopa-induced oromandibular dyskinesia which were controlled by drug holiday. The younger sister of this case developed dystonia at 25 years of age which partially responded to levodopa, but it had to be withdrawn because of dyskinesia; for this case trihexyphenidyl was more effective (Y. Kaji, personal communication).

The case of Ujike *et al.*[23] was a report of two male sibling cases. The elder brother was reported as JPA Yokichi's Type III and the younger brother as HPD. There was consanguinity in this family. The age at onset of the younger brother was 8 years and the older brother was 12.5 years. The clinical course of the younger brother did not contradict that of HPD except for scoliosis. The degree of levodopa effectiveness on this case was not clear enough from the description that the improvement was that daily life was unaffected. The elder brother showed a decreasing response to levodopa and developed levodopa-induced side-effects. The accidental death of the younger brother halted the evaluation of further changes in the clinical course and in the effects of levodopa, which might have taken a different course from HPD.

DISCUSSION

The case of Japanese HPD subjected to this study were divided into two groups: familial and sporadic. The familial cases were further divided into cases with vertical transmission and those with affected siblings without transgenerational involvement.

Probands of familial cases with vertical transmission (i.e. most of the index cases and their affected siblings) and sporadic cases had the characteristic features of HPD described by Segawa[1–3,35,36]. In these cases the clinical onset was in the first decade and mostly started with pes equinovarus of one side. There was marked female predominance. The main symptom was postural dystonia throughout the course. Marked diurnal fluctuation was observed in all cases. There was asymmetry in the severity of dystonia in all cases with the left side more affected. Axial torsion or action dystonia was not observed. Postural tremor developed around the early teens in some cases who had reached this age without treatment. Although, in a few adult cases, transient resting tremor was observed in the leg, no cases showed parkinsonian resting tremor. Deep tendon reflexes were exaggerated in all cases and ankle clonus was observed in some, but none showed Babinski sign. Levodopa showed complete and sustained effects without any side-effects.

Among these proband or index cases, the variations of symptom were small. Only minor variations were observed, depending on the ages at onset and the ages of the patients. The symptoms tended to be milder in later onset cases, and some symptoms and signs were modified by age – that is, postural tremor developed in the 2nd decade in some, but in most after the 4th decade, and diurnal fluctuation reduced its grade with age, becoming almost inapparent by the 5th decade.

Marked variation of clinical features was observed when probands were compared with cases of earlier generations in some of the reported families with vertical transmission. The earlier generations had onset at older ages than the proband, the differences being small in some families, although in others it was more than a few decades and was in the late teens or 30s. In two families, cases in two or three previous generations had ages at onset in the 6th or the 7th decade.

The cases with childhood onset, despite the generation, showed similar clinical features as their probands, although the late onset cases showed slightly different features. The clinical features of these late-onset cases were characterized by the intitial symptoms of gait disturbance and/or tremor with or without postural abnormality. Although it was not described clearly in some cases, the tremor of these cases was postural with higher frequency. The diurnal fluctation of symptoms was not present in most cases. They were often diagnosed as JPA or Parkinson disease. However, the symptoms of these cases were milder with slower progression than their probands and some did not show full-blown symptoms. Moreover, these cases responded markedly and completely to a smaller amount of levodopa with sustained effects without any unfavorable side-effects, which are the characteristics of HPD rather than JPA or Parkinson disease. These observations strongly suggest that these cases must be late-onset HPD or forme fruste of HPD, but not JPA or Parkinson disease.

Thus the variation of symptoms observed in cases of different generations depends, basically, on the ages of onset.

The same pathophysiological basis of this variation of symptoms according to the age of onset is reflected in the natural course of HPD, namely the apparent and marked progression of symptoms in the 1st decade and early part of the 2nd decade, slowing down in the later part of the 2nd to 3rd decade, ceasing in the 4th decade and attaining the steady state thereafter. The diurnal fluctuation of symptoms reduces its amplitude gradually with age and, with progression of the illness, becomes almost unnoticeable when the illness reaches the steady state. We consider this process as a reflection of the age-variation of the activity of the nigrostriatal dopamine (NS–DA) neurons, particularly of their terminals[3,35,37,38].

Tremor may develop in the first part of the teens but it is transient and usually becomes apparent after the fourth decade of age. There are ample clinical observations to suggest that the cerebellar tremor and action myoclonus, with probable involvement of the thalamo-cortical pathway, manifest in the second decade, even though the lesions occur in earlier years. This suggests that the clinical manifestation of tremor is delayed until after the functional maturation of the NS–DA neurons or the specific nuclei of the thalamus, through which tremor becomes clinically apparent. Therefore, cases with onset after the 2nd decade may show tremor from the beginning of the disease.

In the three particular familial cases with affected siblings, index cases developed symptoms of HPD at onset. Older-onset sibling cases showed characteristics of the JPA of Yokochi and Narabayashi[4,5], with more severe clinical courses than younger-onset proband cases, and no complete response to levodopa. Two cases with HPD features initially soon displayed the clinical features of JPA, and the other set of siblings were both males, which is a feature of the JPA of Yokochi's Type III. Thus, these proband cases, whose initial features mimicked HPD, probably belong to the category of the so-called JPA. These observations suggest that JPA can start before 10 years of age and might be a recessive trait with male predominance.

JPA differs from HPD in its progressive course, less marked response to levodopa and tendency to develop levodopa-induced side-effects. It is thought also to have a different pathophysiology from HPD[37]. The onset of JPA Yokochi's Type III is usually in the 2nd decade, and Types I and II in the 4th decade[4,5]. The maturational level of the NS–DA neurons may modify the clinical features. For the full-blown clinical features of JPA to manifest, it is necessary for the NS–DA system and the related structures involved to have reached certain maturational levels.

If JPA manifests before 10 years of age, it will be partial because the neurons responsible are still in an immature state. Furthermore, since the activity of the terminal of NS–DA neurons are physiologically high in the 1st decade, symptoms may be less marked during this period.

The definition of DRD (see Chapter 2) seems to be similar to that of HPD. However, we have experienced dopa-responsive dystonias which differ from HPD. One type is a dystonia associated with marked action dystonia[38] and the other is associated with oculogyric crisis with action retrocollis. The effect of levodopa on the latter case was moderate and needed trihexyphenidyl to obtain the optimal effects. Thus, DRD indicates a group of dystonias with various pathophysiologies which respond to levodopa, including HPD.

In summary, the variation of symptoms of HPD depends on the age. The age-dependent alteration of symptoms is thought to be the reflection of a maturational process of the nervous systems which are involved in the pathophysiology of HPD, either directly or indirectly. In familial cases with transgenerational involvement, the ages of onset tend to be younger in later generations. Only the cases who develop symptoms in the 1st decade show full-blown clinical features and those that develop in later ages show milder features or forme fruste. Taking all these together, HPD is considered to be a disease entity with an autosomal dominant trait, and adult-onset cases represent late-onset HPD, which differs from JPA or Parkinson disease by its milder course, and marked and sustained response to a small dose of levodopa. The clinical course – without progression after a certain stage, and showing a complete and sustained response to levodopa – suggests that the pathophysiology of HPD as a functional abnormality restricted to the NS–DA neurons and degenerative process is unlikely. Furthermore, the clinical features of HPD reflect age-variation of the terminals of the NS–DA neurons. Thus, the pathophysiology of HPD is suspected to be the low level of dopamine in the terminals[3,35,37,38]. Although the experience of the use of BH4 in HPD is limited, its effect was not complete as with levodopa. The case reported by Ishida and colleagues[12] showed accentuation of the effects of levodopa by BH4. The study by Fujita and co-workers[39] on pteridine metabolism in a sporadic case who had been reported by Hiraki and colleagues[25] implied a possible deficiency of guanosine triphosphate –

cyclohydrolase-1. These reports suggest the possible involvement of biopterin in the pathogenesis of HPD.

The case with cerebellar astrocytoma, operated on 3 years before the onset of HPD[13] suggested that the cerebellum was not involved in the pathophysiology of HPD.

The concomitant occurrences of other disease in some patients and a family may be coincidental, but they are informative and may open the avenue for future research, with regard to gene hunting for the cause of hereditary progressive dystonia with marked diurnal fluctuation.

REFERENCES

1. Segawa, M., Ohmi, K., Itoh, S., Aoyama, M. and Hayakawa, H. (1971). A childhood basal ganglia disease with remarkable response to L-Dopa, 'hereditary progressive basal ganglia disease with marked diurnal fluctuation.' *Shinryo* (*Tokyo*), **24**, 667–72 (in Japanese)
2. Segawa, M., Hosaka, A., Miyagawa, F., Nomura, Y. and Imai, H. (1976). Hereditary progressive dystonia with marked diurnal fluctuation. In Eldridge, R. and Fahn, S. (eds.) *Advances in Neurology*: *Dystonia*, Vol. 14, pp. 215–33 (New York: Raven Press)
3. Segawa, M., Nomura, Y. and Kase, M. (1986). Diurnally fluctuating hereditary progressive dystonia. In Vinken, P.J., Bruyn, G.W. and Klawans H.L. (eds.), *Handbook of Clinical Neurology*: *Extrapyramidal Disorders*, Vol. 5, pp. 529–39 (Amsterdam: Elsevier)
4. Yokochi, M. (1979). Juvenile Parkinson's disease, part 1. Clinical aspects. *Adv. Neurol. Sci.* (*Tokyo*), **23**, 1048–59 (in Japanese)
5. Narabayashi, H., Yokochi, M., Iizuka, R. and Nagatsu, T. (1986) Juvenile parkinsonism. In Vinken, P.J., Bruyn, G.W. and Klawans, H.L. (eds.), *Handbook of Clinical Neurology*: *Extrapyramidal Disorders*, Vol. 5, pp. 153–65 (Amsterdam: Elsevier)
6. Sunohara, N., Mano, Y., Ando, K. and Satoyoshi, E. (1985). Idiopathic dystonia – parkinsonism with marked diurnal fluctuation of symptoms. *Ann. Neurol.*, **17**, 39–45
7. Nygaard, T.G. and Duvoisin, R.C. (1986). Hereditary dystonia – parkinsonism syndrome of juvenile onset. *Neurology*, **36**, 1424–8
8. Nygaard, T.G., Marsden, C.D. and Duvoisin, R.C. (1988). Dopa responsive dystonia. In Fahn, S., Marsden, C.D. and Calne, D.B. (eds.) *Advances in Neurology*: *Dystonia 2*, Vol. 50, pp. 377–84 (New York: Raven Press)
9. Kumamoto, I., Nomoto, M., Yoshidome, H., Osame, M. and Igata, A. (1984). Five cases of dystonia with marked diurnal fluctuation and special reference to homovanillic acid in CSF. *Clin. Neurol.* (*Tokyo*), **24**, 697–702 (in Japanese)
10. Tachi, N., Yamazaki, K., Jo, M. and Shinoda, M. (1979). A case of progressive dystonia with marked diurnal fluctuation. *J. Clin. Pediatr.* (*Sapporo*) **27**, 111–7 (in Japanese)
11. Tachi, N., Sasaki, K. and Shinoda, M. (1987). Four cases including identical triplets of progressive dystonia with marked diurnal fluctuation. *J. Jpn. Pediatr. Soc.*, **91**, 1403–6 (in Japanese)
12. Ishida, A., Takada, G., Kobayashi, Y., Higashi, O., Toyoshima, I. and Takai, K. (1988). Serotonergic disturbance in hereditary progressive dystonia – clinical effects of tetrahydrobiopterin and 5-hydroxytryptophan. *No To Hattatsu* (*Tokyo*), **20**, 195–9 (in Japanese)
13. Maeda, Y., Nakayama, H., Kitamoto, I., Mizuno, Y., Ueda, K., Kurokawa, T. and Tomita, S. (1988). Sibling cases of hereditary progressive dystonia – diurnal fluctuation of catecholamine metabolism before and after treatment. *No To Hattatsu* (*Tokyo*), **20**, (Suppl.) S164 (in Japanese)
14. Iwami, O., Kawamura, J., Hashimoto, S., Suenaga, T. and Nakamura, M. (1990). Hereditary progressive dystonia with marked diurnal fluctuation – a report of two siblings, one of them showing age-dependent changes of symptoms. *Clin. Neurol.* (*Tokyo*), **30**, 961–5 (in Japanese)
15. Nomoto, M., Kumamoto, I., Sano, Y., Nakajima, H., Osame, M. and Igata, A. (1984). A family with benign familial Parkinson Disease including a case with marked 'dopa responsive fluctating dystonia' of early childhood onset. *Clin. Neurol.* (*Tokyo*), **24**, 1388 (in Japanese)

16. Nomoto, M. (1991). A family with familial Parkinson disease which include both dopa responsive fluctuating dystonia (Segawa Disease) and Parkinson disease. Presented at the *6th Annual Meeting of the Japan Basal Ganglia Society*, Susono City, Japan, July
17. Morone, A., Suzuki, T., Tezuka, C. and Takahashi, T. (1983). Two cases of hereditary progressive dystonia with marked diurnal fluctuation. *Tohoku Arch. Orthop. Surg. Traumat. (Sendai)*, **26**, 16–19 (in Japanese)
18. Hirasawa, K., Ochiai, Y. and Fukuyama, Y. (1984). Two cases with hereditary progressive dystonia with marked diurnal fluctuation. *J. Jpn. Pediatr. Soc.*, **88**, 708–13 (in Japanese)
19. Shimizu, N., Hara, M., Yoshihara, S., Tateno, A. and Aoki, T. (1986). A family (mother and son cases) with hereditary progressive dystonia with marked diurnal fluctuation. *Jpn. J. Pediatr.* (*Tokyo*), **39**, 1442–6 (in Japanese)
20. Ibi, T., Sahashi, K., Watanabe, K., Morishima, T., Mitsuma, T., Fujishiro, K., Takahashi, A., Hagihara, M., and Nagatsu, T. (1991). Progressive dystonia with marked diurnal fluctuation and tetrahydrobiopterin therapy. *Neurol. Ther.*, **8**, 71–5 (in Japanese)
21. Sahashi, I. (1991). Early onset dopa-responsive dystonia with diurnal fluctuation (HPD); clinical findings and etiological findings in 2 families. Presented at the *6th Annual Meeting of the Japan Basal Ganglia Society*, Susono City, Japan, July
22. Horiguchi, A., Inami, Y., Nagao, H. and Sano, N. (1985). Treatment of dystonia musculorum deformans with L-dopa and the effect of drug holiday. *Psychiatr. Neurol. Paediatr. Jpn.*, **25**, 67–71 (in Japanese)
23. Ujike, H., Nakashima, M., Kuroda, S. and Otsuki, S. (1989). Two siblings of juvenile Parkinson's disease dystonic type (Yokochi type 3) and hereditary progressive dystonia with marked diurnal fluctuation (Segawa). *Clin. Neurol.*, (*Tokyo*), **29**, 890–4 (in Japanese)
24. Hakamada, S., Watanabe, K., Hara, K., and Miyazaki, S. (1982). A case of 'hereditary progressive dystonia with marked diurnal fluctuation.' *No To Hattatsu* (*Tokyo*), **14**, 44–8 (in Japanese)
25. Hiraki, M., Waki, S., Kusano, T., Terashima, H. and Fujita, S. (1982). A case of progressive dystonia with marked diurnal fluctuation. *J. Clin. Pediatr.* (*Sapporo*), **30**, 111–18 (in Japanese)
26. Ishitsu, T., Itai, Y. and Matsuda, I. (1986). A study on catecholamine metabolism in a case with hereditary progressive dystonia with marked diurnal fluctuation associated with hearing deficit. *J. Jpn. Pediatr. Soc.*, **90**, 59–63 (in Japanese)
27. Shimoyamada, Y., Yoshikawa, A., Kashii, H., Kihira, S. and Koike, M. (1986). Hereditary progressive dystonia – an observation of the catecholamine metabolism during L-Dopa therapy in a 9-year-old girl. *No To Hattatsu*, (*Tokyo*), **18**, 505–9 (in Japanese)
28. Nomura, K., Negoro, T., Takaesu, E., Aso, K., Furune, S., Takahashi, I., Yamamoto, N. and Watanabe, K. (1987). Bromocriptine therapy in a case of hereditary progressive dystonia with marked diurnal fluctuation. *Brain Dev.*, **9**, 199
29. Yamashita, S., Kurihara, M., Sugio, Y., Miyake, S., Yamada, M. and Iwamoto, H. (1987). Hereditary progressive dystonia with marked diurnal fluctuation: a case study. *Brain Dev.*, **9**, 203
30. Maekawa, N., Hashimoto, T., Sasaki, M., Oishi, T. and Tsuji, S. (1988). A study on catecholamine metabolites in CSF in a patient with progressive dystonia with marked diurnal fluctuation. *Clin. Neurol.* (*Tokyo*), **28**, 1206–8 (in Japanese)
31. Nakayama, S., Nakasako, H., Momota, K., Kodama, S. and Matsuo, T. (1988). A boy with hereditary progressive dystonia with marked diurnal fluctuation. *J. Jpn. Pediatr. Soc.*, **92**, 835 (in Japanese)
32. Segawa, M., Nomura, Y., Yamashita, S., Kase, M., Nishiyama, N., Yukishita, S., Ohta, H., Nagata, K., and Hosaka, A. (1990). Long-term effects of L-Dopa on hereditary progressive dystonia with marked diurnal fluctuation. In Berardelli, A., Benecke, R., Manfredi, M. and Marsden, C.D. (eds.) *Motor Disturbances II*, pp. 305–18. (London: Academic Press)
33. Kase, M. (1978). Parkinson disease-like disorder *Jpn. Med. J.* (*Tokyo*), **2850**, 3–11 (in Japanese)
34. Nomura, Y., Kase, M., Igawa, C., Ogiso, M. and Segawa, M. (1982). A female case of hereditary progressive dystonia with marked diurnal fluctuation with favorable response to anticholinergic drugs for 25 years. *Clin. Neurol.* (*Tokyo*), **22**, 734 (in Japanese)
35. Segawa, M. (1981). Hereditary progressive dystonia (HPD) with marked diurnal fluctuation. *Adv. Neurol. Sci.* (*Tokyo*), **25**, 73–81 (in Japanese)

36. Segawa, M. and Nomura, Y. (1991). Hereditary progressive dystonia with marked diurnal fluctuation. In Nagatsu, T., Narabayashi, H. and Yoshida, M. (eds.). *Parkinson's Disease. From Clinical Aspects to Molecular Basis.* (*Key Topics in Brain Research*), pp. 167–77 (Wien, New York: Springer–Verlag)
37. Segawa, M., Nomura, Y. and Kase, M. (1986). Hereditary progressive dystonia with marked diurnal fluctuation: clinicopathophysiological identification in reference to Juvenile Parkinson's disease. In Yahr, M.D. and Bergmann, K.J. (eds.) *Advances in Neurology: Parkinson's Disease*, Vol. 45, pp. 227–34 (New York: Raven Press)
38. Segawa, M., Nomura, Y., Tanaka, S., Hakamada, S., Nagata, E., Soda, M. and Kase, M. (1988). Hereditary progressive dystonia with marked diurnal fluctuation – consideration on its pathophysiology based on the characteristics of clinical and polysomnographical findings. In Fahn, S., Marsden, C.D. and Clane, D.B. (eds). *Advances in Neurology: Dystonia 2*, Vol. 50, pp. 367–76 (New York: Raven Press)
39. Fujita, S. and Shintaku, H. (1990). Etiology and pteridin metabolism abnormality of hereditary progressive dystonia with marked diurnal fluctuation (HPD: Segawa disease). *Med. J. Kushiro City Hosp.*, **2**, 64–7 (in Japanese)

7

An analysis of North American families with dopa-responsive dystonia

T.G. Nygaard

INTRODUCTION

The classical phenotype in dopa-responsive dystonia (DRD) is a childhood-onset dystonic disorder[1]. DRD appears to be inherited as an autosomal dominant disorder with reduced penetrance. Large clinical series suggest that DRD occurs three times more frequently in women than in men. The analysis of one large North American family revealed a high penetrance of a spectrum of possible phenotypic manifestations, ranging from minor rigidity to overt parkinsonism[2]. Based on these findings, it was suggested that adult-onset parkinsonism may also be part of the phenotype in DRD. This paper reviews the clinical impressions from my examination of 21 North American probands and their available first-degree relatives. These prior clinical observations are evaluated in an informal segregation analysis.

METHODS

Probands were identified as the first family member who sought treatment for their dystonia (Table 1). All probands had their residence in North America at the time of ascertainment and were included solely on the basis of their dopa-responsiveness, without regard to family history. First-degree relatives (parents, siblings, and children) were examined when available. A detailed history concerning signs or symptoms suggestive of dystonia or parkinsonism was taken for all first-degree relatives and extended to more distant relatives when possible.

All subjects received a standardized clinical evaluation for evidence of dystonia and parkinsonism[2]. Affected status for dystonia was assigned with categories: definite (unequivocal features of dystonia), probable (examination is highly suggestive of dystonia), possible (examination is abnormal but not diagnostic of dystonia), or no dystonia[3]. Parkinsonism was scored by the presence of:

(1) Rest tremor (at least intermittently present at one site);

Table 1 Identification of probands. Prior ID refers to the identification used for each proband in a prior publication[6]

Proband no.	*Prior ID*	*Sex*	*Age at onset* (years)	*Age* (years)	*Duration levodopa* (years)
1	1	F	5	39	14
2	4	M	6	10	3
3	6	F	6	53	23
4	18	F	6	28	9
5	21	F	5	61	17
6	29	F	6	37	6
7	34	F	3	33	4
8	35	F	6	17	3
9	36	M	4	17	4
10	37	F	3	34	4
11	38	F	8	17	2
12	39	F	6	13	1
13	42	F	4	14	1
14	43	F	7	42	13
15	48	F	2	8	1
16	49	F	5	33	19
17	54	M	5	18	10
18	56	M	6	26	12
19	57	F	6	17	3
20	58	F	6	40	4
21	61	F	10	13	2

(2) Bradykinesia (at least moderate in degree);

(3) Postural instability (at least three steps required to recover, on repeated pull tests); and

(4) Rigidity (moderate in degree in at least one site).

The presence of two or more of the above features (including either (1) or (2) was scored *definite* parkinsonism[2]. The presence of either (1) or (2), alone, was scored *probable* parkinsonism. The presence of either (3) or (4), or both was scored as *possible* parkinsonism.

RESULTS

There were 21 probands included in this study. The numbers of available parents, siblings, and children of the probands and numbers examined appear in Table 2. (One set of affected monozygotic twins[2] was counted as a single sibling for this analysis.) Over 150 additional more distant relatives were examined (principally from two large families). At the time of ascertainment, 14 probands reported they were the only affected individual in their family and seven were aware of at least one other affected family member.

Dystonia

Fourteen first-degree relatives had definite dystonia and five had possible dystonia (Table 3). Ten other more distantly related relatives were definitely

Table 2 Number of first-degree relatives and number examined

	Parents	*Siblings*	*Children*	*Total*
Total	42	44	7	93
Deceased	8	2	0	10
Living	34	42	7	83
Examined	30	29	3	62
Percentage of living first-degree relatives examined	88	61	43	75

Table 3 First-degree relatives with dystonia

Proband	*Affected first-degree relative(s)*	*Clinical history*
Definite dystonia		
1	mother	foot dystonia at 12, overt parkinsonism in late adulthood
2	mother	exertional foot dystonia in early teenage
4	3 sisters, mother	mother with torticollis, sisters with generalized dystonia
5	sisters (twins)	monozygotic twins with generalized dystonia
6	sister and daughter	sister generalized dystonia, daughter with exertional foot dystonia
7	father, brother	father with childhood exertional leg dystonia, later parkinsonism, brother with generalized dystonia
10	sister	generalized dystonia
11	mother	writer's cramp, adult parkinsonism
13	brother	generalized dystonia
Possible dystonia		
5	sister	possible foot dystonia with parkinsonism
5	sister	oromandibular movements
8	mother	exertional foot dystonia
12	father	dystonic arm movements
12	brother	action-induced foot inversion and slow foot movements

affected on examination. Reliable examination data from another neurologist established another two distantly related relatives as affected and historical data suggested 11 additional affected relatives. In four instances, a symptomatic relative (three first-degree relatives) was first diagnosed with dystonia on the basis of this study. In another case, two nieces and a second cousin of a proband became affected 12 years after the proband was first identified. This led to a final determination of 13 probands with hereditary disease, nine with affected first-degree relatives (Table 3) and four with more distantly affected relatives (Table 4). There were eight sporadic cases. Autosomal dominant inheritance with male-to-male transmission of disease was evident in six families. In the 12 families in which the parental source of the DRD gene could be inferred, it had paternal origin in six cases and maternal origin in six cases.

Table 4 Relationship of relatives with definite dystonia for probands without affected first-degree relatives

Proband	*Affected relative*	*Clinical history*
3	niece	generalized dystonia
9	paternal grandmother	exertional foot dystonia, parkinsonism
12	paternal grandfather	writer's cramp in teenage, parkinsonism
14	2 nieces and a second cousin	foot dystonia in all three

Table 5 Tabulation of first-degree relatives affected with dystonia. (The differences from the expected values for this model are not significant by χ^2 analysis)

	Male	*Female*	*Total*
Parents (affected/total)	1/21	4/21	5/42 (12%)
Children (affected/total)	0/3	1/4	1/7 (14%)
Siblings (affected/total)	2/14	6/30	8/44 (18%)
Totals	3/38 (8%)	11/55 (20%)	14/93 (15%)

A 3:1 ratio of affected women to men has been observed in DRD suggesting that there is a sex-related difference in penetrance (see Chapter 2). A prior analysis of the extended pedigree of proband 5 estimated the overall DRD penetrance in this family at about 30%[2]. These estimates would suggest sex-related penetrances of 45% in women and 15% in men. In an autosomal dominant condition, half of first-degree relatives (parents, offspring, and children) of a proband are gene carriers. Thus, 7.5% (0.5 × 0.15) of first-degree male relatives and 22.5% (0.5 × 0.45) of first-degree female relatives would be expected to be affected by application of the above estimates. These crude estimates fit well with the observed results (Table 5).

Parkinsonism

Definite parkinsonism was rated in 12 individuals from six families (Table 6) and, historically, was probably present in one member of family 3[4] and one member of family 9. In six individuals, the parkinsonism was preceded by evidence of dystonia which began in childhood but remained mildly symptomatic. Five of these are obligate carriers of the DRD gene.

All possible phenotypes

The analysis of data regarding the finding of definite parkinsonism, possible dystonia, or rigidity reveals that the inclusion of these potential phenotypical elements dramatically increases the estimated penetrance of the disorder, although it is not complete (Table 7). In the 12 instances where both parents of a proband could be examined, they were both found to be normal on three occasions (25%). In two instances, the proband was regarded as a

Table 6 Family members affected with definite parkinsonism

Proband	*Relative*	*Clinical history*	*Levodopa treatment* (*duration*, years)
1	mother	foot dystonia as child. Progressive bradykinesia, rigidity and postural instability after age 45	100 mg/day (8)
	aunt	foot dystonia as child. Progressive bradykinesia, rigidity, postural instability and rest tremor after age 40	100 mg/day (6)
5	cousin	exertional foot dystonia as child. At age 61, onset of intermittent rest and postural tremor of left hand, postural instability, and rigidity	100 mg/day (2)
	cousin	definite foot dystonia as child. At age 57, onset of 'fatigue', rigidity, bradykinesia and postural instability	100 mg/day (8)
	sister	at age 70, onset of hypomimia, bradykinesia, postural instability, and rigidity	none
	sister	at age 57, onset of rest tremor in right hand and rigidity	none
	sister	at age 49, onset of rest tremor in right hand and rigidity	100 mg/day (1)
7	father	dystonic cramps as child. At age 50, onset of bradykinesia, rigidity, and postural instability	150 mg/day (15)
11	mother	writer's cramp as child. At age 45, onset of rigidity and bradykinesia	100 mg/day (1)
12	paternal grandfather	writer's cramp at age 59. At age 77, onset of rest tremor and bradykinesia	375 mg/day (5)
14	mother	at age 50, onset of rest tremor and postural instability	150 mg/day (12)
	maternal great aunt	at age 67, onset of rest tremor	50 mg/day (8)

Table 7 Examination findings in first-degree relatives

	Examined	*Affected*	*Parkinsonism*	*Possible dystonia*	*Rigidity*	*Any finding*
Parents						
male	13	1*	0 (1*)	1	3	5/13
female	17	4†	1 (3†)	1	0	6/17
Siblings						
male	7	2	0	1	1	5/7
female	22	6	3	2	4	15/22
Children						
male	1	0	0	0	1	1/1
female	2	1	0	0	0	1/2
All first-degree relatives						
male	21	3	0 (1)*	2	5	11/21
female	41	11	4 (6†)	3	4	22/41

*One father with dystonia later developed definite parkinsonism. †Two mothers with dystonia later developed definite parkinsonism

sporadic case, and in the third, the father was the 'obligate' gene carrier for DRD. In no case were possible phenotypical elements detected in both parents.

DISCUSSION

The prior analysis of the extended pedigree of one of these probands revealed a high prevalence of tone abnormalities and parkinsonism[2]. The extension of this analysis by the inclusion of 20 nuclear families suggests that these observations may be generalized to all families with DRD. These data are consistent with an autosomal dominant mode of transmission for DRD, with sex-related differences in penetrance. There does not appear to be any influence of the sex of a gene carrier parent on the likelihood of a child becoming affected. Thus, imprinting does not appear to be a factor in gene expression[5].

The reason for the sex-related difference in DRD penetrance is unknown. In addition to this difference in penetrance, there appears to be a greater severity of disability in affected women as a group when compared to men[6]. Within the group studied here, a similar proportion of each sex had some potential phenotypical finding on examination, but these were symptomatic in a higher proportion of women.

Several observations suggest an important influence of the sex hormones (progesterone and estrogen) in this regard. There is a high frequency of premenstrual exacerbation of symptoms in women with DRD and several women have reported a diminished response to levodopa during co-administration of birth control pills[6]. Peak progesterone levels occur premenstrually and progesterone is an important component of most oral contraceptives. While this might suggest a key role for progesterone, a marked decrease in DRD symptom severity has been reported during the second and third trimesters of pregnancy, a period when progesterone levels are rising.

Estrogens are known to influence dopamine receptor sensitivity and the explanations for these phenomena may involve a complex interaction between these hormones, and others, and their relative levels[7].

Parkinsonism with late adult-onset had a surprising frequency within these families. Using only first-degree relatives who were older than age 40 as the population 'at risk' for parkinsonism, 1/19 men (5%) and 6/31 women (19%) had definite parkinsonism. The non-age-adjusted frequency of 14% is far above the prevalence ratio of 0.6% found as the risk of Parkinson disease after age 40[8] ($p < 0.05$, by χ^2 analysis, with Yates' correction).

This observation raises the issue that the DRD gene might represent a risk factor for the development of Parkinson disease. However, seven of the 12 individuals affected with parkinsonism have remained functionally normal with low-dose levodopa treatment for 5 years, or longer. This response to treatment, without the development of the complications of therapy which are common to Parkinson disease, is similar to that observed in typical DRD. Additionally, the sex-related skew in distribution of those affected with parkinsonism is similar to that observed in the childhood-onset dystonia DRD phenotype and would be unexpected in Parkinson disease[8]. This suggests the parkinsonism in these family members is due to the same genetically determined dopamine deficiency that affects other family members with typical DRD. The mild childhood-onset dystonia in several cases, and absence of childhood symptoms in others, may be a reflection of slightly differing childhood dopamine levels in these individuals. The difference in phenotype in children (predominantly dystonic) and adults (predominantly parkinsonian) may represent age-related differences in the expression of this dopamine deficiency. Thus, the DRD gene does not appear to represent a risk factor for idiopathic Parkinson disease. These data give strong support for the inclusion of adult parkinsonism as part of the phenotype of the DRD gene.

ACKNOWLEDGEMENTS

This work was supported in part by the Dystonia Medical Research Foundation, the Parkinson's Disease Foundation, and NIH Grant HD00914-01

REFERENCES

1. Nygaard, T.G., Marsden, C.D. and Duvoisin, R.C. (1988). Dopa-responsive dystonia. In Fahn, S., Marsden, C.D. and Calne, D.B. (eds.) *Advances in Neurology*, Vol. 50, pp. 377–84. (New York: Raven Press)
2. Nygaard, T.G., Trugman, J.M., de Yebenes, J.G. and Fahn, S. (1990). Dopa-responsive dystonia: the spectrum of clinical manifestations in a large North American family. *Neurology*, **40**, 66–9
3. Bressman, S.B., de Leon, D., Brin, M.F., Risch, N., Burke, R.E., Greene, P.E., Shale, H. and Fahn, S. (1989). Idiopathic dystonia among Ashkenazi Jews: evidence for autosomal dominant inheritance. *Ann. Neurol.*, **26**, 612–20
4. Allen, N. and Knopp, W. (1976). Hereditary parkinsonism-dystonia with sustained control

by L-dopa and anticholinergic medication. In Eldridge, R. and Fahn, S. (eds.) *Advances in Neurology*, Vol. 14, pp. 201–13. (New York: Raven Press)

5. Solter, D. (1988). Differential imprinting and expression of maternal and paternal genomes. *Annu. Rev. Genet.*, **22**, 127–46
6. Nygaard, T.G., Marsden, C.D. and Fahn, S. (1991). Dopa-responsive dystonia – long-term treatment response and prognosis. *Neurology*, **41**, 174–81
7. Bedard, P.J., Langelier, P., Dankova, J., Villeneuve, A., DiPaolo, N., Barden, N., Labrie, F., Boissier, J.R. and Euvrard, C. (1979). Estrogens, progesterone, and the extrapyramidal system. In Poirier, L.J., Sourkes, T.J. and Bedard, P. J. (eds.) *Advances in Neurology*, Vol. 24, pp. 411–22. (New York: Raven Press)
8. Schoenberg, B.S., Anderson, D.W. and Haerer, A.F. (1985). Prevalence of Parkinson disease in the biracial population of Copiah County, Mississippi. *Neurology*, **35**, 841–5

SECTION 4

Molecular biology

8

Linkage analysis of hereditary progressive dystonia to the tyrosine hydroxylase gene locus

S. Tsuji, H. Tanaka, T. Miyatake, E. I. Ginns, Y. Nomura and M. Segawa

INTRODUCTION

Hereditary progressive dystonia with marked diurnal fluctuation (HPD) was initially reported by Segawa and colleagues[1]. The age of onset of clinical symptoms ranges from 1 to 9 years with an average of 5.25 ± 2.5 years of age. The initial symptoms in most cases are fatigability and gait disturbance with dystonic posture of foot. The symptoms are aggravated in the evening and markedly alleviated in the morning after sleep. Levodopa produces remarkable and dramatic effects in all cases[1–4].

The tyrosine hydroxylase (TH) activity in the nerve terminals of the nigrostriatal neurons is high in infancy and shows a rapid decline during childhood[5]. The age-dependent changes slow after the third decade. The age of onset and the clinical course, with minimal progression after the third decade, observed in HPD patients correlate quite well with the changes of TH activity in the caudate[3]. Based on these observations, Segawa and colleagues proposed that the pathophysiology of HPD is a functional abnormality in the nerve terminals of the nigrostriatal dopaminergic neurons in the caudate[3]. As TH is the rate-limiting enzyme in catecholamine synthesis, TH deserves consideration as a candidate gene for HPD.

Linkage analysis has been successfully applied to map chromosomal localizations of a number of hereditary neurodegenerative disorders, including torsion dystonia[6,7]. Although TH gene expression is limited to specific organs[8,9], TH cDNA has already been isolated and restriction fragment length polymorphisms have been detected[8–10]. Therefore, it seems feasible to investigate whether HPD is linked to TH gene locus. Furthermore, the availability of a highly polymorphic variable number of tandem repeat (VNTR) markers, that is, Harvey-ras and insulin, adjacent to the TH locus makes linkage analysis more promising. In this paper, we describe the linkage analysis of HPD to the TH locus on chromosome 11p11.5.

PATIENTS AND METHODS

HPD families

Three Japanese HPD families containing six affected individuals were studied. In addition, two sporadic HPD patients were also analysed for the integrity of the TH gene.

Southern blot analysis

High molecular weight genomic DNA was extracted from leukocytes, digested to completion with *Bam*HI, *Eco*RI, *Bgl*II, *Sac*I, or *Dra*I, fractionated by agarose gel electrophoresis and blotted to nitrocellulose membranes[11]. The nitrocellulose filters were hybridized to ^{32}P-labelled TH cDNA. After the hybridization, the filters were washed to a final stringency of 30-min washing, in 0.1 × SSC–0.1% SDS (1 × SSC = 150 mmol/l NaCl and 15 mmol/l sodium citrate) at 55°C, and exposed to X-ray films (Fuji RX®) for 1–3 days with an intensifying screen[12].

DNA probes

The TH gene has been mapped to human chromosome 11p11.5 in the vicinity of the loci for insulin (INS) and for the oncogene Harvey-ras-1 (HRAS). The three probes have been used to detect restriction fragment length polymorphisms (RFLPs); TH (type 2 cDNA) detected a *Pst*I RFLP[13]; INS detected a *Pvu*II RFLP[14] and HRAS detected a *Sca*I RFLP[15].

Simulation studies

SIMLINK is a computer program used to estimate the probability of detecting linkage with given family history on a set of identified pedigrees[16]. This calculation is most usefully undertaken after family history data are gathered, but prior to examination and testing of pedigree members to obtain marker information. We used SIMLINK version 4.0 to estimate if the HPD families were sufficient to demonstrate linkage. The program assumed autosomal dominant inheritance and three linked co-dominant allelic markers with a gene frequency of $p = 0.333$.

Linkage analysis

To evaluate accurately the relative position of the HPD gene and the marker loci, linkage analyses were performed using the LIPED computer program[17] and the LINKAGE program[18] on an IBM PC computer. We used LIPED for the pairwise linkage analysis and the LINKMAP subprogram of LINKAGE for the multipoint linkage analysis. Lod scores were calculated over a range of recombination fractions (θ), assuming the same recombination in both males and females. The location of the HPD gene was varied with respect to a fixed map for the two markers (TH and HRAS). The marker TH was chosen as the arbitrary origin and was set at 0.0 cM. The relative location distance between TH and HRAS was set at 3.8 cM using Haldane's mapping function[19]. It has been demonstrated that the TH and INS genes are contiguous, which indicates that both TH and INS genes are found at the same locus[9].

In HPD families, siblings are affected but their parents do not show any neurological abnormalities. Although autosomal dominant inheritance with incomplete penetrance is most likely in HPD, we cannot calculate the exact penetrance rate with currently available data. Therefore, we used the data only from affected individuals and their parents in the HPD families, treating the parents as being a carrier for the HPD gene.

RESULTS

When genomic DNAs from 8 HPD patients were digested with *Bam*HI, *Eco*RI, *Bgl*II, *Sac*I, or *Dra*I, and subjected to Southern blot hybridization analysis using TH cDNA as a probe, all the HPD patients showed identical patterns to those of normal controls (Figure 1). The results indicate that there are no deletions or rearrangements of the TH gene detectable by Southern blot analysis in HPD patients.

The result of the computer simulation using SIMLINK is shown in Figure 2. As shown, a mean lod score of 2.8 and a maximal lod score of 4.8 can be obtained with given HPD families, suggesting that there is a probability of demonstrating linkage if we have markers closely linked to the HPD locus.

Three markers on chromosome 11p11.5 were used for the linkage analysis of HPD to the TH locus. Figure 3 shows the result of RFLP analyses with INS, HRAS and TH in an HPD family, and Figure 4 shows the result of multipoint linkage analysis using the HPD locus and two loci (HRAS and TH). The lod score never exceeds the critical linkage value of +3.0 at any map position. Linkage was excluded in the 8.4 cM region around the HRAS locus. The lod score at the TH locus was −1.6 suggesting that HPD is less likely to be linked to the TH locus.

DISCUSSION

Since TH is the rate-limiting enzyme in catecholamine biosynthesis and the changes in TH activity in the caudate correlate quite well with the clinical course of HPD[3,5], we have studied the TH gene as a candidate gene for HPD. Southern blot analysis failed to detect any alterations of the TH gene in HPD patients. Furthermore, linkage analysis has suggested that HPD is less likely to be linked to the TH locus, though the lod score of −1.6 cannot completely exclude the linkage. Linkage analysis to the TH locus has been recently performed on a related disorder, dopa-responsive dystonia (DRD),

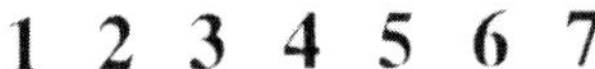

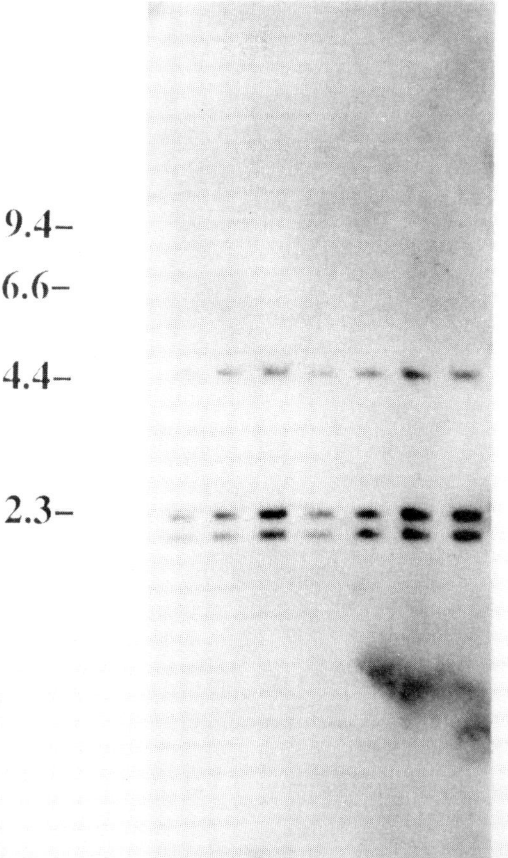

Figure 1 Southern blot hybridization analysis of genomic DNA digested with *Bam*HI using the tyrosine hydroxylase (TH) cDNA as a probe; Lanes 1–3, HPD patients, lanes 4–7, normal controls

which is an extrapyramidal disorder consisting of dystonia, parkinsonism, diurnal fluctuation of symptoms and a dramatic response to levodopa[20]. As with HPD, autosomal dominant inheritance is postulated for DRD. Flecher and colleagues however, reported that there was no evidence for genetic linkage between DRD and the TH locus[20].

A potential problem of linkage analysis of HPD is the penetrance rate, which is not defined precisely, as enough data are not available to calculate it. Nonetheless, development of highly polymorphic markers such as CA repeat polymorphisms[21–24] in addition to VNTR polymorphism probes[25] makes the linkage analysis more promising. Henceforth, it will be necessary to perform linkage analysis using highly polymorphic markers on all other chromosomes.

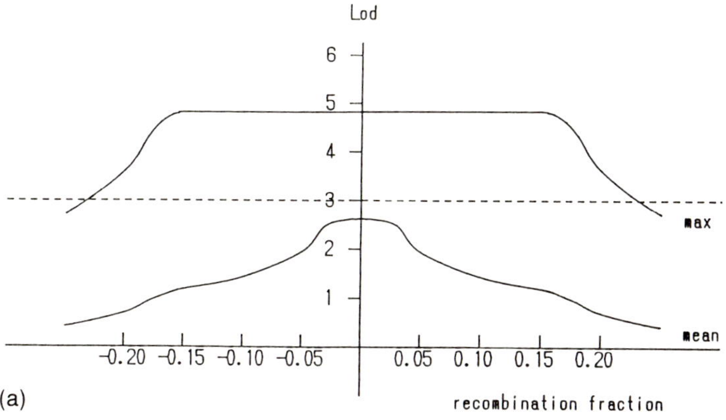

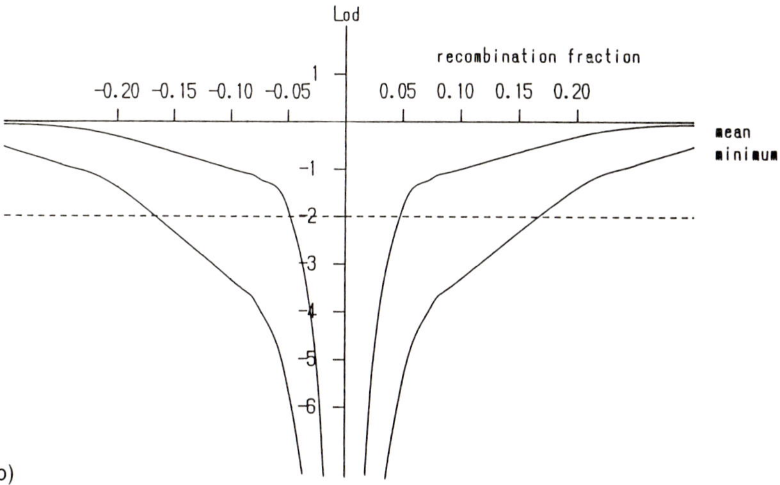

Figure 2 Simulation studies with SIMLINK. For the positive lod scores (a), expected maximal lod scores as well as mean lod scores are plotted for the given families. For the negative lod scores (b), expected mean lod scores as well as minimum lod scores are plotted

Furthermore, factors involved in the regulation of TH activities in the dopaminergic nerve terminals at the caudate should be investigated more intensively, as the regulatory mechanism of TM activity at the caudate seems to be altered in HPD. The regulatory mechanisms of biopterin biosynthesis in HPD should also be analysed carefully. The genes involved in these regulation mechanisms can, therefore, be treated as candidate genes for HPD.

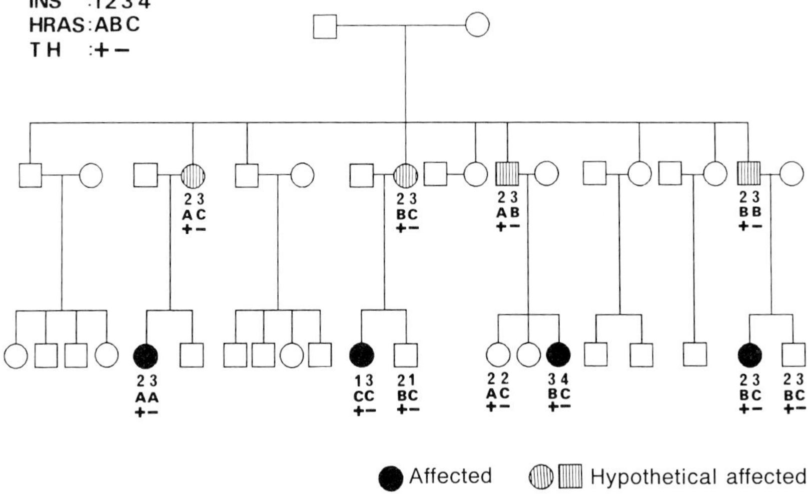

Figure 3 Results of restriction fragment length polymorphism (RFLP) analyses with insulin (INS), Harvey-ras (HRAS) and tyrosine hydroxylase (TH) probes in an HPD family

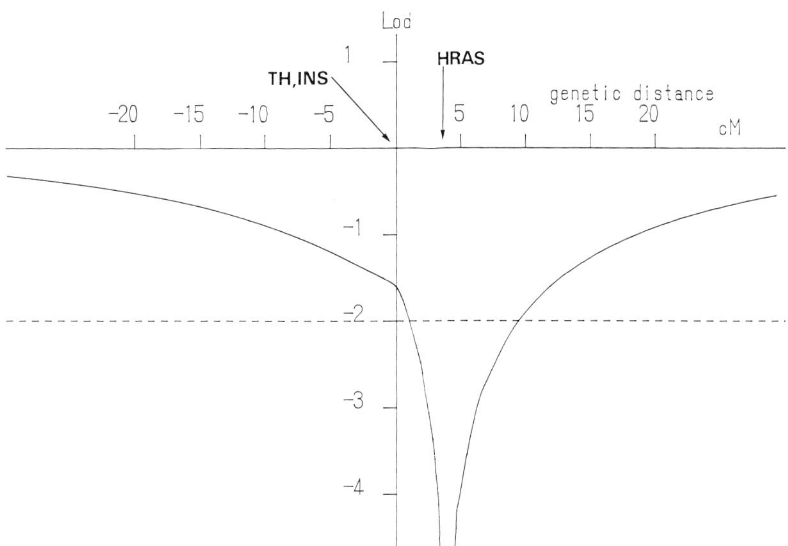

Figure 4 Multipoint linkage analysis using Harvey-ras (HRAS) and insulin (INS) probes. The relative distance between tyrosine hydroxylase (TH), INS and HRAS was set at 3.8 cM. Lod scores were calculated for a range of recombination fractions (θ), assuming the same recombination in both males and females

REFERENCES

1. Segawa, M., Ohmi, K., Itoh, S., Aoyama, M. and Hayakawa, H. (1971). Childhood basal ganglia disease with remarkable response to L-dopa, 'hereditary basal ganglia disease with marked diurnal fluctuation'. *Shinryo*, **24**, 667–72
2. Segawa, M., Hosaka, A., Miyagawa, F., Nomura, Y. and Imai, H. (1976). Hereditary progressive dystonia with marked diurnal fluctuation. In Eldridge, R. and Fahn, S. (eds). *Adv. Neurol.*, Vol. 14, 215–33
3. Segawa, M., Nomura, Y. and Kase, M. (1986). Hereditary progressive dystonia with marked diurnal fluctuation – clinico-pathophysiological identification in reference to juvenile Parkinson's disease. *Adv. Neurol.*, Vol. 45, 227–34
4. Segawa, M., Nomura, Y. and Kase, M. (1986). Diurnal fluctuating hereditary progressive dystonia. In Vinken, P.J., Bruyn, G.W. and Klawans, H.L. (eds.) *Handbook of Clinical Neurology*, 529–39
5. McGeer, E.G. and McGeer, P.L. Some characteristics of brain tyrosine hydroxylase. In Mandel, A. J. (ed.) *New Concepts in Neurotransmitter Regulation*, pp. 53–68. (New York, London: Plenum Press)
6. Ozelius, L. (1989). Human gene for torsion dystonia located on chromosome 9q32–q34. *Neuron*, 2, 1427–34
7. Kramer, P.L., de Leon, D., Ozelius, L. *et al.* (1990). Dystonia gene in Ashkenazi Jewish population is located on chromosome 9q32–34. *Ann. Neurol.*, **27**, 114–20
8. Moss, P.A., Devis, K.E., Boni, C. *et al.* (1986). Linkage of tyrosine hydroxylase to four other markers on the short arm of chromosome 11. *Nucleic Acids Res.*, **14**, 9927–32
9. O'Malley, K.L. and Rotwein, P. (1988). Human tyrosine hydroxylase and insulin genes are contiguous on chromosome 11. *Nucleic Acids Res.*, **16**, 4437–46
10. Grima, B., Lamouroux, A., Boni, C. *et al.* (1987). A single human gene encoding multiple tyrosine hydroxylase with different predicted functional characteristics. *Nature* (*London*), **326**, 707–11
11. Southern, E.M. (1975). Detection of specific sequences among DNA fragments separated by gel electrophoresis. *J. Mol. Biol.*, **98**, 503–17
12. Tanaka, H., Ishikawa, A., Ginns, E.I. *et al.* (1991). Linkage analysis of juvenile parkinsonism to tyrosine hydroxylase gene locus on chromosome 11. *Neurology*, **41**, 719–22
13. Kelsoe, J.R., Stubblefield, B.K. and Ginns, E.I. (1988). Human tyrosine hydroxylase (TH) genomic fragment (pHGTH4) identifies a *Pst*I polymorphism. *Nucleic Acids Res.*, **16**, 7760
14. Chakravarti, A., Elbein, S.C. and Permutt, M.A. (1986). Evidence for increased recombination near the human insulin gene: implication for disease association studies. *Proc. Natl. Acad. Sci. USA*, **83**, 1045–9
15. Detera-Wadleigh, S.D., Berrettini, W.H., Goldin, L.R. *et al.* (1987). Close linkage of c-Harvey-ras-1 and the insulin gene to affective disorder is ruled out in three North American pedigrees. *Nature* (*London*), **325**, 806–8
16. Boehnke, M. (1986). Estimating the power of proposed linkage study: a practical computer simulation approach. *Am. J. Hum. Genet.*, **39**, 513–27
17. Ott, J. (1974). Estimation of the recombination fraction in human pedigrees: efficient computation of the likelihood for human linkage studies. *Am. J. Hum. Genet.*, **26**, 588–97
18. Lathrop, G.M., Lalouel, J.M., Jullier, C. *et al.* (1984). Strategies for multilocus linkage analysis in humans. *Proc. Natl. Acad. Sci. USA*, **81**, 3443–6
19. Haldane, J.B.S. (1919). The combination of linkage values, and the calculation of distances between the loci of linked factors. *J. Genet.*, **8**, 299–309
20. Fletcher, N.A., Holt, I.J., Harding, A.E. *et al.* (1989). Tyrosine hydroxylase and levodopa responsive dystonia. *J. Neurol. Neurosurg. Psychiatry*, **52**, 112–4
21. Litt, M. and Luty, J.A. (1989). A hypervariable microsatellite revealed by *in vitro* amplification of a dinucleotide repeat within the cardiac muscle actin gene. *Am. J. Hum. Genet.*, **44**, 397–401
22. Smeets, H.J.M., Brunner H.G., Roberts, H.H. and Wieringa, B. (1989). Use of variable sequence motifs as genetic markers: application to study of myotonic dystrophy. *Hum. Genet.*, **83**, 245–51
23. Tautz, D. (1989). Hypervariability of simple sequences as a general source for polymorphic markers. *Nucleic Acids Res.*, **17**, 6463–71

24. Weber, J.L. and May, P.E. (1989). Abundant class of human DNA polymorphisms which can be typed using the polymerase chain reaction. *Am. J. Hum. Genet.*, **44**, 388–96
25. Nakamura, Y., Leppert, M., O'Connell, P. *et al.* (1981). Variable number of tandem repeats (VNTR) markers for human gene mapping. *Science*, **275**, 1616–22

SECTION 5

Tetrahydrobiopterin, dystonia and parkinsonism

9

Neurochemical investigations of dystonia: catecholamine neurotransmitter synthesis

P.A. LeWitt

At present, the biological basis for dystonia is unknown and the disorder can be recognized only in its clinical expression[1]. Dystonia's identity as a *syndrome* becomes a more tangible pathophysiological process only when this movement disorder can be linked either to hereditary patterns, to known damage or disease of brain structures, or to neurochemical aberrations. Even when it occurs as a genetic disorder, its clinical manifestations can be indistinguishable from apparently sporadic or acquired (secondary) forms. The markedly heterogeneous character of dystonia is evident from the variety of sites and patterns of dystonic involvement (even among siblings with inherited dystonia derived from the same source). Among the strongest clues to the pathophysiology of dystonia are the results of pharmacological interventions that can either initiate, exacerbate, or else improve its clinical features. While anticholinergic drugs may be among the most effective therapies for the majority of dystonic disorders[2], a small number can be highly responsive to levodopa or other forms of dopaminergic therapy[3-5]. The subgroup of dystonias responsive to levodopa is not distinct from other forms of dystonia in its clinical characteristics. Nevertheless, its relationship to parkinsonism has been of great interest, with some speculation that the levodopa-responsive dystonia might represent an intermediate disorder[3]. Motor impairment, responsive to levodopa, is the hallmark of Parkinson disease, and in many instances parkinsonians present with dystonic features, often years before the onset of more typical resting tremor, rigidity, or bradykinesia[6]. Whether dystonia is a variant or risk factor for the development of parkinsonism has been of considerable interest[7]. The predominance of dystonic parkinsonism among younger individuals has been taken as an indication that age has a strong influence on the development or expression of primary dystonia.

Only a few clues to the pathophysiology of primary dystonia have arisen from neurochemical studies of the brain. While decreased metabolites of dopamine have been reported in cerebrospinal fluid (CSF) specimens from patients with dystonia[8,9], other investigations have not found alterations in brain concentrations of dopamine or its major metabolite homovanillic acid

(HVA)[10]. Among the available studies of the dystonic brain, there have been no findings that would suggest major neuronal changes compatible with alterations in catecholamine systems, as have been found in Parkinson disease. However, two unrelated cases of primary dystonia (one familial) have been examined in which prominent changes of norepinephrine metabolism were identified in several brain stem regions[11]. These findings bear comparison with an autosomally inherited mutation in the rat, which produces dystonic features and which also manifests alterations of norepinephrine[12,13].

An additional line of inquiry into the neurochemical origins for dystonia has come from the investigation of tyrosine hydroxylase co-factor, tetrahydrobiopterin (THB). This has a role in the formation of catecholamines as the obligate co-factor for tyrosine hydroxylase[14–16]. Among other influences, concentrations of THB regulate the hydroxylase reaction, and the rapid turnover of the co-factor to oxidized forms suggests that its reduction may also be an important determinant of THB production. Studies of THB metabolism in a variety of neurological disorders[17] have shown it to be decreased prominently in Parkinson disease[18] as well as in other conditions in which dopaminergic innervation is decreased (e.g. Alzheimer disease[19]). Tetrahydrobiopterin, or its oxidized form biopterin, appears in cerebrospinal fluid and thus, like homovanillic acid, provides a marker of dopamine metabolism. Indeed, THB and homovanillic acid are closely correlated in cerebrospinal fluid[20].

There have been several investigations to assess whether THB metabolism provides any insight on catecholamine synthesis in primary dystonia. The initial studies[15,17,20] used a radioenzymatic assay to detect THB. Later developments in methodology involved development of HPLC separation techniques with fluorometric detection of pterins. These methods require the oxidation of cerebrospinal fluid THB (which is the predominant CSF pterin species) and also permit the detection of other pterin species, such as neopterin. Neopterin is derived from dihydroneopterin triphosphate, an intermediate formed in the synthesis of THB. The action of guanosine triphosphate cyclohydrolase produces dihydroneopterin triphosphate, which yields neopterin through as yet undetermined pathways. Measurements of CSF neopterin and its ratio to biopterin concentration may provide an index for the rate of THB synthesis and turnover[21].

Investigations carried out at the National Institutes of Health (Bethesda, Maryland) discovered[17] and later confirmed[22] the low THB metabolism in some patients with primary dystonia. In a 1986 study, eight patients with primary dystonia of various types were investigated for both CSF biopterin and neopterin concentrations. Three were affected by generalized torsion dystonia, one had adult-onset spasmodic torticollis, and another had hemidystonia that began prior to the development of ipsilateral parkinsonism[22]. The remaining three subjects were sisters, each affected with limb dystonia that fluctuated in severity. Each of these subjects had sustained dystonic posturing that was absent in the morning and gradually worsened over the course of a day, and after prolonged exercise of the affected limbs. This disorder, quite typical of the Segawa type of *diurnally fluctuating dystonia*[23–26], began in their teens and had slowly worsened in each instance. The dystonia responded fully to treatment with levodopa or anticholinergics.

The CSF studies involved the collection of specimens by the same protocol used for unmedicated patients, after subjects had had bedrest overnight. Cerebrospinal fluid aliquots were collected from the same points. While there does not appear to be a major caudal–rostral gradient in CSF concentrations of either biopterin or neopterin, there is a prominent rise of CSF homovanillic acid concentrations[27], so collection techniques need to be standardized with regard to aliquot location. The findings from this study, as previously reported[22], showed that dystonic subjects had a reduction of CSF biopterin concentration to levels approximately half that found with age-matched normal controls. No gender effect was found for measurements of either biopterin or neopterin (only minimal decrease of THB with age has been reported[4,19]). There was some overlap between results in the dystonic and control populations, which were 13.0 ± 0.8 versus 20.6 ± 1.4 pmol/ml ($p < 0.005$), respectively. A highly significant difference between the two groups was also found with respect to CSF neopterin ($p < 0.02$), with dystonic CSF neopterin 12.6 ± 4.8 versus 22.6 ± 1.5 pmol/ml in controls.

For the three subjects with Segawa-type dystonia, determinations of CSF biopterin and neopterin were coupled with studies of homovanillic acid and the major metabolite of serotonin, 5-hydroxyindoleacetic acid (5-HIAA). Their concentrations of homovanillic acid and 5-HIAA were decreased by almost 25%. In fact, the lowest CSF biopterin concentrations among all the dystonic subjects were found in the three subjects affected with diurnally-fluctuating features and whose CSF neopterin was also decreased. After this 1986 publication[22], another study[28,29] investigated Segawa-type dystonia CSF biopterin level in three additional subjects (two of whom were brothers). Again, markedly decreased concentrations were found. The significance of diminished biopterin concentrations is not known, although its high correlation with CSF homovanillic acid[20] would suggest that it reflects central nervous system dopamine metabolism. Reduction of its concentration may be the outcome of one or more pathophysiological scenarios. In the first instance, the decrease may be directly related to a decreased neuronal pool capacity for producing dopamine, as is also the case in Parkinson disease. In the latter disorder, loss of more than 80% of dopaminergic projections to caudate and putamen leads to substantially decreased CSF concentrations of both homovanillic acid[27] and biopterin[18]. Although similar changes in dopaminergic projections are not known to occur in dystonia, it may be that in dystonia there are fewer functional units generating dopamine in nigrostriatal or other dopaminergic pathways.

Another possibility might be that, in dystonia, the biosynthetic apparatus for THB production is intact but down-regulated. This might occur either by regulatory interactions with the dopaminergic system or from feedback inhibition of THB synthesis (which in turn would influence the generation of dopamine). The latter is unlikely to be the major explanation for dystonia, since most forms of this disorder do not improve with dopaminergic supplementation, and may have their clinical features exacerbated by such treatment. Tetrahydrobiopterin, as a rate-limiting cofactor for the synthesis of dopamine, is also involved in the synthesis of norepinephrine. In this context, the decreased tissue concentrations of norepinephrine in two cases of primary dystonia[11] may be related to the other findings of decreased biopterin. Tissue concentrations of the cofactor were not studied in these cases. A third possibility is that the decrease in CSF biopterin concentration is indicative of a primary defect in the synthesis of THB. In support of this possibility, clinical trials carried out with parenteral administrations of THB have provided some evidence.

The first trials of THB therapy involved administration of an intravenous preparation (in a mixed stereoisomer form) for the assessment of dystonia ratings[22]. These trials were carried out in a double-blind, placebo-controlled fashion and involved THB doses of 2.5–10 mg/kg body weight. The compound was administered over 10 min. Of a group of 10 dystonic patients treated with THB, two with diurnally-fluctuating limb dystonia showed improvements. A third patient with hemi-parkinsonism and hemi-dystonia experienced a marked improvement of the involuntary posturing and rigidity of her dystonic foot, but no alteration of parkinsonian signs and symptoms. Another subject affected with familial torsion dystonia reported a subjective improvement from the THB treatment (but not from placebo); his effects came on shortly after the THB infusion and lasted for several hours thereafter. Objective ratings, however, found no changes for this patient after either placebo or THB treatments.

The improvements in dystonic features related to THB administration occurred in only four of the 10 patients, though they were dramatic for three of them. For the two sisters with Segawa-type dystonia, the degree of improvement from THB treatment was comparable to that routinely achieved with levodopa or anticholinergic therapy. In the case of the patient with hemi-dystonia associated with hemi-parkinsonism, she achieved improvement to the degree generally not experienced from each dose of levodopa, which tended to exacerbate dystonic features. From these experiences, it seems likely that the pharmacological effect may have unmasked a primary factor in the pathogenesis of dystonia for these individuals. While an increase in striatal dopaminergic stimulation may have been the final pathway for effecting symptomatic relief (at least for the Segawa-type dystonics), the means by which THB acted indicate that there is an alternative route to augment dopamine synthesis. These findings further support the hypothesis that decreased THB synthesis could be a primary factor in Segawa-type dystonia, and possibly other clinical variants. This is by no means proven. In a later study[29], THB was administered to one of the Segawa-type patients previously treated[22], and a similar response was encountered on this occasion. However, three other patients thought to have a diurnally-fluctuating form of dystonia were reported not to have responded to administration of up to 25 mg/kg body weight. Although a decrease in CSF biopterin was demonstrated, the clinical characteristics of these patients may be at variance with typical features of Segawa-type dystonia. The latter study[29] showed no change in CSF homovanillic acid or 5-HIAA measurements from THB administration, although the initial trials with THB gave a different result[22]. In some instances, rises in both CSF homovanillic acid and 5-HIAA occurred. These results suggest that enhancement of monoamine neurotransmitter synthesis may have occurred as a consequence of treatment with THB.

Although the results were not seen consistently in all patients, the clinical improvements observed are a promising lead for understanding the nature of certain types of primary dystonia. It is of interest that dystonic features, but not parkinsonism, improved in the single example of hemi-dystonia with hemi-parkinsonism. Previous studies of THB administration to parkinsonians showed no symptomatic change[18], despite the responsiveness of such patients to dopaminergic therapy. It would appear that THB administration does not necessarily increase dopamine production, and indeed tyrosine hydroxylase activity is highly regulated by end-product feedback and other factors which might override any stimulatory effect of augmented THB concentrations in the dopaminergic nerve terminal[14–16]. In those neurons of the parkinsonian brain which remain, intra-neuronal THB concentration may be adequate for the purposes of dopamine synthesis. In contrast, the responsiveness of some dystonics to THB might suggest that the deficiency noted in CSF reflects a relative deficiency of the cofactor in the intra-neuronal environment.

Tetrahydrobiopterin may have additional pharmacological properties beyond its role as a cofactor in monoamine synthesis. For example, studies in animals have shown that THB enhances dopamine synthesis[30]. Other investigations have shown that THB can increase the release of striatal dopamine in a manner which is independent of an effect on dopamine biosynthetic rate[31]. The mechanism by which THB (and possibly other pterins) might cause the enhanced release has not been determined. However, these are the first clues that THB may have additional regulatory properties. It would be of particular interest for further studies of the Segawa-type variant of dystonia to know if the mechanisms for worsening and improvement are related to daily cycling in the biosynthesis of THB and, ultimately, production of dopamine. In this regard, another syndrome of diurnally fluctuating neurological impairments has been reported to be due to a defect of dihydrobiopterin synthesis[32].

There has been no further progress with respect to the investigation of catecholamine disturbances in dystonia. While abnormalities of dopamine-β-hydroxylase have been reported as a possible biochemical marker with hereditary dystonia[33,34], these preliminary results have not been confirmed. Furthermore, it is likely that different forms of dystonia have a variety of neurochemical mechanisms, as can be inferred from pharmacological responsiveness.

Further studies of tetrahydrobiopterin (and neopterin) may confirm its use as a marker for the biochemical lesions of dystonia. Whether primary or secondary in origin, the disturbances described (including wide disparity of cerebrospinal fluid neopterin concentrations, in contrast to the range found with normal controls[22]) may be more than just enigmatic neurochemical epiphenomena. One direction for further inquiry would be to determine if some patients with young-onset parkinsonism have features responsive to tetrahydrobiopterin administration. It would be of great interest to learn, for example, if dystonic features occurring in the context of parkinsonism might improve, as was observed in one patient[22]. Although tetrahydrobiopterin administration serves the same neuropharmacological ends as levodopa, response to THB may be an informative screening test for disorders with a primary biopterin deficiency, as is the case for atypical phenylketonuria, which can be due to defects of various types in the synthesis of tetrahydrobiopterin[16,21].

REFERENCES

1. Fahn, S., Marsden, C.D. and Calne, D.B. (eds.) (1988). *Adv. Neurol.*, Vol. 50, Dystonia 2
2. Greene, P., Shale, H. and Fahn, S. (1988). Experience with high dosages of anticholinergic and other drugs in the treatment of torsion dystonia. *Adv. Neurol.*, **50**, 547–56
3. Nygaard, T.G., Marsden, C.D. and Duvoisin, R.C. (1988). Dopa-responsive dystonia. *Adv. Neurol.*, **50**, 377–84
4. Newman, R.P., LeWitt, P.A., Schults, C., Bruno, G., Foster, N.L., Chase, T.N. and Calne, D.B. (1985). Dystonia: treatment with bromocriptine. *Clin. Neuropharmacol.*, **8**, 328–33
5. Lang, A.E. (1988). Dopamine agonists and antagonists in the treatment of idiopathic dystonia. *Adv. Neurol.*, **50**, 561–70
6. LeWitt, P.A., Burns, R.S. and Newman, R.P. (1986). Dystonia in untreated parkinsonism. *Clin. Neuropharmacol.*, **9**, 293–7
7. Gershanik, O. and Nygaard, T.G. (1990). Parkinson's disease beginning before age 40. *Adv. Neurol.*, **53**, 251–8
8. Tabaddor, K., Wolfson, L.I. and Sharpless, N.S. (1978). Diminished ventricular fluid dopamine metabolites in adult-onset dystonia. *Neurology*, **28**, 1254–8
9. Wolfson, L.I., Sharpless, N.S., Thal, L.J., Waltz, J.M. and Shapiro, L. (1983). Decreased ventricular fluid norepinephrine metabolite in childhood-onset dystonia. *Neurology*, **33**, 369–72
10. Kartzinel, R. and Chase, T.N. (1977). Pharmacology of dystonia. *Clin. Neuropharmacol.*, **2**, 43–53
11. Hornykiewicz, O., Kish, S.J. and Becker, L.E. (1988). Biochemical evidence for brain neurotransmitter changes in idiopathic torsion dystonia (dystonia musculorum deformans). *Adv. Neurol.*, **50**, 157–65
12. Lorden, J.F., McKeon, T.W., Baker, H.J., Cox, N. and Walkley, S.U. (1984). Characterization of the rat mutant dystonic (dt), a new animal model of dystonia musculorum deformans. *J. Neurosci.*, **4**, 1925–32
13. Lorden, J.F., Oltmans, G.A., Stratton, S. and Mays, L.E. (1988). Neuropharmacological correlates of the motor syndrome of the genetically dystonic (dt) rat. *Adv. Neurol.*, **50**, 277–97
14. LeWitt, P.A. and Miller, L.P. (1987). Pterin abnormalities in nervous system disease: treatment aspects. In Lovenberg, W. and Levine, R.A., (eds.), *Topics in Neurochemistry and Neuropharmacology*, Vol. 1, pp. 154–71. (London: Taylor and Francis)
15. Levine, R.A., Miller, L.P. and Lovenberg, W. (1981). Tetrahydrobiopterin in the striatum: localization in dopamine nerve terminals and its role in catecholamine synthesis. *Science*, **214**, 919–21
16. Nichol, C.A., Smith, G.K. and Duch, D.S. (1985). Biosynthesis and metabolism of tetrahydrobiopterin and molybdopterin. *Ann. Rev. Biochem.*, **54**, 729–64
17. Williams, A.C., Levine, R.A., Chase, T.N., Lovenberg, W. and Calne, D.B. (1980). CSF hydroxylase cofactor levels in some neurological diseases. *J. Neurol. Neurosurg. Psychiatr.*, **43**, 735–8
18. LeWitt, P.A., Miller, L.P., Newman, R.P., Burns, R.S., Insel, T., Levine, R.A., Lovenberg, W. and Calne, D.B. (1984). Tyrosine hydroxylase cofactor (tetrahydrobiopterin) in parkinsonism. *Adv. Neurol.*, **40**, 459–62
19. LeWitt, P., Levine, R., Lovenberg, W., Pomara, N., Stanley, M., Gurevich, D., Schlick, P. and Roberts, R. (1990). Monoamine neurotransmitter metabolites and hydroxylase cofactor in Alzheimer-type dementia and normals. In Fisher, A., Hanin, I. and Lachman, C. (eds.)

Alzheimer's and Parkinson's Diseases: Strategies for Research and Development, pp. 323–7. (New York: Plenum Press)

20. Williams, A.C., Levine, R.A., Chase, T.N., Lovenberg, W. and Calne, D.B. (1979). Hydroxylase cofactor activity in cerebrospinal fluid of normal subjects and patients with Parkinson's disease. *Science*, **204**, 624–6
21. Nixon, J.C., Lee, C.-L., Milstein, S., Kaufman, S. and Bartholome, K. (1980). Neopterin and biopterin levels in patients with atypical forms of phenylketonuria. *J. Neurochem.*, **35**, 898–904
22. LeWitt, P.A., Miller, L.P., Levine, R.A., Lovenberg, W., Newman, R.P., Papavasiliou, A., Rayes, A., Eldridge, R. and Burns, R.S. (1986). Tetrahydrobiopterin in dystonia: identification of abnormal metabolism and therapeutic trials. *Neurology*, **36**, 760–4
23. Segawa, M., Hosaka, A., Miyagawa, F., Nomura, Y. and Imai, H. (1976). Hereditary progressive dystonia with marked diurnal fluctuation. *Adv. Neurol.*, **14**, 215–33
24. Ouvrier, R.A. (1978). Progressive dystonia with marked diurnal variation. *Ann. Neurol.*, **4**, 412–17
25. Gordon, N. (1982). Fluctuating dystonia and allied syndromes. *Neuropediatrics*, **13**, 152–4
26. Deonna, T. (1986). Dopa-sensitive progressive dystonia of childhood with fluctuations of symptoms – Segawa's syndrome and possible variants. *Neuropediatrics*, **17**, 81–5
27. LeWitt, P.A. and Galloway, M.P. (1990). Neurochemical markers of Parkinson's Disease. In Koller, W.C. and Paulson, G. (eds.) *Therapeutics in Parkinson's Disease*, pp. 63–93. (New York: Marcel Dekker)
28. Fink, J.K., Barton, N.W. and Cohen, W.E. (1988). Dystonia with marked diurnal variation associated with biopterin deficiency. *Neurology*, **38**, 707–11
29. Fink, J.K., Ravin, P. and Argoff, C.E. (1989). Tetrahydrobiopterin administration in biopterin-deficient progressive dystonia with diurnal variation. *Neurology*, **39**, 1393–5
30. Kettler, R., Bartholini, G. and Pletscher, A. (1974). *In vivo* enhancement of tyrosine hydroxylation in rat striatum by tetrahydrobiopterin. *Nature* (*London*), **249**, 476–8
31. Koshimura, K., Miwa, S., Lee, K., Fushiwara, M. and Watanabe, Y. (1990). Enhancement of dopamine release *in vivo* from the rat striatum by dialtyic perfusion of 6-R-*L-erythro*-5,6,7,8-tetrahydrobiopterin. *J. Neurochem.*, **54**, 1391–7
32. Tanaka, K., Yoneda, M. and Nakajima, T. (1987). Dihydrobiopterin synthesis defect: an adult with diurnal fluctuation of symptoms. *Neurology*, **37**, 519–522
33. Wooten, G.F., Eldridge, R., Axelrod, J. and Stern, R.S. (1973). Elevated plasma dopamine-beta-hydroxylase activity in autosomal dominant torsion. *N. Engl. J. Med.*, **288**, 284–7
34. Korczyn, A.P., Rabinowitz, R. and Kahana, E. (1982). Dopamine-beta-hydroxylase (DBH) in idiopathic torsion dystonia (IDT). *J. Neurol. Sci.*, **53**, 91–3

10

Effect of tetrahydrobiopterin and 5-hydroxytryptophan on hereditary progressive dystonia with marked diurnal fluctuation: a suggestion of serotonergic system involvement

A. Ishida and G. Takada

INTRODUCTION

Hereditary progressive dystonia with marked diurnal fluctuation (HPD) was first described by Segawa and colleagues in 1971[1]. Since then, more than 40 cases have been reported. The age of onset of clinical symptoms ranges from 1 to 9 years. The cardinal symptoms are fatigability and gait disturbance with dystonic posture, such as pes equinovarus, which spreads to other limbs in due course. The characteristic feature of the disease is aggravation of symptoms in the evening and the dramatic effect of levodopa without any side-effect, even after long-term administration[2]. The pathogenesis of diurnal fluctuation is not clear. Recently, tetrahydrobiopterin (BH_4) was described as alleviating dystonic symptoms in HPD[3]. To the best of our knowledge, however, there is no paper on 5-hydroxytryptophan (5-HTP) therapy for HPD.

We report here a mother and daughter with HPD who responded favorably to both BH_4 and 5-HTP therapy, which suggests the involvement of the serotonergic system in this disorder.

CASE REPORTS

An 8-year-old Japanese girl was normal till the age of 4, when fatigability, gait disturbance, and a tendency to fall developed. These symptoms were progressive, though slight improvement was noticed after sleep. She was referred to us at age 5. On admission, pes equinovarus was observed in her left ankle. She walked with a wide base and long stride. Tremor, akinesia, torticollis, and trunk torsion were not observed. The symptoms disappeared completely with the therapy of 5 mg/kg per day of levodopa with carbidopa.

The 35-year-old mother of this girl began to feel fatigue in her legs at age 34. Trembling of her arms and slight stiffness of her limbs developed the next year. When writing, dusting, or cutting with a kitchen knife, her right hand tended to turn inward. On admission, ankle rigidity and cog-wheel rigidity and postural tremor of her right arm were observed. There was no apparent gait disturbance, pill-rolling or resting tremor, bradykinesia, or stooped posture. Her symptoms responded thoroughly to 4 mg/kg per day of levodopa with carbidopa.

METHODS

We administered oral levodopa, BH_4 and 5-HTP separately to the patients, who had completed a drug-free period of 4 weeks. Dr T. Noguchi, Suntory Biochemical Institute (Yamazaki, Japan) generously supplied 6R-L-erythro-5,6,7,8-BH_4 and 5-HTP was purchased from Sigma Chemical Company (St Louis, Mo, USA). Doses of each drug are shown in Table 1. Levodopa was given in combination with 5-HTP, at a dose which was not sufficient for removing all the symptoms.

Neurological examinations and videotape recordings of dystonic movements were made at 2-h intervals every day. To evaluate the hand dystonia of the mother, a hand-tapping test was performed, which involved making dots at the indicated point on a paper with a felt pen for 30 s. As the wrist turned inward, the dots made a quarter of a circle. A foot-tapping test for the daughter was to repeat up-and-down movements of her tiptoe as fast as she could, while keeping her heel on the floor. The time needed to repeat the exercise 30 times was measured.

Samples of cerebrospinal fluid (CSF) were obtained by lumbar puncture at noon. The first 2 ml was for 5-hydroxyindoleacetic acid (5-HIAA) and homovanillic acid (HVA) determination, the second 2 ml for amino acid analysis, and the third 2 ml for biopterin. Biopterin, 5-HIAA and HVA were measured with high performance liquid chromatography after Fukushima and colleagues[4] and Wagner and colleagues[5]. Each sampling was done with informed consent.

Table 1 Doses of BH_4, levodopa and 5-HTP (mg/kg per day). Levodopa contains 10% of carbidopa

	5-year-old	*35-year-old*
BH_4	37	37
Levodopa	5	2–6
5-HTP	~7.2	0.3
+ levodopa	3.0	2.0

RESULTS

Clinical evaluation

The effect of BH_4 on the child was obvious in every aspect of the symptoms. She could walk a longer distance normally, and diurnal fluctuations decreased though not completely. The foot-tapping test improved clearly as shown in Figure 1. All the symptoms returned to the extent of pretreatment by day 14. As for the mother, the effect was clearly observed. She felt less fatigue starting on day 1 of the administration. Her hand dystonia improved remarkably as shown by the hand-tapping test (Figure 2). These improvements lasted for 2 weeks with gradual attenuation.

The effect of 5-HTP on the daughter was ambiguous. Her fatigability and gait disturbance improved greatly, but worsened at times without any apparent cause. There was no effect on the foot-tapping test. The dose was increased up to 7.2 mg/kg per day without further improvement. On the other hand, the mother's hand dystonia improved remarkably when 5-HTP supplementing a low dose of levodopa was used, just as observed during BH_4 therapy (Figure 2).

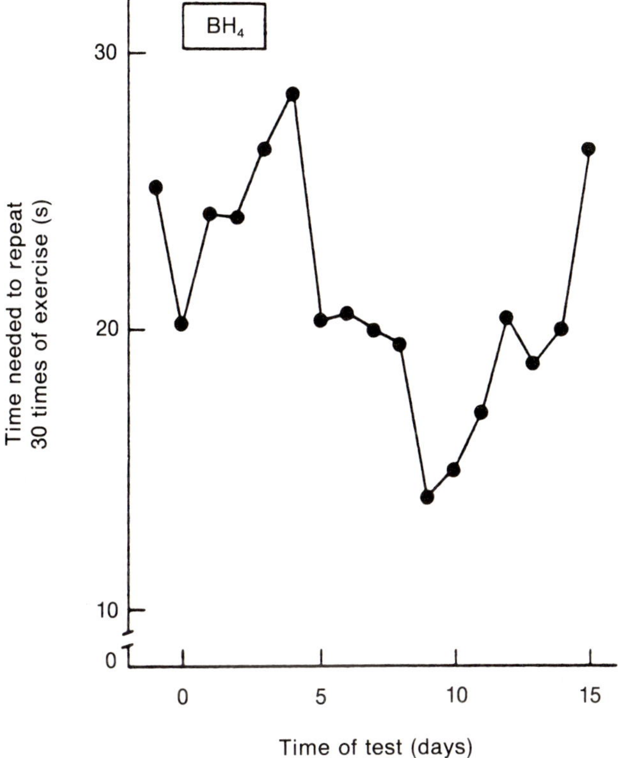

Figure 1 Time course of results of the foot-tapping test of the child. Age-matched normal control results were 10.9 ± 2.0 (mean ± SD, $n = 7$)

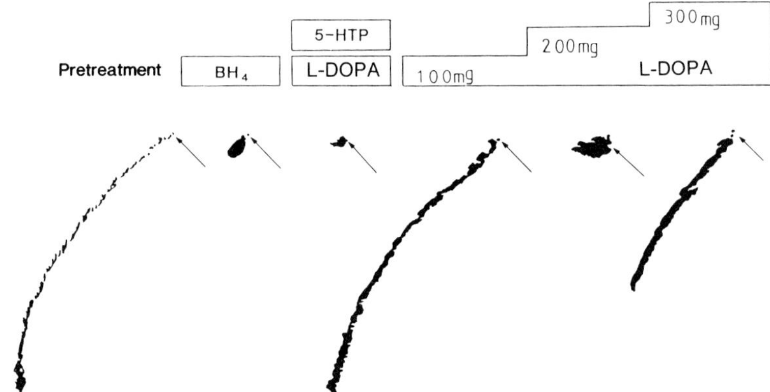

Figure 2 Actual tracing of the hand-tapping test of the parent. See text for the method; ← shows the point indicated for making dots. 5-HTP (0.3 mg/kg/day) was added to low dose (2 mg/kg/day) of levodopa. Each prescription was continued for at least two weeks, except for BH_4. Dots centered at the indicated point when this patient was on BH_4, 5-HTP plus levodopa and 200 mg/day of levodopa therapy, which perceptibly shows the effect of these drugs. Furthermore, it also shows that 5-HTP plus levodopa had the best effect among them, which was not discernible by conventional neurological examination

Biochemical estimation

Total serum biopterin concentrations increased markedly during BH_4 administration with concomitant increase in total CSF biopterin levels in both patients (Figure 3). The rise of biopterin in the daughter was not so high as that of the mother.

There was an apparent response to BH_4 of 5-hydroxyindoleacetic acid in the CSF of the child but not in that of the parent. As for homovanillic acid in CSF, the parent showed a clear response to BH_4 (Figure 4).

COMMENTS

The pathogenesis of HPD is taken to be a dysfunction of the nigrostriatal dopaminergic system[2]. This assumption seems to be based on the following facts:

(1) The dramatic and continuous response to levodopa occurs without any relation to the duration of illness and previous therapy with anticholinergic drugs;

(2) The duration of the disease corresponds to the period when rapid decrease of tyrosine hydroxylase activity in the caudate nucleus physiologically occurs;

(3) An autopsied brain with this disease revealed no neuropathological abnormalities in the basal ganglia and other subcortical neurons except loss of pigmentation of the substantia nigra[6].

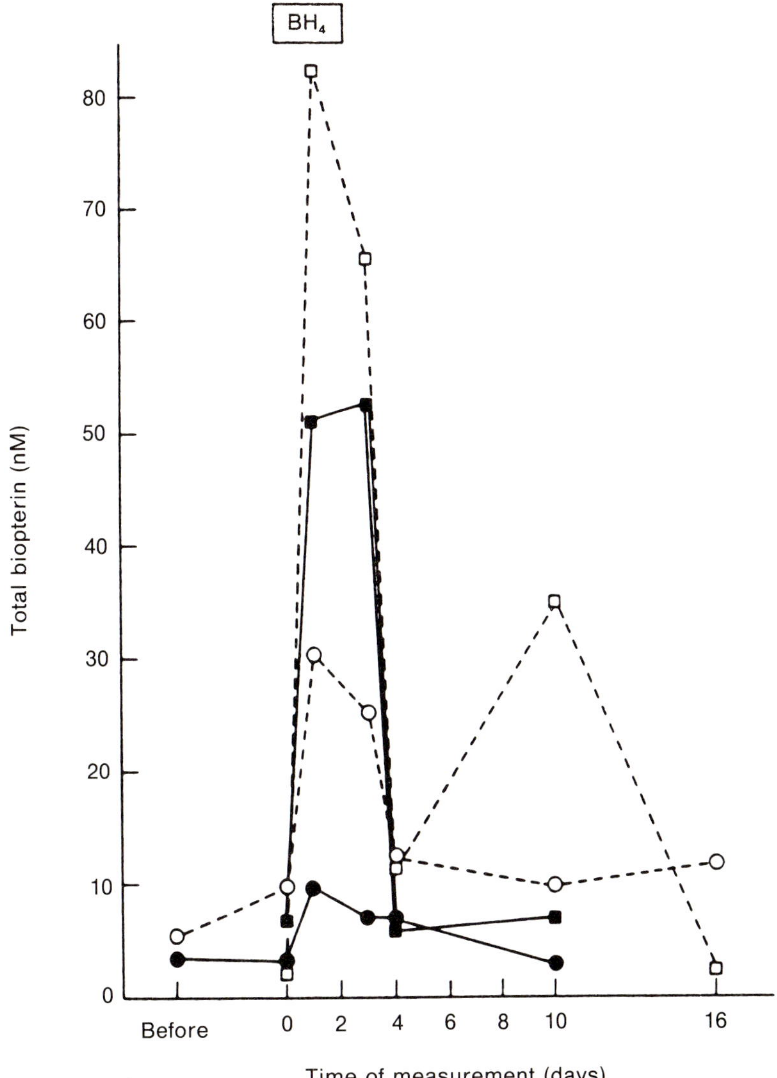

Figure 3 Total biopterin concentration in serum and CSF of our two patients, obtained before, during and after BH_4 therapy. Both serum and CSF concentrations of total biopterin increased markedly during BH_4 administration. ●—●, CSF of the daughter; ○—○, CSF of the mother; ■—■, serum of the daughter; □—□, serum of the mother

The mother described here has developed symptoms of HPD at age 34. She seems to be the first case of adult onset HPD to be reported. We hear that the mother of one of Segawa's cases, too, has been recently diagnosed as having HPD (personal communication). Considering that HPD is regarded as a genetic disorder, it is quite interesting that the age of onset of HPD is

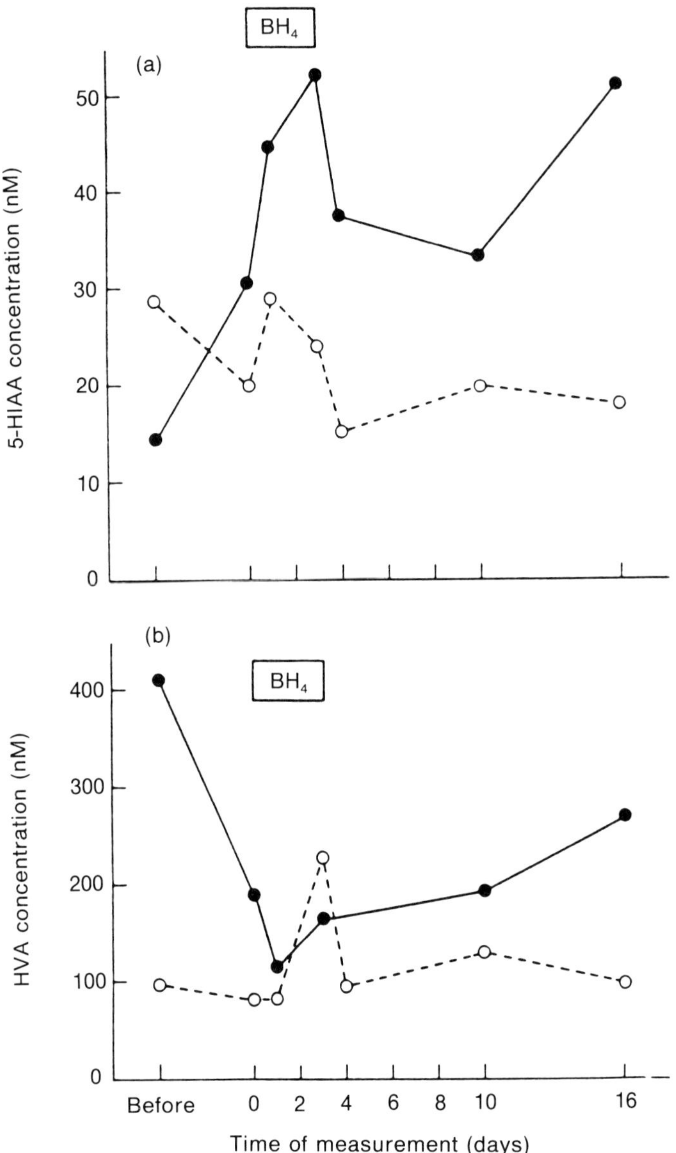

Figure 4 (a) 5-HIAA and (b) HVA concentrations in CSF of the daughter (●—●) and the mother (○—○). Control values for 5-HIAA and HVA, which were obtained from patients with neurological disease without dystonia or parkinsonism, are 39.9 ± 18.9 nM ($n = 8$) and 367.9 ± 165.0 nM ($n = 8$), respectively. Values are mean ± SD

far apart even within a family.

In other studies BH_4 seemed to be more effective on the patients who were less severely affected[3,7]. Although the daughter in this report was severely affected and the mother was an adult-onset type, the effects of BH_4

were apparent. Intravenous infusion of low-dose BH_4 was reported to produce greater clinical improvement than high-dose infusion, where CSF biopterin exceeded normal levels[7]. Oral administration of BH_4 might be more suitable for maintaining the CSF biopterin level within the normal range.

Loci of the nigrostriatal system are found to show distinctive biochemicl changes with age, such as the diminution of tyrosine hydroxylase activity in the terminals of nigrostriatal neurons with increasing age[8,9]. The tyrosine hydroxylase activity in that system is also thought to be decreased in HPD[2]. The differential response of HVA and 5-HIAA to BH_4, and that of the clinical symptoms to 5-HTP, between our two patients could partially be ascribed to both the difference in their present ages and the ages of onset.

Although an inhibitory serotinin receptor at the terminals of dopaminergic neurons in the striatum has been found to modulate dopamine release[10], the functional reciprocal relation between serotonergic and dopaminergic neurons is quite obscure at present.

There has been no evidence in the literature which suggests the involvement of the serotonergic system in the HPD. As shown in our patients who were treated with, and responded well to, both BH_4 and 5-HTP, the serotonergic system might play some role in the pathogenesis of HPD, particularly in dystonia. Much work has to be done along this line.

ACKNOWLEDGEMENT

This work was partly supported by a grant-in-aid for new drug development from the Ministry of Health and Welfare, Japan.

REFERENCES

1. Segawa, M., Ohmi, K., Itoh, S., Aoyama, M. and Hayakawa, H. (1971). Childhood basal ganglia disease with remarkable response to L-dopa, 'hereditary basal ganglia disease with marked diurnal fluctuation'. *Shinryou* (Tokyo), **24**, 667–72
2. Segawa, M., Nomura, Y. and Kase, M. (1986). Diurnal fluctuating hereditary progressive dystonia. In Vinken, P.J., Bruyn, G.W. and Klawans, H.L. (eds.) *Handbook of Clinical Neurology*, pp. 529–39. (Amsterdam: Elsevier Science)
3. LeWitt, P.A., Miller, L.P., Levine, R.A., Lovenberg, W., Newman, R.P., Papavasiliou, A., Rayes, A., Eldridge, R. and Burns, R.S. (1986). Tetrahydrobiopterin in dystonia: Identification of abnormal metabolism and therapeutic trials. *Neurology*, **36**, 760–4
4. Fukushima, T. and Nixon, J.C. (1980). Analysis of reduced forms of biopterin in biological tissues and fluids. *Ann. Biochem.*, **102**, 176–88
5. Wagner, J., Vitali, P., Palfreyman, M.G., Zraika, M. and Hout, S. (1982). Simultaneous determination of 3,4-dihydroxyphenylalanine, 5-hydroxytroptophan, dopamine, 4-hydroxy-3-methoxyphenylalanine, norepinephrine, 3,4-dihydroxyphenylacetic acid, homovanillic acid, serotonin, and 5-hydroxyindoleacetic acid in rat cerebrospinal fluid and brain by high-performance liquid chromatography with electrochemical detection. *J. Neurochem.*, **38**, 1241–54
6. Yokochi, M., Narabayashi, H., Iizuka, R. and Nagatsu, T. (1984). Juvenile parkinsonism – some clinical, pharmacological and neuropathological aspects. In Hassler, R.G. and Christ, J.F. (eds.) *Advances in Neurology*, *Vol.* 40, pp. 407–13. (New York: Raven Press)
7. Fink, J.K., Ravin, P., Argoff, C.E., Levine, R.A., Brady, R.O., Hallett, M. and Barton, N.W. (1989). Tetrahydrobiopterin administration in biopterin-deficient progressive dystonia with diurnal variation. *Neurology*, **39**, 1393–5

8. McGeer, E.G. and McGeer, P.L. (1973). Some characteristics of brain tyrosine hydroxylase. In Mandel, J. (ed.) *New Concepts in Neurotransmitter Regulation*, pp. 53–68. (New York: Plenum Press)
9. McGeer, P.L., McGeer, E.G. and Suzuki, J.S. (1977). Aging and extrapyramidal function. *Arch. Neurol.*, **34**, 33–5
10. Ennis, C., Kemp, J.D. and Cox, B. (1981). Characterization of inhibitory 5-hydroxytryptamine receptors that modulate dopamine release in the striatum. *J. Neurochem.*, **36**, 1515–20

11

Tetrahydrobiopterin therapy for juvenile parkinsonism

T. Kondo, H. Miwa, Y. Furukawa, Y. Mizuno and H. Narabayashi

INTRODUCTION

The reduction of dopamine content and lowering of tyrosine hydroxylase (TH) activity in the nigrostriatal system associated with parkinsonism may be attributable to the degeneration of the neurons.

Tetrahydrobiopterin is a co-factor of tyrosine hydroxylation, the rate-limiting step of catecholamine synthesis *in vivo*[1]. The reductions of biopterin content and of the activity of GTP cyclohydrolase I, the enzyme of the first step of biopterin synthesis, in the striatum of parkinsonian brain have been reported[2,3]. The reduction of biopterin content in the striatum is noted to parallel the decrease in TH activity in the region of the disease[2].

Juvenile parkinsonism is defined by Yokochi as onset of the disease before the age of 40. Pathobiochemical analysis of the cases of juvenile parkinsonism has been poorly carried out. Only two cases have been analyzed by Yokochi and colleagues[5]. The analysis suggests that the level of reduction of TH activity of the brain in cases of juvenile parkinsonism is not uniform.

Therapeutic use of tetrahydrobiopterin in parkinsonism has been tried by several authors. The findings regarding the efficacy of this substance on the disease are conflicting.

According to recent reports on the action mechanism of tetrahydrobiopterin, the substance activates TH and enhances the release of dopamine from dopaminergic neurons[6,7]. Therefore, patients who have more preserved dopaminergic nerve terminals and greater TH activity in the striatum may be expected to show a more favorable response to tetrahydrobiopterin therapy.

In this paper, the authors add biochemical data of three cases of juvenile parkinsonism, and describe their previous experience of tetrahydrobiopterin administration in cases of juvenile parkinsonism.

PATHOBIOCHEMISTRY OF THE BRAIN IN JUVENILE PARKINSONISM

The data of pathological and biochemical analysis have been reported in

Table 1 Comparison of TH activity between the clinical types of juvenile parkinsonism and Parkinson disease. Case T.M. and case T.O. indiicate the cases reported by Yokochi and colleagues[5]. Values are expressed as the percentage of the mean values for each respective control group

		Brain region		
	Clinical type	*Substantia nigra*	*Head of caudate nucleus*	*Putamen*
Juvenile parkinsonism				
Case 1	Ia	37.6	30.0	52.2
Case 2	Ia	30.6	24.2	46.1
Case 3	Ia	59.4	33.3	5.6
Case T.M.	Ib	4.7	0	0.1
Case T.O.	II	84.1	12.8	26.4
Parkinson disease ($n = 11$)		9.9	12.5	4.9
Range	—	0–44.8	0–35.6	0–10.0

two cases of juvenile parkinsonism by Yokochi and colleagues[5]. In one case, the clinical manifestations and response to levodopa therapy were similar to those of late-onset parkinsonism, with classical pathological features. The other case, showing dystonia of the feet, dramatic response to levodopa therapy with severe diurnal fluctuations and choreic dyskinesia, exhibited a poor cell population including fewer neuromelanin-containing neurons and neurons suggesting immature development in the substantia nigra compacta[8]. The TH activities in the substantia nigra and the striatum were severely reduced in the former case, but were similar to those in late-onset Parkinson disease. In the latter case, the TH activity in the substantia nigra was within the normal range and that in the striatum was decreased.

Recently we analyzed TH activity and total biopterin content in the substantia nigra and striatum in three cases of juvenile parkinsonism[9]. These cases had been subgrouped as type Ia by Narabayashi and colleagues from the clinical features and response to levodopa therapy[10]. The TH activity in the substantia nigra of these patients was fairly well preserved. These values seemed to be intermediate between the values of the two cases reported by Yokochi and colleagues[5]. The reduction in TH activity in the putamen was modest in two out of the three cases. The values for TH activity in the head of the caudate nucleus were observed to be within the range found in Parkinson disease (Table 1). The reductions of total biopterin content in the substantia nigra and the striatum seem to parallel the reduction in TH activity in the respective brain regions (Figure 1). The previous report and our present data indicate that the biochemical pathology of juvenile parkinsonism is not uniform. The TH activity may be partially preserved in some cases. From the viewpoint of tetrahydrobiopterin therapy, fairly well-preserved dopamine nerve terminals and TH activity in the striatum might be favorable for improving parkinsonism.

EFFECT OF TETRAHYDROBIOPTERIN THERAPY ON PARKINSONISM

Several conflicting results on the response to tetrahydrobiopterin administration in parkinsonism have been reported. Narabayashi and co-workers

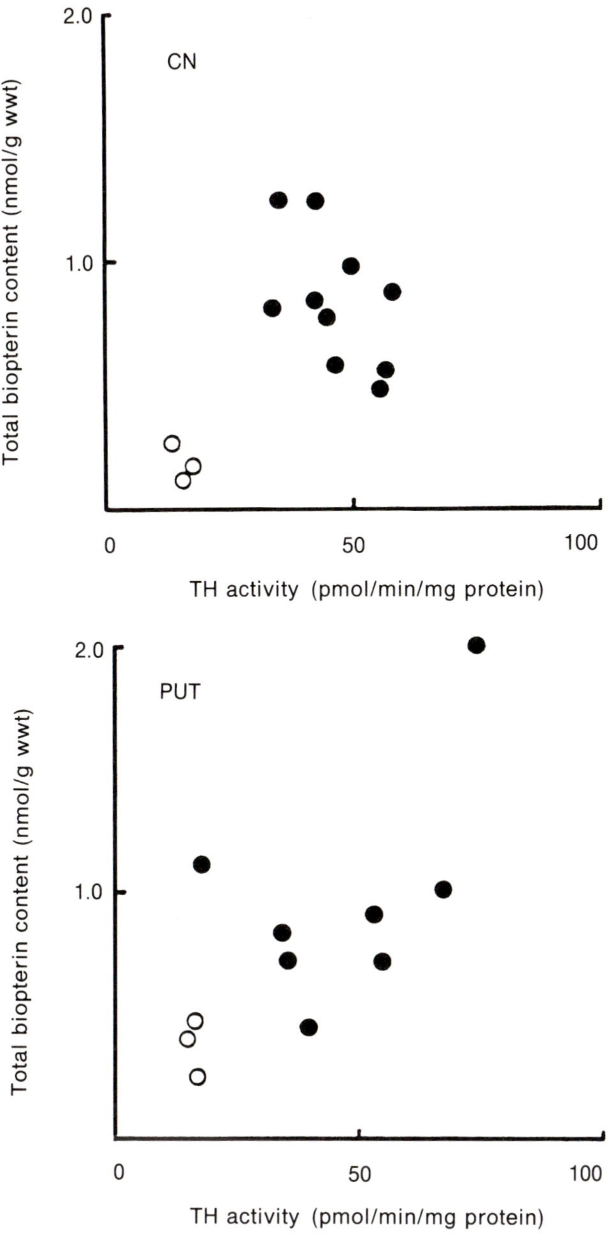

Figure 1 Correlation between TH activity and total biopterin content (nmol/g wet weight) in the head of the caudate nucleus (CN) and in the putamen (PUT). ○ = juvenile parkinsonian subjects; ● = normal subjects

observed a mild or moderate effect of single doses of 300–600 mg of (6R,S)-L-erythro-5,6,7,8-tetrahydrobiopterin on Parkinson disease, after one-week withdrawal of antiparkinsonians including levodopa[11]. Curtius and colleagues reported two cases of Parkinson disease which showed full improvement in hypokinesia and rigidity after administration of a 1 g dose of tetrahydrobiopterin two days after withdrawal of levodopa and bromocriptine[12]. The effect of tetrahydrobiopterin appeared within 4 and 5 hours, respectively after treatment and continued for 5 hours. LeWitt and colleagues administered 10 mg/kg or 2.5 mg/kg of diastereoisomer of tetrahydrobiopterin, intravenously, to two Parkinson disease patients with long duration of the illness. This was done 24 hours after withdrawal of conventional therapy, including levodopa, but no effect on parkinsonism was observed[13]. Moore and co-workers observed four cases of Parkinson disease who received a low dose (200 mg) of tetrahydrobiopterin in a double-blind manner, but did not note any beneficial effect on parkinsonism[14]. Dissing and colleagues also failed to find any effect on parkinsonism during administration of 1000 mg/day of (6R,S)-L-erythro-5,6,7,8-tetrahydrobiopterin for 3 or 5 days, in two cases of Parkinson disease, 5 days after withdrawal of levodopa, and in one case who had not been treated by levodopa[15].

What is the cause of discord in these results? The most probable cause might be the severity of the disease in the brain, because the effect of tetrahydrobiopterin is dependent on the function of remaining dopamine nerve terminals in the striatum. A second possible cause might be the period of levodopa withdrawal, because the effect of levodopa decreases in 2 or 3 days after administration is stopped, but residual effects continue to diminish over a week, and the effect of tetrahydrobiopterin may not be enough to surpass the effect of levodopa. According to the authors' experience, it seems to be easier to observe the effect of tetrahydrobiopterin in patients who show milder clinical symptoms under the condition of levodopa withdrawal or in cases where there is no history of levodopa therapy.

EFFECT OF TETRAHYDROBIOPTERIN THERAPY ON JUVENILE PARKINSONISM

A method for the synthesis of (6R)-L-erythro-5,6,7,8-tetrahydrobiopterin (R-THBP), the natural form of tetrahydrobiopterin, has been developed[16]. The natural (6R) form of tetrahydrobiopterin may be more effective than the unnatural (6S) form. A therapeutic trial of the substance in parkinsonism has been carried out. Seven cases of juvenile parkinsonism were examined in the trial (Table 2). The criterion for juvenile parkinsonism was based on onset of the disease before the age of forty, according to the definition by Yokochi[4].

All cases were withdrawn from antiparkinsonians including levodopa and dopamine agonist for at least 7 days, and started on administration of R-THBP. On the first day of R-THBP administration, an 800 mg single dose of the substance was administered orally, and the pharmacokinetics were observed in five patients. The levels of total biopterin in the plasma became

Table 2 Cases of juvenile parkinsonism treated with (6R)-L-erythro-5,6,7,8-tetrahydrobiopterin (R-THBP). Symptoms improved by administration of R-THBP. 0, symptom not observed before therapy; +, improved by therapy; −, no improvement was seen

	Case no.						
	1	*2*	*3*	*4*	*5*	*6*	*7*
Age	38	52	42	42	52	38	21
Sex	m	m	m	m	f	f	f
Duration of illness (years)	2	17	6	3	28	12	7
Yahr's stage	I	IV	III	III	III	II	IV
History of levodopa therapy	no	no	yes	yes	yes	yes	yes
Dose of R-THBP (mg)	800, 1000	800	800	800	800	800	800
Symptoms improved							
akinesia in general	+	+	+	−	−	−	−
rigidity	+	+	+	−	+	+	−
tremor	−	+	+	0	−	−	−
gait disturbance	+	+	−	−	−	−	−

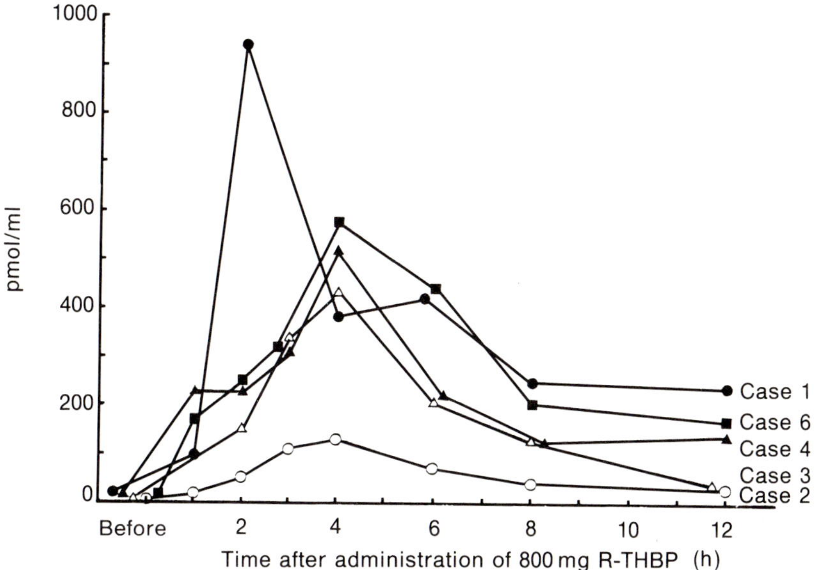

Figure 2 Total biopterin levels in the plasma before and after administration of 800 mg of R-THBP. Each patient took the substance in the morning after overnight fasting

elevated to at least 10 times higher than those prior to administration. The high levels of total biopterin persisted for about 6 hours. The total biopterin level peaked between 2 and 4 hours after administration (Figure 2).

Following pharmacokinetic examination, administration of R-THBP was continued for one or two weeks in five patients, and 18 months in one patient (case no. 1). One patient (case no. 2) was examined after only a single administration.

Clinical improvement, measured by movement time in one patient (case no. 2) appeared 2 hours after administration and persisted for 6 hours (Figure 3). Rigidity and tremor, that is, levels of stretch reflex and grouping discharge recorded by surface electromyography also improved. Rolling over and rising from a supine position, movements impossible before administration of R-THBP, were improved. In this patient, the severity of the disease was Hoen-Yahr's stage IV before treatment, and the duration of illness was 17 years. The patient had never received levodopa or dopamine agonist therapy. The improvement of parkinsonism in this patient was impressive; however, the improvement was not sufficient to perform daily activities.

The patient treated for 18 months (case no. 1) received 1000 mg once a day in the morning. This patient had unilateral parkinsonism in the right extremities and experienced difficulty in writing and walking to his job before starting the therapy. The difficulties were alleviated for the period of the therapy without any adverse effect.

Clinical improvement was observed in five out of seven patients. The symptoms improved were: rigidity in five patients; akinesia in general, in three patients; gait disturbance in two out of seven patients, and tremor in two out of six patients (Table 2). In comparison with the levodopa effect on parkinsonism, the effect of R-THBP may not be dramatic.

Total biopterin content and amine metabolites in cerebrospinal fluid were measured before and during administration of R-THBP in three patients in this series. Although poor permeability of tetrahydrobiopterin through the blood-brain barrier has been reported[17], all cases examined showed elevation of total biopterin in cerebrospinal fluid during the treatment, in comparison to that before. Homovanillic acid content during treatment increased

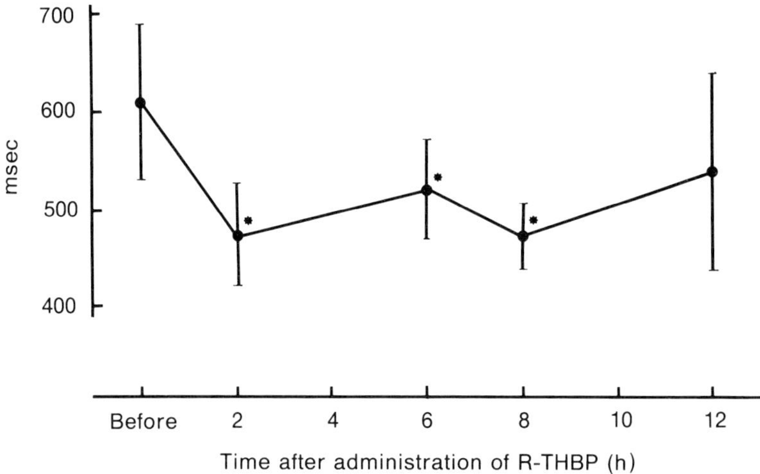

Figure 3 The mechanical movement time measured in one patient (Case no. 2) using two separated on–off switches. Statistic analysis was done by paired *t*-test. $*p < 0.01$

Table 3 Total biopterin (T-BP), homovanillic acid (HVA) and 5-hydroxyindolacetic acid (5-HIAA) concentrations, in cerebrospinal fluid, before and during administration of R-THBP

	T-BP (pmol/ml)		*HVA* (ng/ml)		*5-HIAA* (ng/ml)	
Case no.	*Before*	*During*	*Before*	*During*	*Before*	*During*
1	10.5	26.5	17.6	25.0	9.3	9.0
		283.0		39.5		12.0
3	8.0	17.8	27.0	32.0	18.0	17.4
5	7.7	40.5	17.3	24.0	7.4	12.5

conspicuously in the patient treated for 18 months; however, it was equivocal in the other two cases (Table 3). The level of 5-hydroxyindolacetic acid was unchanged.

As mentioned before, the efficacy of R-THBP in parkinsonism may mainly depend on the remaining dopamine nerve terminals in the striatum. In this sense, there is no value in discussing the efficacy in Parkinson disease and juvenile parkinsonism separately. In Parkinson disease, decrease in TH activity in the striatum may result from degeneration of the neurons in the substantia nigra. Reduction of total biopterin content in the striatum was paralleled by decrease in the TH activity in the disease. Our limited biochemical analyses in three cases of juvenile parkinsonism suggest that the decrease in TH activity is parallel to the reduction of total biopterin in the striatum. This may indicate that the reduction of total biopterin in the striatum is secondary to the degeneration of dopamine neurons in the substantia nigra. However, as indicated by the clinical features and response to levodopa therapy, cases of juvenile parkinsonism may not be uniform, suggesting multiplicity of the pathophysiology of the disease. Further pathobiochemical analyses are needed.

CONCLUSIONS

Although levodopa is a most potent substance in the treatment of parkinsonism, postponement of the start of its administration during the course of therapy, and reduction of its dosage by combining it with other antiparkinsonian agents, have recently become accepted practices because of its adverse effects during the long courses of the disease, and in order to reduce its ill effects in the prognosis of the disease.

One characteristic feature of juvenile parkinsonism is severe diurnal fluctuation of symptoms and dyskinesia under levodopa therapy.

The effects of R-THBP seem to be mild when compared with the effects of levodopa. Patients with juvenile parkinsonism in early stages, or patients who had never received levodopa seem to respond to treatment with R-THBP. Therefore, it may be concluded that R-THBP or tetrahydrobiopterin is an introductory agent for the treatment of parkinsonism, not only juvenile parkinsonism but also Parkinson disease in early stages, providing a better prognosis for the disease.

REFERENCES

1. Levine, R.A., Miller, L.P. and Lovenverg, W. (1981). Tetrahydrobiopterin in striatum: localization in dopamine nerve terminals and role in catecholamine synthesis. *Science*, **214**, 919–21
2. Nagatsu, T., Yamaguchi, T., Kato, T., Sugimoto, T., Matsuura, S., Akino, M., Nagatsu, I., Iizuka, R. and Narabayashi, H. (1981). Biopterin in human brain and urine from controls and parkinsonian patients: application of a new radioimmunoassay. *Clin. Chim. Acta*, **109**, 305–11
3. Nagatsu, T., Horikoshi, T., Sawada, M., Nagatsu, I., Kondo, T., Iizuka, R. and Narabayashi, H. (1986). Biosynthesis of tetrahydrobiopterin in parkinsonian human brain. In Yahr, M.D. and Bergmann, K.J. (eds.) *Advances in Neurology*, Vol. 45, pp. 223–6. (New York: Raven Press)
4. Yokochi, M. (1979). Juvenile Parkinson's disease. 1. Clinical aspects. *Adv. Neurol. Sci.*, **23**, 1048–59
5. Yokochi, M., Narabayashi, H., Iizuka, R. and Nagatsu, T. (1986). Juvenile parkinsonism. Some clinical, pharmacological, and neuropathological aspects. In Hassler, R.G. and Christ, J.F. (eds.) *Advances in Neurology*, Vol. 40, pp. 407–13. (New York: Raven Press)
6. Miwa, S., Watanabe, Y. and Hayaishi, O. (1985). 6R-L-erythro-5,6,7,8-tetrahydrobiopterin as a regulator of dopamine and serotonin biosynthesis in the rat brain. *Arch. Biochem. Biophys.*, **239**, 234–41
7. Koshimura, K., Miwa, S., Lee, K., Fujiwara, M. and Watanabe, Y. (1990). Enhancement of dopamine release *in vivo* from the rat striatum by dialytic perfusion of 6R-L-erythro-5,6,7,8-tetrahydrobiopterin. *J. Neurochem.*, **54**, 1391–7
8. Mizutani, Y., Yokochi, M. and Oyanagi, S. (1991). Juvenile parkinsonism: A case report with neuropathological findings suggesting a new pathogenesis. *Clin. Neuropathol.*, **10**, 91–7
9. Kondo, T., Yokochi, M., Sugita, H., Mizutani, Y. and Mizuno, Y. (1990). Tyrosine hydroxylase activity in the nigrostriatal region in patients with juvenile parkinsonism. *Movement Disorders*, **5**, Suppl. 1, 29
10. Narabayashi, H., Yokochi, M., Iizuka, R. and Nagatsu, T. (1986). Juvenile parkinsonism. In Vinken, P.J., Bruyn, G.-W. and Klawans, H.L. (eds.) *Handbook of Clinical Neurology*, Vol. 5(49), *Extrapyramidal Disorders*, pp. 153–65. (Amsterdam: Elsevier Science Publishers)
11. Narabayashi, H., Kondo, T., Nagatsu, T., Sugimoto, T. and Matsuura, S. (1982). Tetrahydrobiopterin administration for parkinsonian symptoms. *Proc. Jpn. Acad.*, **58**, Ser. B., 283–7
12. Curtius, H.-Ch., Niederwieser, A., Levine, R. and Muldner, H. (1984). Therapeutic efficacy of tetrahydrobiopterin in Parkinson's disease. In Hassler, R.G. and Christ, J.F. (eds.) *Advances in Neurology*, Vol. 40, pp. 463–6. (New York: Raven Press)
13. Lewitt, P.A., Miller, L.P., Newman, R.P., Burns, R.S., Insel, T., Levine, R.A., Lovenberg, W. and Calne, D.B. (1984). Tyrosine hydroxylase cofactor (tetrahydrobiopterin) in parkinsonism. In Hassler, R.G. and Christ, J.F. (eds.) *Advances in Neurology*, Vol. 40, pp. 459–62. (New York: Raven Press)
14. Moore, A.P., Behan, P.O., Jacobson, W. and Armarego, W.L.F. (1987). Biopterin in Parkinson's disease. *J. Neurol. Neurosurg. Psychiatr.*, **50**, 85–7
15. Dissing, I.C., Guttler, F., Pakkenberg, H., Lou, H., Gerdes, A.-M., Lykkelund, C. and Rasmussen, V. (1989). Tetrahydrobiopterin and Parkinson's disease. *Acta Neurol. Scand.*, **79**, 493–9
16. Matsuura, S., Sugimoto, T., Hasegawa, H., Imaizumi, S. and Ichiyama, A. (1980). Studies on biologically active pteridines. III. The absolute configuration at the C-6 chiral center of tetrahydrobiopterin cofactor and related compounds. *J. Biochem.*, **87**, 951–7
17. Kapatos, G. and Kaufman, S. (1980). Peripherally administered reduced biopterins do enter the brain. *Science*, **212**, 955–6

SECTION 6

Clinical neurophysiology of hereditary progressive dystonia, dystonia and parkinsonism

12

Polysomnographical studies on hereditary progressive dystonia with marked diurnal fluctuation

M. Segawa and Y. Nomura

INTRODUCTION

The marked improvement of symptoms after sleep is one of the cardinal signs of hereditary progressive dystonia with marked diurnal fluctuation (HPD) and suggests the involvement of a certain sleep mechanism in the pathophysiology of this disorder. On the other hand, most parents of children with HPD noticed a lack of, or scanty, body movements during sleep. This evidence urged us to study the polysomnography (PSG) of HPD to clarify not only the background physiology of the remedial effects of sleep but also the pathophysiology of HPD.

In this chapter, we review the results of our polysomnographical investigations on HPD and other basal ganglia diseases and discuss the pathophysiology of HPD from the standpoint of sleep mechanism.

MATERIALS AND METHODS

A total of 12 cases of HPD were examined in this study. Our pathological controls included: three cases of idiopathic dystonia, one with action retrocollis and the other two with action retrocollis and oculogyric crisis; eight cases of symptomatic torsion dystonia, with four unilateral and four bilateral lesions of the basal ganglia detected by computerized tomography (CT) or magnetic resonance imaging (MRI), and one patient with unilateral Parkinson disease, or hemi-Parkinson disease. Besides these, six normal children were used as controls. The findings of brain imaging in the eight cases with symptomatic torsion dystonia are shown in Table 1.

PSG was performed with a 21-channel electroencephalograph (EEG) according to the method previously reported[1]. Besides the three channels for EEG, the two channels for electro-oculogram (EOG) of the horizontal eye movement, one each for an electromyogram (EMG) of the mentalis muscle, an electrocardiogram (ECG) and monitoring of respiration for

Table 1 Computerized tomography (CT) or magnetic resonance imaging (MRI) findings of cases with unilateral and bilateral basal ganglia lesions

Patient	*Age* (years)	*Sex*	*CT, (MRI) findings*
Unilateral lesions			
TM	7	male	left-putaminal lesion, due to focal infarction that occurred at the age of 10 months
JS	5	male	cystic low density area, localized in the caudal part of the left putamen and the external globus pallidus.
KS	11	male	low density area expanding from the putamen to the thalamus on the right side through the internal capsule, with dilatation of the ipsilateral lateral ventricle
TH	39	male	focal infarction in the left putamen (MRI)
Bilateral lesions			
KH	9	male	multiple high density area (calcification) in the bilateral globus pallidus as well as the bilateral frontal lobe
SO	8	female	dilatation of the bilateral anterior horn due to atrophy of the caudate nucleus and linear low density area in the right putamen
RM	5	female	low density area in the bilateral putamen and in the left caudate nucleus
KK	17	male	prominent calcification in the bilateral basal ganglia, most prominent in the putamen

evaluating the sleep stages, another 12 channels were used for EMG to record activities from 12 muscles, six on each side. Eye movements exceeding the rising angle of 30° with the paper speed of 15 mm per second were defined as rapid eye movements (REMs). The sleep stages were evaluated according to the criteria of the Association of Psychophysiological Study of Sleep[2]. Two kinds of body movement, gross movement (GM) and twitch movement (TM) were also evaluated. GM is a diffuse sequential muscle activity of the upper and lower extremities, including that of the trunk muscle (rectus abdominalis), lasting more than two seconds. TM is a short EMG activity localized to one muscle that lasts less than 0.5 second.

The total number of REMs in REM stage (sREM) was counted. Also the number of REMs towards the right or left were counted separately, and the ratio of REMs towards the right against those toward the left (R/L ratio) was calculated. The numbers of GMs and TMs of each muscle were counted. The numbers of both movements occurring in one hour of each sleep stage were also calculated and their sleep stage-dependent modulation (the pattern of each body movement against sleep stages) was evaluated. As for TMs, their number in sREM was calculated on both sides for each muscle and their side difference was evaluated. The side difference of the number of TMs was also correlated with that of the direction of the horizontal REMs. Besides these, the ratio of the number of TMs of the mentalis muscle in sREM against the number of REMs (mentTM$_{sREM}$/REMs) was calculated.

In each case, the PSG was performed once, but in patients with HPD and a patient with action dystonia with or without oculogyric crisis, it was performed twice or more, before and after levodopa.

POLYSOMNOGRAPHICAL FINDINGS IN HPD

In HPD no abnormalities were observed in the ratio of sleep stages, REM–non-REM (NREM) cycles or in the sleep structures, (that is, the nocturnal variation of each sleep stage, with a significantly high amount of slow wave sleep (SWS) in the first one-third of sleep and a relatively high amount of sREM in later cycles towards morning). Thus the main abnormalities were observed in the phasic components of sleep, that is, body movements and REMs.

In HPD, GMs were reduced in number and also showed abnormality in their sleep stage-dependent modulation, with an increase in the rate of occurrence in sleep stage 2 (S2) and a decrease in their rate in sleep stage 1 (S1) and sREM[1,3–6]. After levodopa, the number increased to normal range and their pattern against sleep stages also improved to normal, showing the highest rate of occurrence in S1, next in sREM, and low in the other NREM stages[1,3–6]. The number of TMs also decreased markedly, but their sleep stage-dependent modulation remained normal, where their rate of occurrence was highest in sREM, next in S1 and low in the other NREM stages[1,3–6]. The number of TMs was decreased more markedly in the muscles more affected. When comparing the side difference of each muscle, the side of the sternocleidomastoid (SCM) more affected, or less in number of TMs, was contralateral to the side of the limb muscles predominantly involved. After levodopa, the number of TMs of each muscle was increased to normal range with improvement in clinical features[1,3–6].

In one patient, who had a clinical onset at the age of three years and had been treated with anticholinergics for 24 years since the age of nine, the PSG performed at the age of 33 showed features identical to those observed in childhood cases before levodopa[7]. On the other hand, in an adolescent patient who was experiencing a feeling of ineffectiveness of levodopa (see Chapter 3) a decrease of TMs reappeared in the muscle of the lower limb initially affected, but there was no recurrence of abnormalities in the TMs of the other muscles, nor in the number and pattern of GMs[7].

The number of REMs in sREM was increased in HPD but it was decreased after levodopa, showing the reverse feature to TMs[1,4,5,8,9]. So the ratio of mentTM$_{sREM}$/REMs was lower than normal before treatment, but it increased to normal range (0.4 ± 0.2) after levodopa[4–6,8,10].

The number of REMs shows a marked variation among subjects. However, there is a side preference towards the right in the direction of horizontal REMs, so normally the R/L ratio reveals a rather constant value of 1.26 ± 0.24[9]. In our studies on the four cases with HPD, the R/L ratio showed significantly lower values, revealing an increase in the rate of REMs towards the left[9]. In three patients in whom the left extremities were more affected, the reduction in the R/L ratio was more marked and, after levodopa, the ratio increased. In one case with a right side predominance the decrease in the R/L ratio was slight, and it reduced further after levodopa. It was revealed that in HPD the REMs tended to direct towards the side with the more affected limbs, which showed a smaller number of TMs, this also being towards the less affected SCM side, where the number of TMs was larger.

The rate of TMs occurring in a given hour of sleep has shown a nocturnal variation[11]. In normal volunteers TMs tend to increase their rate with the course of sleep. This tendency is observed most clearly in sREM. The nocturnal alteration of the number of GMs shows intersubject variation, that is, some show incremental, while others show decremental, variations[11].

Although in HPD the number of TMs in the whole sleep period was decreased, the nocturnal variation of TMs was observed to be normal[3,12]. That is, in the early period of sleep the number of TMs was markedly reduced in all the muscles examined, while the numbers tended to increase with the passage of sleep. With the progression of the disease the number of TMs decreased further throughout the sleep periods and only a small number of TMs was observed in the later period of sleep.

GMs in HPD showed a nocturnal variation of GMs with an increase in number in the later sleep cycles, but they also showed a variation in the pattern of movement[12]. That is, in the early period of sleep the pattern of rolling over was abnormal, being initiated in the lower extremities, but in the later period it became normal beginning with the turning of the neck and the upper extremities, followed by the rotation of the trunk and lower extremities. After levodopa, the number of TMs increased throughout the course of sleep, a moderate amount of TMs being observed even in the first period of sleep[3,12], and the pattern of rolling over became normal from the earliest period of sleep[12].

POLYSOMNOGRAPHIC FINDINGS IN MOVEMENT DISORDERS OTHER THAN HPD

In a patient with hemi-Parkinson disease, PSG of GMs showed a marked decrease in their number in all stages of sleep with only a few movements in S2 (Figure 1), so their sleep stage-dependent modulation disappeared[10]. The same feature has already been reported in the PSG of cases with Parkinson disease[11]. On the other hand, in Huntington disease GMs were shown to increase their number in all sleep stages without alteration of the pattern of occurrence against sleep stages[11].

In a female patient with dystonia, with clinical characteristics identical to HPD except for action retrocollis, GMs showed a particular abnormal deviation in the pattern against sleep stages which was different from that of HPD, that is, their rate of occurrence decreased in sREM leaving those in other stages within normal range. This pattern abnormality did not improve after levodopa though complete recovery was obtained clinically[6,10]. Similar abnormalities in the modulation of GMs were observed in cases with action dystonia or oculogyric crisis, whether or not they responded to levodopa[13].

In the PSG of the four cases of symptomatic hemidystonia, with unilateral basal ganglia lesions revealed by brain imaging, GMs showed an abnormal modulation in three cases. One of these had a wide low density area on the right including the putamen, pallidum and thalamus (KS), and the other two had a large low density area in the left putamen (TM, TH). The fourth case, with a lacunar infarct on the caudal border of the putamen and the globus

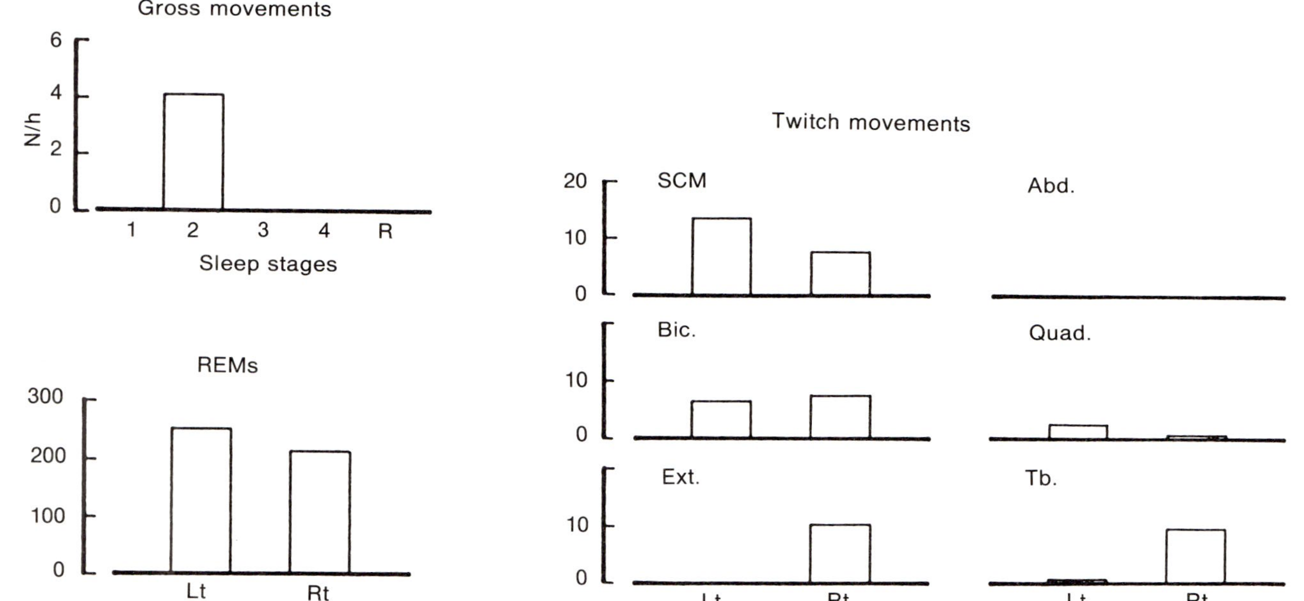

Figure 1 Results of PSG on a case with left hemi-Parkinson disease. The top left graph shows the sleep stage-dependent modulation of gross movements (GMs); ordinate shows number of GMs per hour of each sleep stage; abscissa shows sleep stages. The bottom left illustration shows the number of REMs toward the left (Lt) and right (Rt). The right-hand illustration shows the number of twitch movements (TMs) per hour of stage REM on each side of muscles examined; ordinate shows the number of TMs per hour of sREM; abscissa shows the side of the muscle, left (Lt) and right (Rt). SCM, sternocleidomastoid; Bic, biceps brachii; Ext, forearm extensor; Abd, rectus abdominalis; Quad, quadriceps femoris; and Tb, tibialis anterior

pallidus (JS), showed minimal abnormalities in the modulation of GMs[10] (Figure 2). Among the four cases with symptomatic dystonia with bilateral basal ganglia lesions, shown on the X-ray CT scan or MRI, two cases showed a marked abnormality in the pattern of GMs, with a decrease in their rate of occurrence in S1 and sREM, similar to HPD. One of these had a large low density area in the bilateral putamen and the left caudate nucleus (RM), and the other had a high density area in the putamen, bilaterally (KK). One patient, with multiple high density areas in the bilateral globus pallidus (KH), and another with atrophy of the bilateral caudate nucleus with a low density area in the right putamen (SO), revealed another pattern of abnormality, with a decrease in the rate of GMs in sREM[10] (Figure 2).

It was shown that in Parkinson disease TMs were reduced markedly in number in all sleep stages[11], and in hemi-Parkinson disease only a few TMs were observed in the muscles of the affected limbs throughout the course of sleep. Thus in Parkinson disease there is no sleep stage-dependent modulation nor nocturnal variation of TMs[10]. On the other hand, in Huntington disease, TMs increased their number markedly in all sleep stages[11].

In idiopathic dystonia with action dystonia or oculogyric crisis, TMs showed a decrease in number, and abnormality in the pattern against sleep stages[12]. In unilateral symptomatic dystonia, TMs of the affected muscles also showed a decrease in number with an abnormal pattern, but in the unaffected side they were normal. In cases with bilateral basal ganglia lesions, TMs also revealed a marked decrease in number in all stages, and abnormalities in pattern in all patients, except for one with a high density area in the bilateral putamen, in whom TMs showed an increase in number in S1 though they decreased in other sleep stages[10].

The side difference in the rate of occurrence of TMs in sREM was examined in each muscle, and on the side predominantly affected a comparison was made between the muscles of the extremities and the SCM. As already mentioned in hemi-Parkinson disease and symptomatic hemi-dystonia with unilateral basal ganglia lesion, the number of TMs decreased markedly in the muscle of the affected side. However, in hemi-Parkinson disease the side of the SCM with a reduced number of TMs was contralateral to the side of the limb predominantly affected (Figure 1) while in cases with hemi-dystonia it was ipsilateral to the side of the extremities involved (Figure 3).

All the three cases with action dystonia showed asymmetry in involvement. In two of them, the side with the more affected SCM was contralateral to that of the more affected extremities while in one it was ipsilateral. Levodopa was effective in the former two but not in the latter case[1].

The ratio of $mentTM_{sREM}$/REMs was observed to be nearly zero in the case with hemi-Parkinson disease[10] and those of patients with idiopathic dystonia with action retrocollis were also revealed to be significantly lower than normal range[1]. In symptomatic dystonia, this ratio was also below normal range, both in cases with unilateral and in those with bilateral lesions (Figure 4).

In patients with unilateral or asymmetrical lesions in the nigrostriatal system, the horizontal REMs exhibited a side preference, depending on the side of the affected or predominantly affected extremities[8]. The patient with

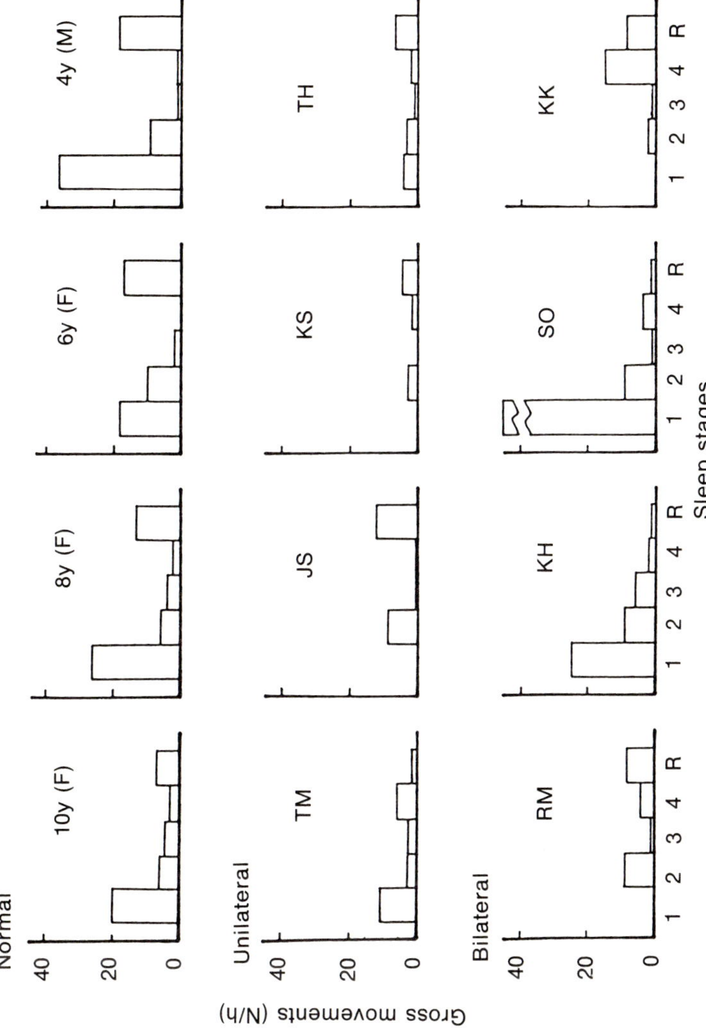

Figure 2 Sleep stage-dependent modulation of gross movements (GMs) in symptomatic torsion dystonia. Normal, normal control, sex and age, shown in graph; Unilateral, cases with unilateral basal ganglia lesion; Bilateral, cases with bilateral basal ganglia lesion; ordinate, number of GMs per hour of each sleep stage; abscissa, sleep stages

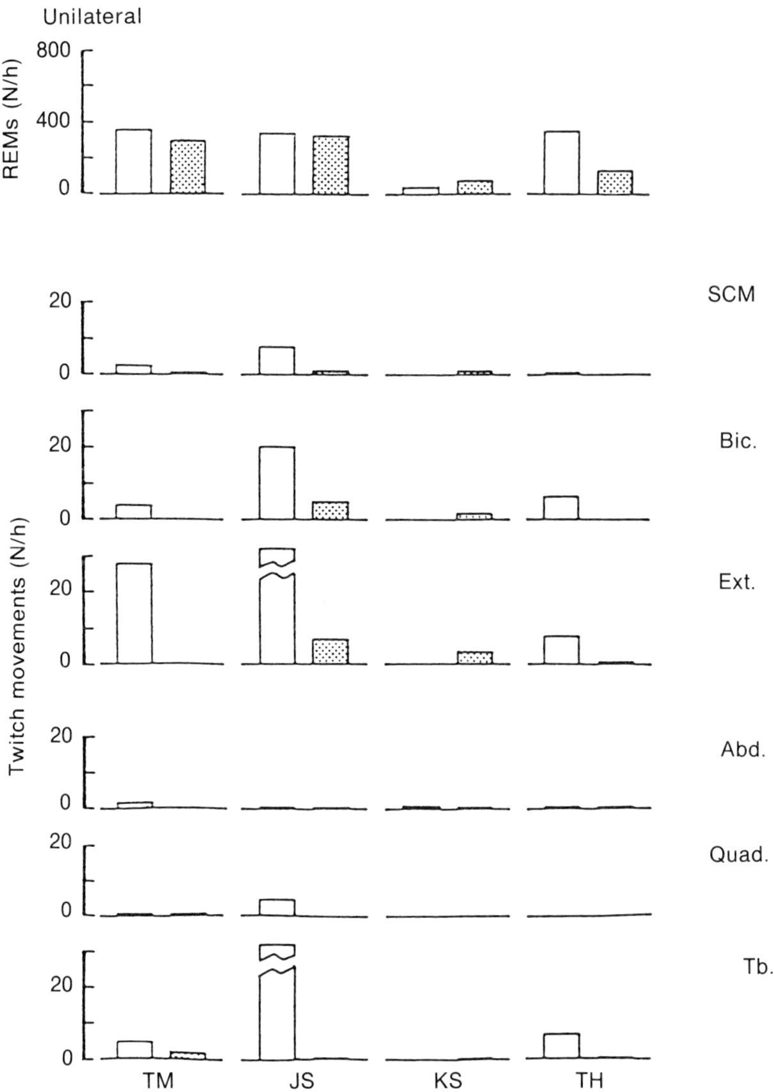

Figure 3 Correlation of the side preference of direction of REMs and that of twitch movements (TMs) of stage REM (sREM) in each muscle in symptomatic torsion dystonia with unilateral basal ganglia lesion. Open columns, REMs directed towards the left or TMs of the muscle of the left side; hatched columns: REMs directed towards the right or TMs of the muscle of the right side; ordinate: number of REMs or TMs per hour of sREM. SCM, sternocleidomastoid; Bic, biceps brachii; Ext, forearm extensor; Abd, rectus abdominalis; Quad, quadriceps femoris; Tb, tibialis anterior

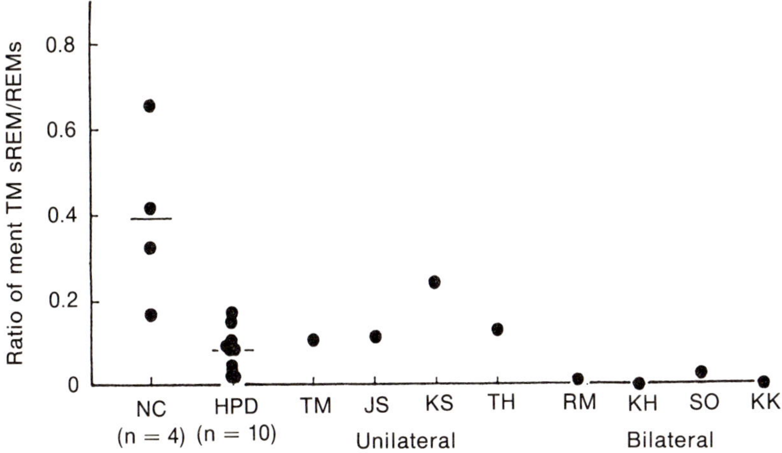

Figure 4 Ratio of ment TMsREM/REMs of HPD and symptomatic torsion dystonia. NC, normal controls; HPD, hereditary progressive dystonia with marked diurnal fluctuation; Unilateral, symptomatic torsion dystonia with unilateral basal ganglia lesion; Bilateral, symptomatic torsion dystonia with bilateral basal ganglia lesion

the left hemi-Parkinson disease showed an increase in the ratio of REMs towards the left (Figure 1). On the other hand, in right hemi-dystonia with lesion in the left basal ganglia (TM, JS, TH), REMs preferred to direct towards the left and the R/L ratio was decreased (Figure 5). In contrast, in the patient with left hemi-dystonia with lesion on the right (KS), REMs showed a reverse feature with an increase in their number towards the right, resulting in a significant increase in the R/L ratio (Figure 5).

When correlating the side preference of the REMs to the side of the limbs predominantly affected in each disorder, the REMs tended to direct towards the dominantly affected side of limbs in hemi-Parkinson disease (Figure 1), while they preferred to direct towards the side of the non-affected limbs in cases with symptomatic dystonia with unilateral lesions of the basal ganglia (Figure 3). As the relation of the side of the more-affected SCM to that of the more-affected limb muscles was different between hemi-Parkinson disease and symptomatic dystonia, horizontal REMs tended to direct towards the side of SCM less-affected, both in hemi-Parkinson disease and symptomatic hemi-dystonia.

PATHOPHYSIOLOGICAL CONSIDERATIONS

PSG showed various, but particular, abnormalities in movement disorders of various etiologies. The results of PSG on HPD revealed abnormalities of the phasic components, but normal preservation of the tonic components. That is, the abnormalities were restricted to body movements and REMs, while the ratio of sleep stages, REM–NREM rhythm, and nocturnal variation of the sleep stages (sleep structures) were not affected. Moreover, there was

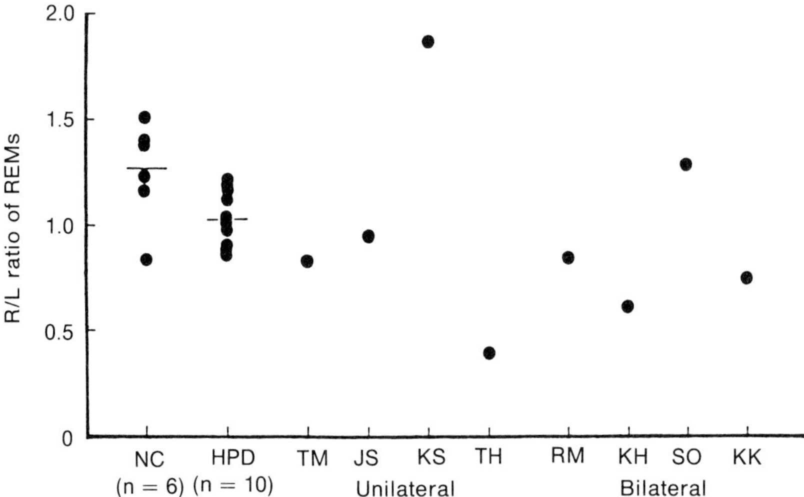

Figure 5 Side preference in the direction of REMs in HPD and symptomatic torsion dystonia. Ordinate illustrates the ratio of the number of REMS towards the right against those towards the left (R/L ratio). NC, normal controls; HPD, hereditary progressive dystonia with marked diurnal fluctuation; Unilateral, symptomatic torsion dystonia with unilateral basal ganglia lesion; Bilateral, symptomatic torsion dystonia with bilateral basal ganglia lesion

no leakage of components of sREM into NREM stages, that is, REMs or axial atonia were not observed in NREM stages, though the tone of the mentalis muscle was relatively lower in NREM stages. On the other hand, in two of the three patients with idiopathic dystonia and in patients with symptomatic dystonia, there were abnormalities in the ratio of sleep stages and sleep structures, besides disturbance in the phasic components[1]. Parkinson disease also showed abnormalities in these parameters.

Most of the sleep components are controlled by brainstem structures. The REM-NREM rhythm is generated by reciprocal firing of the noradrenergic neurons of the locus ceruleus and the cholinergic neurons of the giant cellular area of the pontine reticular formation[13,14]. The cholinergic neurons have a role in executing most of the components of REM stage[15], and the locus ceruleus and the serotonergic neurons of the dorsal raphe nucleus increase their activities to produce the NREM stage, and they prevent the occurrence of components of REM stage by inhibiting the cholinergic neurons[15]. The serotonergic neurons of the dorsal raphe nucleus have important roles in generating slow wave sleep[16].

When taking these data into account, PSG findings of HPD imply that the monoaminergic and cholinergic neurons of the brainstem are preserved normally, or have no significant roles in the pathogenesis of this disorder, while the results of PSG in Parkinson disease, and some cases with idiopathic dystonia, suggest the involvement of these brainstem neurons besides basal ganglia lesions. Noradrenergic and serotonergic neurons are thought to be involved in Parkinson disease, and neurohistochemical examination of a patient with idiopathic torsion dystonia with onset in childhood, has also revealed the involvement of noradrenergic and serotonergic neurons[17].

Polysomnographical studies on HPD and other dopa-responsive movement disorders have shown that the number of TMs reduces before treatment and increases to normal range after levodopa, with clinical improvement[6,7]. Thus the increase and decrease in dopamine activity seems to be reflected in the increase and decrease in the number of TMs. The number of TMs is also shown to correlate with the levels of homovanillic acid in the cerebrospinal fluid[18]. Moreover, in rats the activities of the tyrosine hydroxylase in the caudate nucleus show circadian oscillation, decrement during the night time and increment during the daytime, while the activities of the neurons in the substantia nigra pars compacta are steady without any sleep stage-dependent alteration[19]. As rats are nocturnal animals, their active (night) and resting (day) phases correspond to the day and night time of humans, respectively. So the nocturnal fluctuation of TMs with increment in their number in humans is considered as a reflection of the incremental variation of tyrosine hydroxylase activities in the striatum, that is, the terminal of the nigrostriatal dopamine neurons.

Examinations on symptomatic hemi-dystonia showed that the number of TMs decreased in all the muscles affected, that is, contralateral to the basal ganglia with the striatal lesion. In Huntington disease, with involvement of the striatal projection to the lateral segment of the globus pallidus, they showed an increase in number, while in Parkinson disease, with involvement of all the striatal projections, the TMs revealed a marked decrease in their number in all sleep stages. These suggest the importance of the components of the striatum on the generation of TMs and also imply that the nigrostriatal dopamine neurons modulate TMs via the striatofugal pathways.

The results of the PSG in HPD have also revealed that the nigrostriatal dopamine neurons regulate the number of REMs and, in contrast to TMs, an increase in their activity seems to decrease the number of REMs[1,9]. Thus hyperactivity of the nigrostriatal dopamine neurons causes an increase in the number of TMs, while it decreases the number of REMs, and vice versa. These features are reflected in the increment and decrement of the ratio of menTM$_{sREM}$/REMs in correlation with hyper- and hypofunction of the nigrostriatal dopamine neurons. Among basal ganglia diseases this reciprocal modulation between these two parameters was observed only in responders to levodopa[9]. On the other hand, the characteristic side preference of REMs in basal ganglia diseases with lesions in the nigrostriatal dopamine neurons or the striatum, revealed the roles of certain striatal projections in REMs. It suggested that the nigrostriatal dopamine neurons regulate the REMs via the striatofugal pathways, particularly those projecting to the superior colliculus via the substantia nigra pars reticulata with double GABAergic inhibitory neurons[1,8], that is, the same pathway involving the voluntary saccade[20]. As TMs and REMs have shown reciprocal responses to the activities of the dopamine neurons, TMs are also thought to be modulated by this striatal projection to the substantia nigra pars reticulata[8].

The PSG of HPD has revealed that the dopamine system is involved in the modulation of GMs against sleep stages[1,6]. The abnormality of the GM pattern shown in Parkinson disease was marked, though it was partly improved by levodopa as well as thalamotomy[11]. Studies on symptomatic dystonia have shown that the nucleus of the basal ganglia, the striatum, particularly the putamen, has a role in the modulation of GMs, similar in features to HPD[1]. With additional lesions in the pallidum or in the thalamus, the abnormalities in the modulation of GMs becomes marked. The pallidal lesion could also cause abnormalities, though the pattern is different from those in putaminal lesions. Parkinson disease with the involvement of all the components of striatal projections showed marked reduction of GMs with loss of sleep stage-related modulation[11]. In Huntington disease, the pattern of GMs against sleep stages was preserved, though their number increased markedly[11]. Unilateral lesions in the basal ganglia could cause fundamentally similar abnormalities in GMs to those observed with bilateral lesions. The number or modulation of the pattern of GMs showed no relation to the number and direction of REMs[1]. In one of the cases with a left putaminal lesion the pattern abnormality of GMs improved with a relatively low dose of levodopa, while the abnormality of TMs of the right extremities, and also the clinical features of the hemi-dystonia remained unchanged[1,6,10]. These data suggest that GMs are controlled by components of the basal ganglia different from those related to TMs or REMs[1].

These PSG findings imply that the basal ganglia modulate GMs, and that the components connected to the pallidofugal thalamic pathway are considered as the main intra-basal ganglia pathway related to GMs[1]. They further suggest that, among the input systems to the medial globus pallidus, the striatofugal direct pathway might be involved mainly in GMs, and the indirect pathway via the subthalamic nucleus might have no role, at least in the sleep stage-dependent modulation of GMs.

In HPD the numbers of TMs and REMs are affected and these abnormalities completely improve after levodopa, with preservation of the reciprocal relation between TMs and REMs. These features suggest the involvement of the striatofugal nigral pathway without irreversible lesions and with preservation of the functional interaction between the dopamine (TMs) and cholinergic (REMs) neurons.

Side preference of horizontal REMs, observed in cases with asymmetrical involvement, showed the difference between cases with lesions in the nigrostriatal dopamine neurons (hemi-Parkinson disease) and those with lesions in the basal ganglia (symptomatic hemi-dystonia). In the former, the REMs tended to direct towards the affected limbs, that is, the nonlesion side of the basal ganglia, while in the latter they preferred to direct to the non-affected limbs, that is, the side of basal ganglia lesion. On the other hand, the REMs preferred to direct to the less-affected side of the SCM in both disorders. Furthermore, the pattern of side preference observed in idiopathic dystonia with axial torsion, which did not respond to levodopa, is similar to that observed in symptomatic torsion dystonia with lesion in the basal ganglia, while those observed in levodopa-responsive cases have the pattern seen in hemi-Parkinson disease, whether they have action dystonia or not[1].

The features observed in the PSG of HPD are identical to those observed in hemi-Parkinson disease, and suggest that the lesion of HPD is in the nigrostriatal dopamine neuron and not in the basal ganglia. This also relates to the responsiveness to levodopa and the absence of axial torsion. Moreover, the presence of nocturnal variation of body movements in HPD, with alleviation towards morning, implies a reflection of incremental variation of tyrosine hydroxylase, in the resting phase, at the terminal of dopamine neurons, suggesting the lesion to be at this terminal. The decremental variation of the enzyme in the active phase could cause diurnal fluctuation of symptoms with aggravation towards the evening.

However, the pattern of GMs in HPD differed from that observed in cases with action dystonia or oculogyric crisis, which clinically responded to levodopa[1,6]. This pattern is considered as the reflection of synaptic supersensitivity[1,6] because it is similar to that observed in particular cases of turberous sclerosis with subependymal nodule at the thalamostriatal sulcus on the left caudate nucleus. These cases had rotatory seizures towards the right which were modulated by the dopamine agonist and antagonist[10,21]. This suggests that synaptic supersensitivity does not exist in the terminal of dopamine neurons in HPD and correlates with the lack of action dystonia or oculogyric crisis and with the persistence of favorable response to levodopa without side-effects.

The pattern of abnormalities of GMs and TMs in HPD did not alter with the progression of the disease or long-term administration of the anticholinergics, and those of GMs did not recur if once improved by levodopa, even in the period of subjective decrease of the effect of levodopa[8]. This evidence suggests that the lesions of HPD are functional without morphological alteration, and that among the components of the basal ganglia, those involved in GMs are less affected than those involved in TMs.

Thus, in HPD, the terminals of the nigrostriatal dopamine neurons which are connected to the striatal projection to the substantia nigra pars reticulata are mainly affected; those connected to the striatal projection to the medial segment of the globus pallidus might be mildly affected, and the projection to the lateral segment of the globus pallidus might be preserved. The lesion is reversible or functional, and no receptor supersensitivity develops at the dopamine receptors throughout the course of the illness.

CONCLUSION

The polysomnography of HPD revealed abnormalities restricted to the phasic components of sleep, which showed nocturnal variation with alleviation towards morning. These abnormalities aggravated with the progression of the disease, but did not alter their characteristics or quality, and were alleviated completely after levodopa. In reference to the PSGs of other basal ganglia diseases and the basic mechanism of sleep, the pathophysiology of HPD is suggested to be functional lesions in the terminals of the nigrostriatal dopamine neurons which are mainly connected to the striatal projection to the substantia nigra pars reticulata. Those which are connected to the striatal projection of the medial portion of the globus pallidus might also be affected but this might not be the dominant lesion. At these terminals, the synapses might be preserved normally in function, without the development of synaptic supersensitivity. These hypotheses explain well the clinical characteristics of HPD (see Chapter 1).

REFERENCES

1. Segawa, M., Nomura, Y., Hikosaka, O., Soda, M., Usui, S. and Kase, M. (1987). Roles of the basal ganglia and related structures in symptoms of dystonia. In Carpenter, M.B. and Jayaraman, A. (eds.) *Basal Ganglia II Structure and Function*, pp. 489–504. (New York: Plenum Press)
2. Rechtschaffen, A. and Kales, A.H. (1968). *A Manual of Standardized Terminology, Techniques and Scoring System for Sleep Stages of Human Subjets*. (Washington, DC: US Government Printing Office)
3. Segawa, M., Hosaka, A., Miyagawa, F., Nomura, Y. and Imai, H. (1976). Hereditary progressive dystonia with marked diurnal fluctuation. In Eldridge, R. and Fahn, S. (eds.) *Advances in Neurology, Vol. 14: Dystonia*, pp. 215–33. (New York: Raven Press)
4. Segawa, M. (1981). Hereditary progressive dystonia (HPD) with marked diurnal fluctuation. *Adv. Neurol. Sci. (Tokyo)*, **25**, 73–81
5. Segawa, M., Nomura, Y. and Kase, M. (1986). Diurnally fluctuating hereditary progressive dystonia. In Vinken, P.J., Bruyn, G.W. and Klawans, H.L. (eds.) *Handbook of Clinical Neurology*, Vol. 5 (49), *Extrapyramidal Disorders*, pp. 529–39. (Amsterdam: Elsevier Science)
6. Segawa, M., Nomura, Y., Tanaka, S., Hakamada, S., Nagata, E., Soda, M. and Kase, M. (1988). Hereditary progressive dystonia with marked diurnal fluctuation: consideration on its pathophysiology based on the characteristics of clinical and polysomnographical findings. In Fahn, S., Marsden, C.D. and Calne, D.B. (eds.) *Advances in Neurology*, Vol. 50, *Dystonia 2*, pp. 367–76. (New York: Raven Press)
7. Segawa, M., Nomura, Y., Yamashita, S., Kase, M., Nishiyama, N., Yukishita, S., Ohta, H., Nagata, K. and Hosaka, A. (1990). Long term effects of L-dopa on hereditary progressive dystonia with marked diurnal fluctuation. In Berardelli, A., Benecke, R.M., Manfredi, M. and Marsden, C.D. (eds.) *Motor Disturbances II*, pp. 305–18. (London: Academic Press)
8. Segawa, M. and Nomura, Y. (1991). Rapid eye movements during Stage REM are modulated by nigrostriatal dopamine (NS-DA) neurons? In Bernardi, G., Carpenter, M.B. and Di Chiara, G. (eds.) *Basal Ganglia III*, pp. 663–71. (New York: Plenum Press)
9. Segawa, M. (1985). Body movement during sleep: its significance in neurology. *Shinkei Naika (Tokyo)*, **22**, 317–25
10. Uchiyama, A., Nomura, Y. and Segawa, M. (1987). Roles of cerebral basal ganglia in the modulation of body movements during sleep. *Rinsho Noha (Osaka)*, **29**, 782–7
11. Shima, F., Imai, H. and Segawa, M. (1974). Polygraphic study on body movements during sleep in cases with involuntary movements. *Clin. Electroencephalogr. (Tokyo)*, **16**, 229–35
12. Segawa, M. (1982). Catecholamine metabolism in neurological diseases in childhood. In Wise, G., Blaw, M.E. and Procopis, P.G. (eds.) *Topics in Child Neurology*, Vol. 2, pp. 135–50. (New York: Spectrum Publications, Inc.)
13. Hobson, J.A., McCarley, R.W. and Wyzinski, P.W. (1975). Sleep cycle oscillation: Reciprocal discharge by two brainstem neuronal groups. *Science*, **189**, 55–8
14. McCarley, R.W. and Hobson, J.A. (1975). Neuronal excitability modulation over the sleep cycle: a structural and mathematical model. *Science*, **189**, 58–60
15. Sakai, K. (1984). Central mechanisms of paradoxical sleep. In Borbely, A. and Valatx, J.L. (eds.) *Sleep Mechanisms. Experimental Brain Research, Suppl.* 8, pp. 3–18. (Berlin, Heidelberg: Springer–Verlag)
16. Hartman, E.L. (1976). *The Mechanism of Sleep*. (New Haven, London: Yale University Press)
17. Horneykiewicz, O., Stephen, J., Becker, L.E., Farley, I. and Shannak, K. (1986). Brain neurotransmitters in dystonia musculorum deformans. *N. Engl. J. Med.*, **315**, 347–53
18. Suzuki, H., Shimohira, M., Koyama, J., Hayashi, M., Ogiso, M. and Iwakawa, Y. (1986). Correlative studies between sleep parameters and monoamine metabolites in CSF in age dependent epileptic encephalopathy. Presented at the 28*th Annual Meeting of the Japanese Association of Child Neurology*, Matsue, Japan, June

19. McGeer, E.G. and McGeer, P.L. (1973). Some characteristics of brain tyrosine hydroxylase. In Mandel, J. (ed.) *New Concepts in Neurotransmitter Regulation*, pp. 53–68. (New York, London: Plenum Press)
20. Hikosaka, O., Sakamoto, M. and Usui, S. (1989). Functional properties of monkey caudate neurons. I. Activities related to saccadic eye movements. *J. Neurophysiol.*, **61**, 780–98
21. Tanaka, S., Igawa, C., Ogiso, M., Nomura, Y. and Segawa, M. (1983). Epileptic seizure with rotational behavior in tuberous sclerosis – Pathophysiological consideration. *Folia Psychiatrica et Neurologica Japonica* (*Tokyo*), **37**, 331–32

13

Deficits in saccadic eye movements in hereditary progressive dystonia with marked diurnal fluctuation

O. Hikosaka, H. Fukuda, M. Kato, K. Uetake, Y. Nomura and M. Segawa

INTRODUCTION

Eye movement precedes action. Guided by eye movement, we direct our attention to an object of interest before reaching it. Most important among different types of eye movement is the saccade which brings our gaze quickly from one location in space to another[1]. Without saccades, we would be hindered from performing purposive actions efficiently. It is not surprising therefore that a number of brain areas, including the basal ganglia, contribute to the initiation and control of saccades[2]. Dysfunction of any of these oculomotor structures would lead to deficits in saccadic eye movement. Observation of saccades, therefore, can be a powerful, non-invasive means of investigating functional changes of the brain. In this article we describe a preliminary attempt to investigate the pathophysiology of human basal ganglia diseases using voluntary saccade tasks. We used a modified version of the behavioral paradigms for trained monkeys, and the interpretation of the observations is based on the physiological properties of basal ganglia neurons obtained in the animal experiments[3,4] which are summarized below.

The basal ganglia system controls the initiation of saccadic eye movements via its efferent connection to the superior colliculus[5] which provides the brainstem reticular formation with burst signals necessary for the generation of saccades[6]. One of the most powerful inputs to the output neurons of the superior colliculus originates in the substantia nigra pars reticulata, an output nucleus of the basal ganglia[3]. This connection is unique in that it is inhibitory and that it has a high, sustained activity. Neurons in the substantia nigra pars reticulata have high background spike activity, but decelerate or stop firing before saccadic eye movements[7], thus removing the inhibition of the superior colliculus[5]. This disinhibition is induced by another inhibition at least partly originating in the caudate nucleus, one of the recipient structures of the basal ganglia[4]. In short, two serial inhibitory connections, both GABAergic, constitute the skeleton of the oculumotor control mechanism in the basal ganglia. The basal ganglia could thus control saccadic eye movement in two ways: by changing the background level of the nigrocollicular inhibition, and by removing the inhibition transiently. A similar mechanism may also underlie the skeletomotor functions of the basal ganglia, which are largely mediated by the equivalent serial inhibitory pathways originating in the putamen through the internal segment of the globus pallidus to the thalamus[8].

A remarkable feature of the basal ganglia oculomotor mechanism is its strong dependency on memory, expectation, or attention[9,10]. The presaccadic changes in spike activity in the substantia nigra or caudate are frequently dependent on how the saccade is initiated rather than where the saccade is to be directed. Presaccadic activity occurs only before purposive saccades which are made during the behavioral tasks in order to obtain reward; no activity changes are seen during spontaneous, automatic saccades. Unique to the basal ganglia is the presence of neurons that change their activity only before saccades to remembered targets[4,11]; saccades which are visually guided are associated with much less activity. These characteristics predict that oculomotor deficits in basal ganglia diseases could be conditional, depending on how saccades are made. In order to reveal such conditional deficits, we need to test voluntary saccades of the patients using a set of paradigms, each of which aims at inducing different types of saccades.

This article describes the characteristics of voluntary saccades, in addition to hand movements, in a patient having hereditary progressive dystonia with marked diurnal fluctuation (HPD)[12,13]. This disease develops in early childhood and is characterized by generalized postural dystonia with lower extremity predominance which shows notable aggravation towards the evening and which markedly responds to levodopa. In our study special emphasis was placed on the changes of saccades before and after starting levodopa therapy. We found that the deficits in saccades and the slowness of manual reaction were ameliorated considerably after starting levodopa therapy, along with improvements of other motor functions.

METHODS

Recording procedures and testing apparatus

The outline of the experimental procedures is illustrated in Figure 1[14,15]. The subject sat in front of a dome-shaped screen with her head fixed on a chin rest. She held a microswitch button which allowed her to initiate and terminate a task trial. Small red spots of light were used for visual targets. The target was chosen by the signal from the computer out of 49 possible locations: eccentricities of 5, 10, 15, 20, 30 and 40° in eight directions plus a central spot. At each location was a pinhole through which light from a light-emitting diode (LED) located at the back of the screen was seen. The room was dim so that the unlit pinholes were not seen. The behavior of the subject, especially movements in the face, was videotaped.

DC electro-oculography (EOG) was used for eye movement recording.

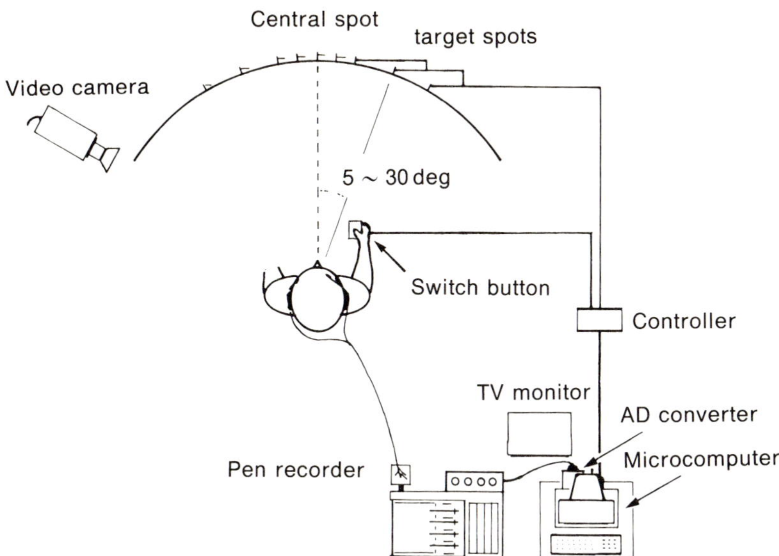

Figure 1 A computer-controlled system for analysis of voluntary saccadic eye movements

Horizontal eye movements were recorded with a pair of electrodes placed on the lateral sides of the orbits. Vertical eye movements were recorded for the right eye.

Computer system for eye movement analyses

The computer system used for this research was originally developed for behavioral and physiological studies using trained animals. A microcomputer (NEC PC9801RA) controls behavioral paradigms for a human or animal subject in an interactive manner, stores analog (for example, eye movement) and digital (for example, press and release of switch button) data, and displays selected data, such as trajectories of eye movement. Eye movement data were amplified, low-pass filtered (DC-20Hz), digitized (500 Hz), and stored in the computer memory. Eye movements were displayed on a computer monitor screen in two ways: firstly, horizontal and vertical components were shown separately against time aligned on a task event, such as the turning off of the fixation point, and secondly, trajectories of saccades on a two dimensional plane were displayed.

Behavioral paradigms

Three kinds of behavioral paradigms were used (Figure 2). The *saccade task* (Figure 2a) was designed to induce visually guided saccades. Shortly after the subject pressed the button, a central spot of light came on upon which

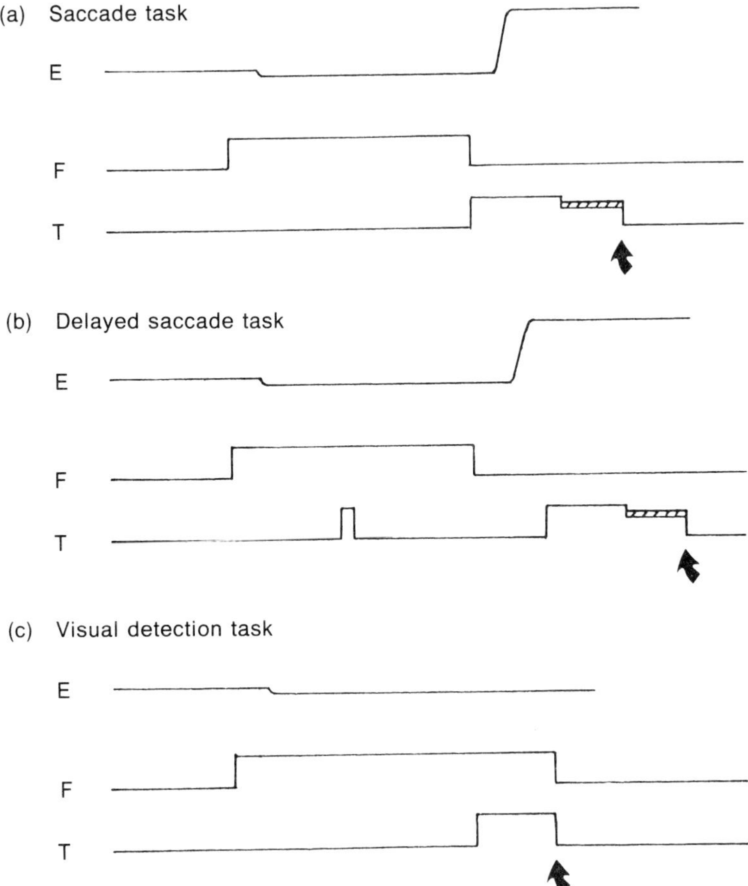

Figure 2 Paradigms to test saccadic eye movements, visual detection, and hand movements. (a) saccade task to test visually guided saccades; (b) delayed saccade task to test memory-guided saccades; (c) visual detection task. F and T indicate central fixation spot and peripheral target spot; E, schematic eye position. Shaded portion of T indicates the dimming of the target, to which the subject had to respond (curved arrow). In visual detection task, the subject responded to the turning on of the target spot

she was required to fixate. After a random period of time (1.2–2.0 s) the spot went out and at the same time another spot (target point) came on at a location which was randomly selected by the computer. The subject was instructed to shift her gaze to the target as quickly as possible. After another random period of time the target became dim. The subject had to release her finger from the button immediately after the dimming. If the button release was early enough (0.5–1.0 s, depending on the performance of individual subjects), a comfortable sound occurred to encourage the subsequent performance of the subject. The goal-directed nature of this, and the following tasks, helps maintain the alertness and volition of the subjects and frequently attracts the great enthusiasm of younger children. The eye movement made in the saccade task was a saccade guided by visual information derived from the target light; we call this a 'visually guided saccade' or simply 'visual saccade'.

The *delayed saccade task* (Figure 2b) was designed to induce memory-guided saccades. While the subject was fixating the central spot, another spot of light was flashed (duration, 50 ms) to indicate the future location of the saccade target. The subject was required to maintain fixation for another period of time (3 s) until the fixation spot went off. The subject was asked to shift her gaze toward the remembered and predicted location of the target immediately after the fixation spot went off. The target came on 0.6 s after the fixation spot went off. It was natural for the subject to make a saccade before the target actually came on. The resultant saccade was therefore guided by visual spatial memory. Interestingly, most subjects were unaware of the difference between their own saccades, whether they were visually guided or memory-guided. The subject terminated each task trial by releasing the button in response to the dimming of the target spot, as in the saccade task.

The *visual detection task* (Figure 2c) was designed to test simple visual perception or spatial attention, especially the presence of its asymmetry or hemineglect. Each trial started with the appearance of the central fixation spot. After a random period of time while the subject was fixating, another spot came on. The subject was required to release her finger from the button as quickly as possible.

An experimental session was usually divided into five blocks, each comprising 20–25 trials, the sequence being: saccade task, delayed saccade task, visual detection task, saccade task and delayed saccade task. We also asked the patient to use a finger of each hand in an alternating fashion across the task blocks: if the right hand was used in the first block of saccade tasks, the left hand was used in the next block of the same saccade task. Between the blocks of trials the patient was allowed to relax to minimize fatigue.

Calibration of eye movements

Before the test session, we asked the subject to perform a task for eye movement calibration. This was the same as the saccade task, except that the target was presented at 20° to the right and to the left in an alternating manner. While the subject was performing the task, we adjusted the gain of the EOG so that the current eye position displayed on the computer monitor screen was aligned on the target position which was simultaneously displayed on the screen. EOG signals were found to be roughly linear so that the calibration was performed usually only for 20°. To prevent possible changes of the gain of EOG during the test session, the patient was adapted to the dim light condition for at least 10 minutes before starting the examination. However, we still noted slight changes in the EOG gain, which were normalized at the time of off-line analyses. EOG signals for vertical eye movements, however, were strongly non-linear and subject to artifacts due to eyelid movements. Therefore, vertical eye movements were examined only qualitatively. An eye blink was associated with a characteristic transient potential, which we also examined.

Off-line analyses

The stored data were composed of two sets of files, an event-data file and an analog-data file. The off-line analyses were performed in two stages. First, eye movement-related parameters for each task trial were determined, and secondly, statistical analyses and displays of the parametric data were produced.

The main function of the off-line analyses was to determine the time of saccade. Parameters used for this determination were eye velocity, acceleration, and duration. The onset of an eye movement was determined if velocity and acceleration exceeded threshold values (28°/s and 90°/s, respectively). The eye movement was accepted as a saccade, depending on its velocity and duration. After the onset, the velocity had to exceed 88°/s and this suprathreshold velocity had to be maintained for at least 10 ms. The total duration had to be more than 30 ms. The end of the eye movement was determined if the velocity became lower than 40°/s. The above process was performed automatically by the computer.

However, EOG signals could contain a significant amount of noise, which varied between different subjects. The above threshold values were determined on a trial-and-error basis, so as to be appropriate for most subjects. Small, slow saccades could be omitted whereas large fluctuations due to body movements could be judged to be a saccade. Therefore, the final judgement of saccades was made by visually inspecting the traces of eye movements. By inspecting each eye movement trace, the investigator judged whether or not the saccade determined by the computer was real; if not, the next candidate saccade was provided by the computer.

For each trial we collected a saccade that occurred first after each task event (that is, turning off of fixation point or coming on of target point). In the present study we focused on the first saccade after the turning off of the fixation point, the main saccade aiming at the visual or remembered target. Parameters of saccade produced by the computer analyses were amplitude, duration, peak velocity, time to peak velocity, accuracy in amplitude, accuracy in angle and fixation instability. Reaction time of button release was also measured.

In the second stage of the off-line analyses, these data were analyzed using a commercial database program (EXCEL®) together with the information about the target position and the side of the hand used. Statistical analyses were also performed.

RESULTS

Clinical observations

A 10-year-old girl came to our clinic with the complaint of disability of the extremities in the evening. She was born to unconsanguineous parents with no family history of neurological diseases. Pregnancy had been uneventful and her birth weight was 2450 g at 41 weeks' gestation. Past history revealed nothing of note.

At 7 years of age, her parents noticed that she was prone to falling. From 8 years, her right foot began to adduct. The adduction was observed also in her left foot and arm, then her feet showed pes equinovarus. These symptoms were more prominent in the evening than in the morning, and naps improved the motor functions temporarily.

Physical examination revealed postural dystonia, bilateral pes equinovarus and mild lumbar lordosis while standing and walking. Dysdiadochokinesis was observed, but interlimb coordination on crawling was well preserved. Mild rigidity was observed in tensive exercise. Stretch reflexes revealed mild rigidity, but resting or postural tremor was not recognized. Although deep tendon reflexes in the arms were normal, patellar tendon reflexes were exacerbated bilaterally and the pseudo-Babinski sign was observed in the right foot. The Westphal phenomenon and Myerson's sign were noticed. These symptoms had marked diurnal fluctuation, showing aggravation towards the evening and alleviation in the morning after taking sleep. Even naps improved symptoms moderately, but she had retrocollis and could not stand by herself in the evening.

After starting levodopa (400 mg divided into two doses a day, 8 mg/kg per day), she soon became able to walk by herself in the evening (Table 1). She did not feel any disturbance in her ordinary life with levodopa 600 mg, divided into three doses a day, though mild pes equinovarus of the left foot, slight dystonic pronation of the left forearm and Westphal phenomenon were still observed. After levodopa was increased to 800 mg/day, almost all

Table 1 Clinical course of a case of hereditary progressive dystonia. Examination before levodopa took place on 22nd December, 1990; examinations 1, 2 and 3 after levodopa therapy were on the 26th January, 23rd February and 30th March, 1991. —, not recognized; ↑, exacerbated; N, normal; ±, present to a slight extent; +, mild; + +, moderate; + + +, severe; /, right versus left

	Before levodopa	*After levodopa* 1	2	3
Dosage (mg/kg per day)	0.0	12.0	14.0	16.0
Dystonia				
arm	+ +/+ + +	+/+ +	—/±	—/— ~ ±
leg	+ + +/+ +	—/+	+/+	—/—
Patellar tendon reflex	↑	N	N	N
Pseudo-Babinski's sign	±/—	—/—	—/—	—/—
Diurnal fluctuation	+ + +*	±	±	—
Myerson's sign	+	±	±	— ~ ±
Westphal phenomenon	+ +/+	+/+	—/±	±/±

*Retrocollis and could not stand by herself in the evening

symptoms disappeared except minimal induced rigidity of the left upper extremity.

Visually guided and memory-guided saccadic eye movements

Figure 3 compares eye movements of the HPD patient before and after starting levodopa therapy. Before levodopa, visually guided saccades (Figure 3a) tended to be hypometric, especially for the peripheral targets, as indicated by the presence of frequent corrective saccades. The hypometric tendency disappeared after levodopa. The latencies were about 200 ms or less, for both before and after levodopa. No obvious changes were seen in velocity.

A qualitative change is seen in memory-guided saccades (Figure 3b). Before the therapy, saccades often occurred after the target came on; memory-guided saccades were unlikely to occur. Their amplitudes were nearly normometric, however. Memory-guided saccades became consistent after levodopa therapy. Their latencies became shorter and less variable. No differences were noted for velocity.

Even after the therapy, memory-guided saccades were slower with longer latencies than visually guided saccades. Such differences are seen in normal human[16] and monkey[17] subjects. In short, the oculomotor performance of this patient after levodopa was not significantly different from normal subjects, except that visually guided saccades were occasionally delayed.

Quantitative analyses

In this section we will describe some quantitative changes in saccadic eye movements and hand movements during the course of levodopa therapy. Figure 4 shows the changes in latencies of saccades and reaction times of button release. The latencies tended to become longer for visually guided saccades but shorter for memory-guided saccades. Interestingly, in second and third post-levodopa examinations latencies of visually guided saccades were more variable than before levodopa, sometimes as great as 800 ms (as indicated by the much larger SD values). At the second post-levodopa examination, the general condition of the patient was worse because she forgot to take the medicine. This may partly explain the variable latencies. The explanation would not hold, however, for the third post-levodopa test in which the same tendency was seen. There was no systematic asymmetry in terms of the direction of saccade.

The changes in manual reaction time were striking. The reaction time became shorter by more than 150 ms on average at the first post-levodopa examination. Here we can compare the data when the subject used her right hand for button press/release. At the second post-levodopa examination the reaction times of her left hand were longer, which was in line with the changes in general clinical symptoms described above. Since trials of every task were terminated by the button release, we were able to compare the reaction times in different situations. We noted no differences between the tasks or between the sides of target positions. For the visual detection task we checked whether the reaction times were different for different targets which might suggest perceptual asymmetry, but found nothing significant.

Figure 5 shows that the likelihood of memory-guided saccade increased monotonically. In the pre-levodopa examination, the patient showed memory-guided saccades in only about half of the trials; in the other half, she waited for the target to appear for the period of the time gap after the fixation point went out. In the later examinations after levodopa, saccades were made more consistently in a predictive mode based on the memory of the target cue. This effect was clearer for leftward saccades. Along with the shortening of their latencies, this result may suggest that levodopa was beneficial for this type of eye movement.

Levodopa also had an effect on the accuracy of saccades, as seen in Figure 6. The degree of hypometricity in visually guided saccades tended to decrease for saccades to both sides, except for the leftward saccades at the second post-levodopa test. The effects on memory-guided saccades were more complex. Leftward saccades tended to be less hypometric, whereas rightward saccades showed a decline in accuracy in the second post-levodopa test. As indicated above, she did not take the medicine on this day. Together with the highly variable latencies of visually guided saccades (Figure 4a), the results might suggest specific, perhaps transient, reactions to on/off of dopamine in this disease state.

Overall, the effect of levodopa was more significant on leftward saccades. There was also lengthening of visually guided saccade latencies (Figure 4a); shortening of memory guided saccade latencies (Figure 4b); increase in the probability of occurrence of memory-guided saccades (Figure 5), and improvement in the accuracy of both visually guided and memory-guided saccades (Figure 6). No clear correlation was found between this result and clinical findings.

DISCUSSION

Voluntary saccade task as a tool for clinical assessment of higher brain functions

Neural mechanisms of saccadic eye movement have been investigated extensively. A saccade is produced by a quick, simultaneous contraction and relaxation of antagonistic extraocular muscles which are the outcomes of pulse-like increase and decrease of activity in the respective motorneurons[18]. In the brainstem reticular formation 'burst neurons' are found that provide the motorneurons specifically with the pulse-like inputs, either activating or inhibiting them[19]. The bursts in the burst neurons are produced by two kinds of input, an excitation, mainly from the superior colliculus, and a removal of inhibition (disinhibition) from 'omnipause neurons' in the brainstem midline structure[19].

The superior colliculus is a key structure for the initiation of saccades[6]. It receives inputs from visual areas, directly from the retina and indirectly from the visual cortical areas[20], and emits motor outputs to the saccadic

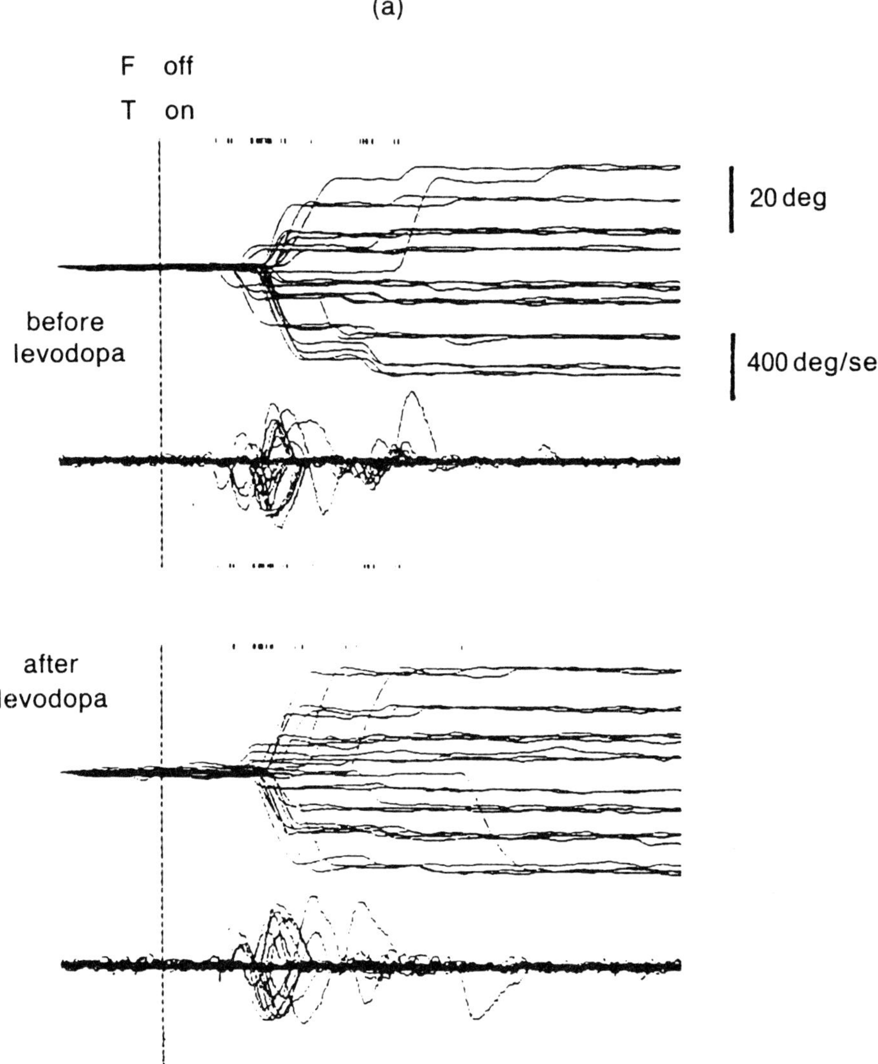

Figure 3 Deficits and improvement by levodopa of voluntary saccadic eye movements in a HPD patient. Visually guided saccades (a) and memory-guided saccades (b) recorded before (upper) and after (lower) starting levodopa therapy (first examination after levodopa). Each record shows superimposed traces of eye position (upper) and eye velocity (lower) for saccades to the targets on the horizontal meridian (5, 10, 20, and 30°; right side upward, left side downward). The vertical lines indicate the turning off of the central fixation point and the onset of the peripheral target points. Tick marks at the top and bottom indicate the onsets of saccades detected by the computer. Changes in the DC level, which were present in the original records, were removed by assuming that the subject was fixating at the central spot at the beginning of the records. The velocity records were smoothed using a median filter method based on three successive data points

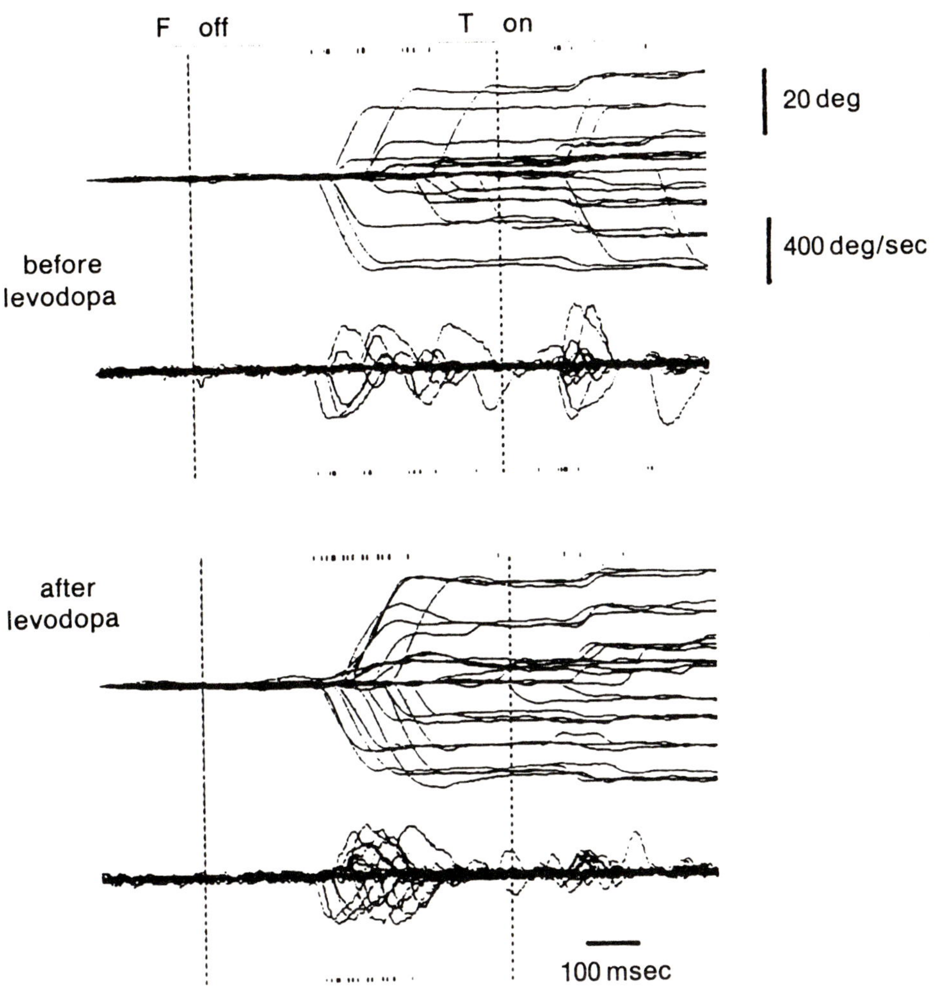

Figure 3 *(continued)*

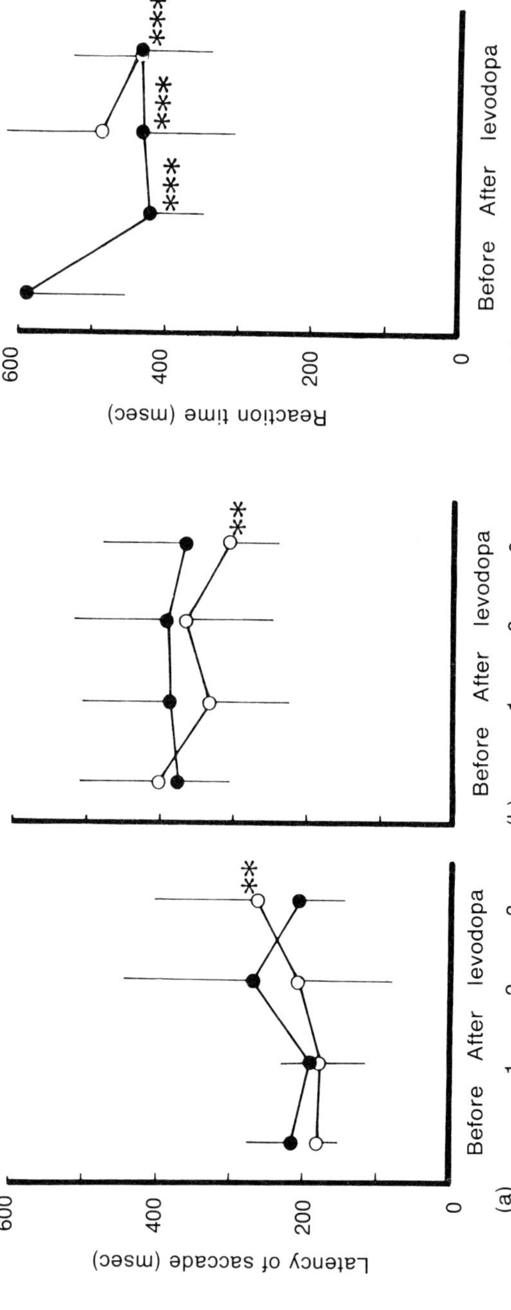

Figure 4 Latencies of saccades and hand movements. The results obtained in four examinations (one before levodopa, and three after starting levodopa) are compared. The mean latencies of visually guided saccades (a) and those of memory-guided saccades (b) are shown for the right targets (filled circles) and the left targets (open circles) separately. The mean reaction times of button release (c) are shown separately for the hand used: right (filled squares) and left (open squares). Standard deviations are indicated by vertical lines. A statistical analysis using the *t*-test was performed for the difference in means between each of the pre- and post-levodopa values for each parameter; $^{**}p < 0.01$; $^{***}p < 0.0001$

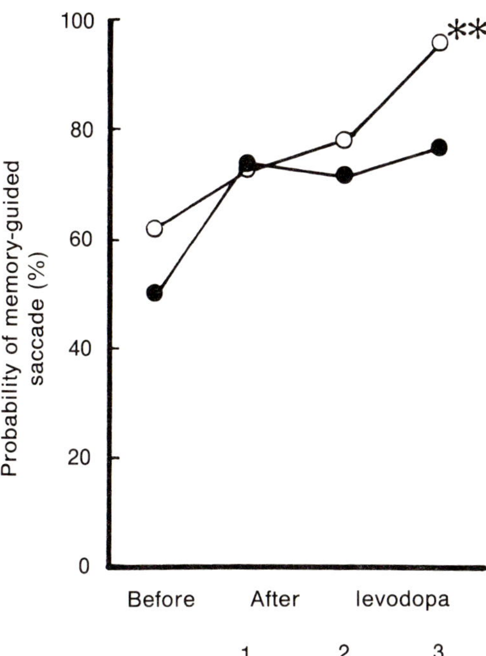

Figure 5 Probability of occurrence of memory-guided saccade. The percentage of the trials of the delayed saccade task in which the first saccade occurred based on the memory of target location is shown for each examination. Data for the right (filled circles) and left (open circles) are shown separately. The difference in the probability was analyzed using the χ^2 test; **, $p < 0.01$

oculomotor[21] and neck/trunk motor systems[22]. Most important in the cerebral cortex for the initiation of saccades is the frontal eye field[23,24] which provides heavy fiber projections to the superior colliculus[25,26]. Other cortical areas such as the posterior parietal cortex[27], prestriate visual cortex[28], and supplementary eye field[29] are also involved either in parallel with, or prior to, the frontal eye field. The information from these cortical areas is largely mediated by the superior colliculus through activation of its output cells. The convergence of the excitatory inputs might lead to chaotic activity in the superior colliculus. A critical function of the basal ganglia would be to prevent chaotic overexcitation through the inhibitory outputs arising from the substantia nigra pars reticulata. A similar mechanism would be at work for skeletal movements, but mainly through another basal ganglia output, the internal segment of the globus pallidus.

Given the detailed functional scheme for saccadic eye movement, we are prepared for studying pathological changes of the saccadic system. Simple reaction time tasks may be insufficient to reveal the dysfunction of the basal ganglia, in view of the context-dependent nature of basal ganglia neuronal activity. We need to compare saccades which are physically the same but are different in terms of the background behavioral context, yet, as far as possible, the clinical examination should not be stressful or tiring. This

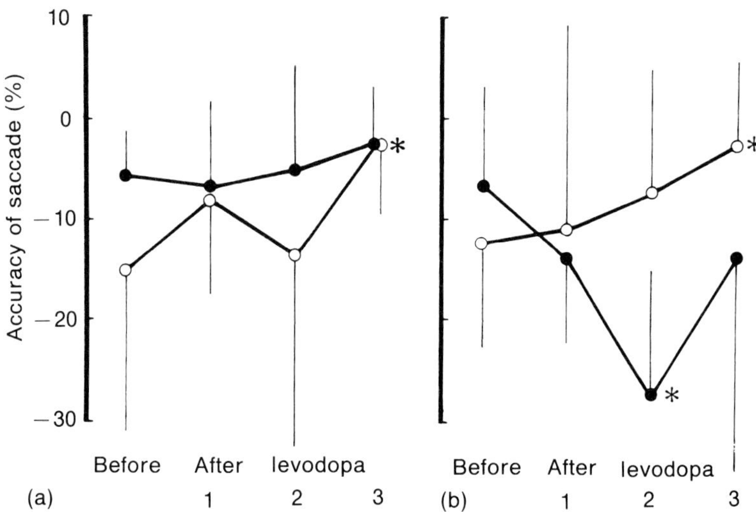

Figure 6 Accuracy of saccades. The ordinate indicates by how much the saccades overshot (+) or undershot (−) relative to the eccentricity of the target. For visually guided saccades (a) and memory-guided saccades (b), the averaged data for each examination are shown for the right (filled circles) and left (open circles) targets separately. Only saccades to the 20 and 30 degree targets were included, because 5 or 10 degree saccades contained relatively greater noise which was judged to be inappropriate. The difference in mean between the pre- and post-levodopa values was analyzed using the t-test; *, $p < 0.05$. For visually guided saccades, statistical significance was found only for the value of the third post-levodopa examination

requirement is especially critical if the patients are children. The set of tasks which we currently employ (saccade task, delayed saccade task, and detection task) was designed to fulfil this requirement. Completely naive patients may not show their full capabilities at the outset of the examination. We therefore repeated the same saccade tasks twice. Finally, we tried to make the examination interesting so that most child patients regarded it as a game. If the patient was successful in releasing the button switch in response to the dimming of the light target, he/she was rewarded by sound. Interestingly, the reward value of the sound was immediately comprehended by almost every patient without any verbal explanation. Such manipulation of the tasks is important not only for the sake of the patients, but also for fully investigating the functional state of voluntary behavior to which the basal ganglia and a large part of the cerebral cortex contribute.

Our computer program is powerful in controlling the tasks and in displaying and storing the data. The data were stored virtually continuously, allowing us to calculate any parameters of eye movements in/outside the tasks. The off-line analyses have been largely automatized so that all necessary parameters for one patient are produced within 20 minutes.

Saccadic eye movements in hereditary progressive dystonia with diurnal fluctuation

The etiology of HPD is thought to be dopamine deficiency in the striatum[12]. Two lines of evidence support this hypothesis. First, classified as dystonia, the motor deficits of HPD are similar to other types of basal ganglia-induced dystonia. Second, the motor symptoms virtually disappear shortly after commencing the levodopa therapy. The required dose is much smaller than that needed for Parkinson disease and is free from any side-effects. These observations suggest that dopaminergic cells in the substantia nigra pars compacta are present but functionally underactive. If this is true, it is unclear why the motor deficits in HPD are considerably different from the deficits in adult Parkinson disease. It is unlikely that the behavioral difference is derived from whether the blocking of the dopaminergic functions is structural or functional. Instead, the difference may be related to the functional changes of the basal ganglia system along with developmental maturation. The dysfunction of the same basal ganglia structure may lead to different symptoms depending on the age of the patient. This is not just an issue of pediatric neurology. Principles of organization of the brain may be revealed by investigating functional changes.

The HPD patient examined in this study showed deficits in saccadic eye movements: both visually guided and memory-guided saccades were hypometric, and memory-guided saccades were infrequent. These features were common to other HPD patients we have examined. However, most of the patients were under levodopa therapy so that the deficits tended to be unclear. In this patient we had a good opportunity to follow the course of the illness before and after starting the drug therapy. The improvement of eye movements was considerable, if not complete. This was in parallel with the decrement of other motor symptoms. In fact, the most remarkable change we noticed was the shortening of manual reaction times. The shortening of saccade latencies were comparatively small. This raised the question of whether the oculomotor region of the basal ganglia (caudate and substantia nigra) is relatively intact compared with the skeletomotor region (putamen and globus pallidus). Here we need to compare HPD with two other types of dopamine deficiency: Parkinson disease of adult human and 1-methyl-4-phenyl-1,2,3,6-tetrahydropyridine (MPTP)-induced dopamine deficiency in monkeys.

Relation to Parkinson disease

There have been a number of studies on parkinsonian eye movements[30–36]. Most studies have examined only one type of saccade, the visually guided saccade, indicating hypometricity, long latency and slight slowness. The deficits revealed in these examinations were usually small compared with overall motor disturbances experienced by the patients in their daily lives. Recent studies, however, have revealed the conditional nature of parkinsonian eye movements. Typically, memory-guided saccades or anti-saccades were devastated, even if visually guided saccades were relatively intact[14,37,38]. In the above two types of saccades the patients had to rely on the internal image or memory information. This is actually the situation in which many of the basal ganglia neurons become active[3,4]. Furthermore, the deficit fits well with the phenomenon of 'akinesia paradoxica'[39] in which immobile parkinsonian patients can move swiftly if appropriate external stimuli are provided or unusual emotional stress is imposed.

The eye movement deficits in the HPD patient were similar to the adult parkinsonian deficits in that memory-guided saccades were infrequent. Some differences should also be noted. Visually guided saccades were relatively more hypometric in HPD, whereas memory-guided saccades were relatively more hypometric in adult parkinsonism. We are far from firm conclusions, however, because the data samples are still small and the experimental situations were not identical.

Relation to MPTP-induced dopamine deficiency in monkeys

The nature of dopamine deficiency in HPD may be examined by comparison with experimentally induced dopamine deficiency in monkeys. The research group of one of the authors (O.H.) has conducted a series of experiments in which voluntary saccades of monkeys were investigated before and after local infusion of MPTP in the caudate nucleus or the putamen.

The MPTP injection into the caudate was aimed at the central part of the head–body junction of the caudate[40,41] where presaccadic neurons are clustered[4]. Tyrosine hydroxylase activity, visualized using a immunohistochemical method, was decreased locally around the injection site with some effects extending into the ipsilateral putamen. These caudate-MPTP monkeys remained active, performed the oculomotor tasks regularly, and showed hardly any skeletomotor deficits, postural changes, tremor, or rigidity. The manual reaction time for lever release was not changed. However, these monkeys showed clear deficits in voluntary saccades. Interestingly, the deficits were selective for memory guided saccades; visually guided saccades remained brisk.

In another series of experiments, MPTP injection was aimed at the rostral part of the putamen[42]. The area decrease in tyrosine hydroxylase activity included the putamen and, to a lesser extent, the caudate. These monkeys initially showed strong contralateral visual hemineglect in addition to parkinsonian motor symptoms (rigidity, tremor, akinesia) in the contralateral extremities. Deficits in saccades were also severe; both visually guided and memory-guided saccades were impaired, in addition to strong ipsilateral deviation of eye position. These oculomotor deficits, however, could be corrected by daily training of the saccade tasks.

That visually guided saccades in the HPD patient were hypometric might suggest that dopamine deficiency in this disease includes the putamen. The abnormally long manual reaction times of this patient support this view. We should be careful, however, before drawing any conclusion from this comparison, because we are dealing with individuals at different ages: a human child compared with adult monkeys. The caudate might perform different roles depending on age.

Dopaminergic system as a modulator in the basal ganglia

The effects of dopamine inside the basal ganglia are still far from clear. Dopamine may be excitatory, inhibitory, or modulatory, depending on the target cells or even depending on the ongoing biophysical events in the cells[43–47]. What is clear is that dopaminergic neurons do not send signals out of the basal ganglia. Any effects of dopamine must be mediated by the output neurons which are GABAergic. Furthermore, the final outcome of the basal ganglia information appears to be created by heterogeneous neural circuits in the basal ganglia. In addition to the serial inhibitory connections (direct pathway) mentioned above, more polysynaptic circuits (indirect pathway) play a role of considerable importance, perhaps antagonistic to the direct pathway[48]. The indirect pathway involves the external segment of the globus pallidus and the subthalamic nucleus[49,50–53]. Saccadic activities have recently been found in the subthalamic nucleus[54]. How the dopaminergic system interacts with the complex neural circuits in the basal ganglia is an open question. Correlation of findings in behavioral experiments using trained monkeys with those obtained in the behavioral examination of human patients with basal ganglia diseases appears most promising for clarifying the role of dopamine. The present study may be the first step in this direction of research.

REFERENCES

1. Westheimer, G. (1989). History and methodology. In Wurtz, R.H. and Goldberg, M.E. (eds.) *The Neurobiology of Saccadic Eye Movements*, pp. 3–12. (Amsterdam: Elsevier Science)
2. Wurtz, R.H. and Goldberg, M.E. (eds.) (1989). *The Neurobiology of Saccadic Eye Movements*. (Amsterdam: Elsevier Science)
3. Hikosaka, O. and Wurtz, R.H. (1989). The basal ganglia. In Wurtz, R.H. and Goldberg, M.E. (eds.) *The Neurobiology of Saccadic Eye Movements*, pp. 257–81. (Amsterdam: Elsevier Science)
4. Hikosaka, O., Sakamoto, M. and Usui, S. (1989). Functional properties of monkey caudate neurons. I. Activities related to saccadic eye movements. *J. Neurophysiol.*, **61**, 780–98
5. Hikosaka, O. and Wurtz, R.H. (1983). Visual and oculomotor functions of monkey substantia nigra pars reticulata. IV. Relation of substantia nigra to superior colliculus. *J. Neurophysiol.*, **49**, 1285–301
6. Sparks, D.L. and Hartwich-Young, R. (1989). The deep layers of the superior colliculus. In Wurtz, R.H. and Goldberg, M.E. (eds.) *The Neurobiology of Saccadic Eye Movements*, pp. 213–55. (Amsterdam: Elsevier Science)
7. Hikosaka, O. and Wurtz, R.H. (1983). Visual and oculomotor functions of monkey substantia nigra pars reticulata. I. Relation of visual and auditory responses to saccades. *J. Neurophysiol.*, **49**, 1230–53
8. Penny, J.B. and Young, A.B. (1983). Speculations on the functional anatomy of basal ganglia disorders. *Annu. Rev. Neurosci.*, **6**, 73–94
9. Hikosaka, O. and Sakamoto, M. (1986). Neural activities in the monkey basal ganglia related to attention, memory and anticipation. *Brain Dev.*, **8**, 454–62
10. Hikosaka, O., Sakamoto, M. and Usui, S. (1989). Functional properties of monkey caudate

neurons. II. Visual and auditory responses. *J. Neurophysiol.*, **61(4)**, 799–813

11. Hikosaka, O. and Wurtz, R.H. (1983). Visual and oculomotor functions of monkey substantia nigra pars reticulata. III. Memory-contingent visual and saccade responses. *J. Neurophysiol.*, **49**, 1268–84
12. Segawa, M., Nomura, Y. and Kase, M. (1986). Hereditary progressive dystonia with marked diurnal fluctuation: clinicopathophysiological identification in reference to juvenile Parkinson's disease. *Advances in neurology, Vol.* 45, pp. 227–34. (Amsterdam: Elsevier Science)
13. Segawa, M., Nomura, Y. and Kase, M. (1986). Diurnally fluctuating hereditary progressive dystonia. In Vinken, P.J., Bruyn, G.W. and Klawans, H.L. (eds.) *Handbook of Clinical Neurology, Vol.* 5, *Extrapyramidal Disorders*, pp. 529–38. (Amsterdam: Elsevier Science)
14. Hikosaka, O., Segawa, M. and Imai, H. (1987). Voluntary saccadic eye movement: application to analyze basal ganglia disease. In Ishikawa, S. (ed.) *Highlights in Neuro-Ophthalmology*, pp. 133–8. (Amsterdam: Aeolus Press)
15. Nomura, Y., Segawa, M., Soda, M. and Hikosaka, O. (1987). Voluntary saccadic eye movements in basal ganglia disorders. In Ishikawa, S. (ed.) *Highlights in Neuro-Ophthalmology*, pp. 139–45. (Amsterdam: Aeolus Press)
16. Smit, A.C., van Gisbergen, J.A.M. and Cools, A.R. (1987). A parametric analysis of human saccades in different experimental paradigms. *Vision Res.*, **27**, 1745–62
17. Hikosaka, O. and Wurtz, R.H. (1985). Modification of saccadic eye movements by GABA-related substances. I. Effect of muscimol and bicuculline in the monkey superior colliculus. *J. Neurophysiol.*, **53**, 266–91
18. Becker, W. (1989). Metrics. In Wurtz, R.H. and Goldberg, M.E. (eds.) *The Neurobiology of Saccadic Eye Movements*, pp. 13–67. (Amsterdam: Elsevier Science)
19. Hepp, K., Henn, V., Vilis, T. and Cohen, B. (1989). Brainstem regions related to saccadic generation. In Wurtz, R.H. and Goldberg, M.E. (eds.) *The Neurobiology of Saccadic Eye Movements*, pp. 105–212. (Amsterdam: Elsevier Science)
20. Wurtz, R.H. and Albano, J.E. (1980). Visual-motor function of the primate superior colliculus. *Annu. Rev. Neurosci.*, **3**, 189–226
21. Moschovakis, A.K., Karabelas, A.B. and Highstein, S.M. (1988). Structure-function relationships in the primate superior colliculus. II. Morphological identity of presaccadic neurons. *J. Neurophysiol.*, **60**, 263–302
22. Grantyn, A. and Grantyn, R. (1982). Axonal patterns and sites of termination of cat superior colliculus neurons projecting in the tecto-bulbo-spinal tract. *Exp. Brain Res.*, **46**, 243–56
23. Robinson, D.A. and Fuchs, A.F. (1969). Eye movements evoked by stimulation of frontal eye fields. *J. Neurophysiol.*, **32**, 637–48
24. Bruce, C.J. and Goldberg, M.E. (1985). Primate frontal eye fields. I. Single neurons discharging before saccades. *J. Neurophysiol.*, **53**, 603–35
25. Stanton, G.B., Goldberg, M.E. and Bruce, C.J. (1988). Frontal eye field efferents in the macaque monkey: II. topography of terminal fields in midbrain and pons. *J. Comp. Neurol.*, **271**, 493–506
26. Huerta, M.F., Krubitzer, L.A. and Kaas, J.H. (1986). Frontal eye field as defined by intracortical microstimulation in squirrel monkeys, owl monkeys, and macaque monkeys: I. Subcortical connections. *J. Comp. Neurol.*, **253**, 415–39
27. Andersen, R.A. and Gnadt, J.W. (1989). Posterior parietal cortex. In Wurtz, R.H. and Goldberg, M.E. (eds.) *The Neurobiology of Saccadic Eye Movements*, pp. 315–35. (Amsterdam: Elsevier Science)
28. Weber, H. and Fischer, B. (1990). Effect of a local ibotenic acid lesion in the visual association area on the prelunate gyrus (area V4) on saccadic reaction times in trained rhesus monkeys. *Exp. Brain Res.*, **81**, 134–9
29. Schlag, J. and Schlag-Rey, M. (1987). Evidence for a supplementary eye field. *J. Neurophysiol.*, **57**, 179–200
30. Corin, M.S., Elizan, T.S. and Bender, M.B. (1972). Oculomotor function in patients with Parkinson's disease. *J. Neurol. Sci.*, **15**, 251–65
31. DeJong, J.D. and Melvill-Jones, G. (1971). Akinesia, hypokinesia, and bradykinesia in the oculomotor system of patients with Parkinson's disease. *Exp. Neurol.*, **32**, 58–68
32. Melvill-Jones, G. and DeJong, J.D. (1971). Dynamic characteristics of saccadic eye movements in Parkinson's disease. *Exp. Neurol.*, **31**, 17–31

33. Shibasaki, H., Sadatoshi, T. and Kuroiwa, Y. (1979). Oculomotor abnormalities in Parkinson's disease. *Arch. Neurol.*, **36**, 360–4
34. Teravainen, H. and Calne, D.B. (1980). Studies of parkinsonian movement: 1. Programming and execution of eye movements. *Acta Neurol. Scand.*, **62**, 137–48
35. White, O.B., Saint-Cyr, J.R., Tomlinson, R.D. and Sharpe, J.A. (1983). Ocular motor deficits in Parkinson's disease. II. Control of the saccadic and smooth pursuit systems. *Brain*, **106**, 571–87
36. Yamazaki, A. and Ishikawa, S. (1972). The eye movement abnormality in Parkinson's disease. *Jpn. J. Clin. Ophthalmol.*, **26**, 619–23
37. Carl, J.R. and Wurtz, R.H. (1985). Asymmetry of saccadic control in patients with hemi-Parkinson's disease. *Invest. Ophthalmol. Visual Sci., Suppl.*, **26**, 258
38. Crawford, T.J., Henderson, L. and Kennard, C. (1989). Abnormalities of non-visually guided eye movements in Parkinson's disease. *Brain*, **112**, 1573–86
39. Schwab, R.S. and Zieper, I. (1965). Effects of mood, motivation, stress and alertness on the performance in Parkinson's disease. *Psychiatr. Neurol.*, **150**, 345–57
40. Usui, S., Kato, M., Kori, A., Matsumura, M., Miyashita, N. and Hikosaka, O. (1990). Deficits in spontaneous eye movements induced by unilateral infusion of MPTP in the monkey caudate nucleus. *Soc. Neurosci. Abstr.*, **16**, 235
41. Miyashita, N., Matsumura, M., Usui, S., Kato, M., Kori, A., Gardiner, T.W. and Hikosaka, O. (1990). Deficits in task-related eye movements induced by unilateral infusion of MPTP in the monkey caudate nucleus. *Soc. Neurosci. Abstr.*, **16**, 235
42. Usui, S., Kato, K., Miyashita, B., Imai, H., Matsumura, M., Kori, A. and Hikosaka, O. (1991). Deficits in saccadic eye movements in hemi-parkinsonian monkeys induced by unilateral intraputaminal infusion of 1-methyl-4-phenyl-1,2,3,6-tetrahydropyridine. *Brain Res.*, in press
43. Akaike, A., Ohno, Y., Sasa, M. and Takaori, S. (1987). Excitatory and inhibitory effects of dopamine on neuronal activity of the caudate nucleus neurons *in vitro*. *Brain Res.*, **418**, 262–72
44. Bergstrom, D.A. and Walters, J.R. (1984). Dopamine attenuates the effects of GABA on single unit activity in the globus pallidus. *Brain Res.*, **310**, 23–33
45. Calabresi, P., Mercuri, N., Stanzione, P., Stefani, A. and Bernardi, G. (1988). Intracellular studies on the dopamine-induced firing inhibition of neostriatal neurons *in vitro*: evidence for D_1 receptor involvement. *Neuroscience*, **20**, 757–71
46. Calabresi, P., Benedetti, M., Mercuri, N.B. and Bernardi, G. (1988). Endogenous dopamine and dopaminergic agonists modulate synaptic excitation in neostriatum: intracellular studies from naive and catecholamine-depleted rats. *Neuroscience*, **27**, 145–57
47. Creese, I. (1982). Dopamine receptors explained. *Trends Neurosci.*, **5**, 40–3
48. Alexander, G.E. and Crutcher, M.D. (1990). Functional architecture of basal ganglia circuits: neural substrates of parallel processing. *Trends Neurosci.*, **13**, 266–71
49. Kanazawa, I., Marshall, G.R. and Kelly, J.S. (1976). Afferents to the rat substantia nigra studied with horseradish peroxidase, with special reference to fibres from the subthalamic nucleus. *Brain Res.*, **115**, 485–91
50. Kita, H., Chang, H.T. and Kitai, S.T. (1983). Pallidal inputs to subthalamus: intracellular analysis. *Brain Res.*, **264**, 255–65
51. Kita, H. and Kitai, S.T. (1987). Efferent projections of the subthalamic nucleus in the rat: light and electron microscopic analysis with the PHA-L method. *J. Comp. Neurol.*, **260**, 435–52
52. Mitchell, I.J., Jackson, A., Sambrook, M.A. and Crossman, A.R. (1989). The role of subthalamic nucleus in experimental chorea. *Brain*, **112**, 1533–48
53. Parent, A. and Smith, Y. (1987). Organization of efferent projections of the subthalamic nucleus in the squirrel monkey as revealed by retrograde labeling methods. *Brain Res.*, **436**, 296–310
54. Matsumura, M., Kojima, J., Gardiner, T.W. and Hikosaka, O. (1991). Visual and oculomotor functions of monkey subthalamic nucleus. *J. Neurophysiol.*, in press

SECTION 7

Neuroimaging: positron-emission tomography scanning

14

Positron-emission tomography scanning in dopa-responsive dystonia, parkinsonism-dystonia, and young-onset parkinsonism

B.J. Snow, A. Okada, W.R.W. Martin, R.C. Duvoisin and D.B. Calne

INTRODUCTION

The lesion responsible for most cases of dystonia is unknown[1]. Evidence implicating the nigrostriatal dopaminergic system includes the induction of dystonia by dopamine agonists, the common involvement of the putamen in cases of secondary dystonia[2], the frequent occurrence of focal dystonia in patients with Parkinson disease, and the dramatic therapeutic response to levodopa in patients with dopa-responsive dystonia (DRD)[3–5].

DRD often presents as an identifiable syndrome with onset around 6 years, initial progressive dystonia involving the feet, legs and then the arms, parkinsonian features including tremor, rigidity, hypomimia and impaired postural reflexes, diurnal variation, and a marked, sustained response to low doses of levodopa. This syndrome was described by Segawa as hereditary progressive dystonia with diurnal variation (HPD)[3]. The response to levodopa and the parkinsonian features of DRD have led to speculation that this condition is a variant of young-onset parkinsonism (juvenile parkinsonism)[6].

Dystonia often occurs in association with otherwise typical Parkinson disease, including patients with a later age of onset[7]. While the dystonia is usually focal, some patients may have hemidystonia. In these patients with parkinsonism-dystonia, the dystonia responds poorly, if at all, to levodopa.

There are no reported postmortem studies of unequivocal DRD, and few of young-onset parkinsonism. An understanding of the relationships between these disorders and between parkinsonism and dystonia in general requires a method that studies the integrity of the nigrostriatal dopaminergic system *in vivo*.

Positron-emission tomography (PET) using the tracer 6-fluorodopa (6FD) is the only direct method for studying the nigrostriatal dopaminergic system in living subjects[8]. The tracer crosses the blood–brain barrier, is decarboxylated to fluorodopamine by L-aromatic amino acid decarboxylase, and remains in the nerve terminals for the 2-hour duration of the typical scan. Neuronal uptake of 6FD is reduced in parkinsonism caused by presynaptic lesions[9–11]. PET is sufficiently sensitive to show asymptomatic dopaminergic deficits[12,13].

We used PET to study the dopaminergic system of patients with DRD, parkinsonism-dystonia and young-onset parkinsonism.

PATIENTS AND METHODS

Patients were recruited through the Movement Disorders Clinic at the University of British Columbia (UBC). One patient with DRD conforming to Segawa's description of hereditary progressive dystonia[3] came from Japan specifically for this study. Characteristics of the dystonic and parkinsonism-dystonia patients are summarized in Table 1. We separated patients with DRD from parkinsonism-dystonia on the basis of whether or not the dystonia responded to levodopa.

The young-onset parkinsonism group consisted of 17 patients who had typical features of Parkinson disease including tremor, bradykinesia and rigidity and a therapeutic response to levodopa in the 14 patients on treatment. None had taken neuroleptic medication, and other conditions associated with parkinsonism were excluded as far as possible. All had experienced their first symptoms before 40 years of age, with a mean age at onset of 32 years (standard deviation, 4.0), and three had shown onset below the age of 30 (23, 27 and 29 years). One patient had onset of symptoms at 11 years; her clinical features are summarized in Table 1.

We used the UBC/TRIUMF PETT VI system in the high resolution mode. The patients stopped their medications the night before scanning. All subjects received 100 mg of carbidopa 1 h before scanning. The 6FD (2.0–3.5 mCi) was prepared as described previously[14] and administered intravenously. During the scanning period 29 sequential blood samples were drawn from an indwelling radial artery catheter, and the total radioactivity in each was determined in a well counter. Twelve sequential emission scans were performed, each of 10 min duration.

We used a graphical method to calculate the steady-state 6FD uptake rate constant for the whole striatum[7]. The method incorporates both the measured blood radioactivity and the corrected striatal radioactivity.

RESULTS AND DISCUSSION

Figure 1 shows the 6FD uptake rate constants for each group. Both patients with parkinsonism-dystonia had lower uptake on the side contralateral to the side with more severe parkinsonism.

We have shown that 6FD PET scans are normal in DRD despite the clinical evidence for dysfunction of the dopaminergic system. Our findings must be interpreted in the light of the processes studied by PET with 6FD (Figure 2). The 6FD uptake rate constant is determined by the transfer of

Table 1 Clinical features of patients studied are listed in the order in which they developed. DCI indicates concomitant decarboxylase inhibitor

Patient number	*Sex*	*Age* (years)	*Age of onset* (years)	*Family history*	*Dose of levodopa* (mg/day)	*Diurnal variation*	*Clinical description*
Dopa-responsive dystonia							
1	F	47	9	No	600	Yes	Japanese patient. Postural dystonia of right leg, right arm, left arm, left leg. Mild hypomimia and rigidity. Marked response to levodopa
2	M	43	5	Yes	150 (DCI)	Yes	Dystonia of right arm then left arm. Torticollis and writer's cramp. Moderate response to levodopa
3	F	34	5	Yes	300	No	Dystonia of left leg, then right leg then generalized. Torticollis. Mild hypomimia and rigidity. Marked response to L-dopa
4	F	42	5	No	500 (DCI)	Yes	Dystonia of left foot, then right foot, arms. Bed-bound for 2 years before starting levodopa, now independent
Parkinsonism-dystonia							
5	M	53	45	No	200 (DCI)	No	Dystonia affecting left arm and leg. Torticollis. Simultaneous parkinsonism affecting left side of body. Only the parkinsonism responded to levodopa
6	F	41	37	No	300 (DCI)	No	Dystonia affecting right arm and leg. Torticollis. Parkinsonism of left side, responsive to levodopa (dystonia non-responsive)
Young-onset parkinsonism							
7	F	27	11	No	400 (DCI)	No	Generalized, mild parkinsonism. Responsive to levodopa

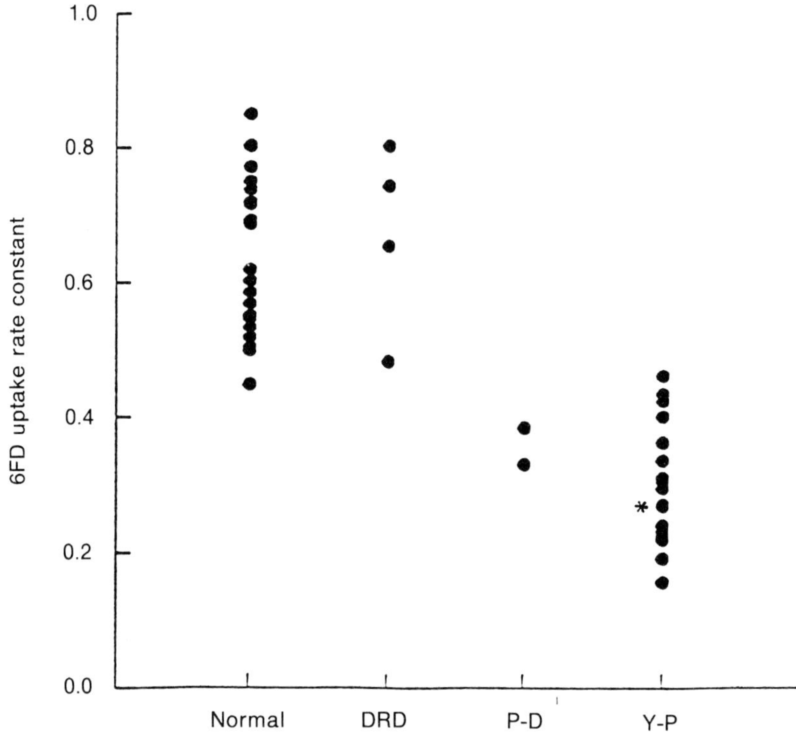

Figure 1 Scatter plots showing 6-fluorodopa (6FD) uptake rate constants (ml/striatum/minute) for each patient group. DRD = dopa-responsive dystonia, P-D = parkinsonism and dystonia, Y-P = young-onset parkinsonism. The asterisk marks patient 7 (see Table 1)

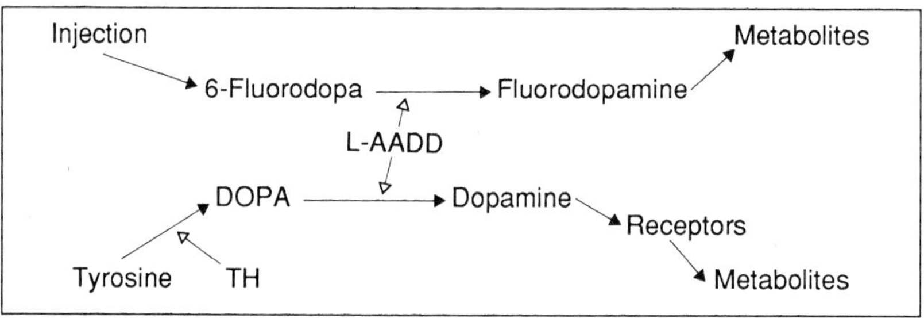

Figure 2 Metabolism of 6FD and endogenous dopamine showing at which steps the two pathways are parallel; L-AAAD = L-aromatic amino acid decarboxylase, TH = tyrosine hydroxylase.

6FD across the blood–brain barrier, decarboxylation to 6-fluorodopamine and its retention in the striatal nerve terminals. The endogenous dopamine pathway differs from the 6FD pathway in that it begins with the metabolism of phenylalanine to tyrosine. Tyrosine is then metabolized to dopa by the rate-limiting enzyme tyrosine hydroxylase. Therefore, a lesion at the level of the hydroxylation of tyrosine may result in a functional dopaminergic deficit and normal 6FD PET. Our PET findings in DRD are consistent with those of cerebrospinal fluid studies that have shown reduced levels of homovanillic acid and tetrahydrobiopterin, the pteridine cofactor of tyrosine hydroxylase[5].

Although 6FD does not completely trace the endogenous dopamine pathway, it is metabolized in a similar way to therapeutic levodopa. Patients with DRD often respond to doses of levodopa that are low compared with those taken by parkinsonian patients[3]. The normal 6FD uptake of our DRD patients implies that their capacity for taking up the levodopa and metabolizing it to dopamine is much higher than in patients with Parkinson disease. Thus the low doses of therapeutic levodopa taken by DRD patients may result in similar, or even greater, levels of dopamine for release into the synaptic cleft than are available to patients with Parkinson disease on standard doses of levodopa.

If DRD patients require such levels of dopamine, why do untreated patients not have more prominent parkinsonism? There is an increased frequency of mild parkinsonism without dystonia in older relatives of patients with DRD[5]. Presumably these patients have the same genetic and dopaminergic deficit as the younger, dystonic patients, and the clinical presentations may relate to different responses to dopamine deficiency at different ages. The basis for these different responses is unclear; although an abnormality at the level of the dopamine receptors would be consistent with the PET and clinical presentations.

The normal 6FD PET findings in DRD patients also explain why they do not develop long-term motor fluctuations on levodopa treatment. The intact vesicular storage mechanism in the nigrostriatal dopaminergic terminals would permit gradual release and steady levels of dopamine in the synaptic cleft. This contrasts with the fluctuating levels that would be experienced by parkinsonian patients with reduced vesicular storage.

To date, the literature has been unclear on whether DRD and young-onset, or juvenile parkinsonism, particularly with onset below 20 years, are distinct conditions[4,15]. Our findings suggest that they are different. The low 6FD uptake in young-onset parkinsonism is consistent with the cell loss from the substantia nigra seen in cases that have come to postmortem examination[15].

Some patients with DRD have more prominent parkinsonism than our subjects. While it is possible that these patients would have low 6FD uptake, we feel this is unlikely. Substantial loss of dopaminergic function is necessary before clinical parkinsonism develops[16]. PET can show even asymptomatic dopaminergic loss[12,13]. We would expect the mild parkinsonism of patients 1 and 3 to be associated with low 6FD uptake if the lesion involved integrity of the dopaminergic pathway, as in Parkinson disease.

The patients with parkinsonism-dystonia had reduced 6FD uptake. The reduction was greater in the striatum contralateral to the more severe parkinsonism, and only the parkinsonian signs responded to levodopa. These findings suggest that the dopaminergic deficit was related to the parkinsonism and not the dystonia. The dystonia of these patients remains to be explained. The suggestion of abnormal dopamine receptor function in DRD is also relevant to this condition.

ACKNOWLEDGEMENTS

The scans were performed with the kind cooperation of the UBC/TRIUMF PET team. Dr Masahiro Nomoto recruited patient 1 for scanning. The studies were supported by the Dystonia Medical Research Foundation and the Medical Research Council of Canada

REFERENCES

1. Rothwell, J.C. and Obeso, J.A. (1987). The anatomical and physiological basis of torsion dystonia. In Marsden, C.D. and Fahn, S. (eds.) *Movement Disorders 2,* pp. 313–31. (London: Butterworths)
2. Marsden, C.D., Obeso, J.A., Zarranz, J.J. and Lang, A.E. (1985). The anatomical basis of symptomatic hemidystonia. *Brain*, **108**, 463–83
3. Segawa, M., Nomura, Y., Tanaka, S., Hakamada, S., Nagata, E., Soda, M. and Kase, M. (1988). Hereditary progressive dystonia with marked diurnal fluctuation – consideration on its pathophysiology based on the characteristics of clinical and polysomnographical findings. In Fahn, S., Marsden, C.D. and Calne, D.B. (eds.) *Advances in Neurology*, Vol. 50, pp. 367–76. (New York: Raven Press)
4. Nygaard, T., Trugman, J.M., de Yebnes, J.G. and Fahn, S. (1990). Dopa-responsive dystonia: the spectrum of clinical manifestations in a large North American family. *Neurology*, **40**, 66–9
5. Nygaard, T.G., Marsden, C.D. and Duvoisin, R.C. (1988). Dopa-responsive dystonia. In Fahn, S., Marsden, C.D. and Calne, D.B. (eds.) *Advances in Neurology*, Vol. 50, pp. 223–9. (New York: Raven Press)
6. Segawa, M., Nomura, Y. and Kase, M. (1986). Hereditary progressive dystonia with marked diurnal fluctuation: clinicopathophysiological identification in reference to juvenile Parkinson's disease. In Yahr, M.D. and Bergman, K.J. (eds.) *Advances in Neurology*, Vol. 45, pp. 227–233. (New York: Raven Press)
7. Rivest, J., Quinn, N. and Marsden, C.D. (1990). Dystonia in Parkinson's disease, multiple system atrophy and progressive supranuclear palsy. *Neurology*, **40**, 1571–8
8. Martin, W.R.W., Palmer, M.R., Patlak, C.S. and Calne, D.B. (1989). Nigrostriatal function in man studied with positron emission tomography. *Ann. Neurol.*, **26**, 535–42
9. Nahmias, C., Garnett, E.S., Firnau, G., Lang, A. (1985). Striatal dopamine distribution in parkinsonian patients during life. *J. Neurol. Sci.*, **69**, 223–30
10. Bhatt, M.H., Snow, B.J., Martin, W.R.W., Cooper, S. and Calne, D.B. (1990). Positron emission tomography in Shy Drager syndrome. *Ann. Neurol.*, **28**, 101–3
11. Guttman, M., Yong, V.W., Kim, S.U., Calne, D.B., Martin, W.R.W., Adam, M.J. and Ruth, R.J. (1988). Asymptomatic striatal dopamine depletion: PET scans in unilateral MPTP monkeys. *Synapse*, **2**, 469–73
12. Calne, D.B., Langston, J.W., Martin, W.R.W., Stoessl, A.J., Ruth, T.J., Adam, M.J., Pate, B.D. and Schulzer, M. (1985). Positron emission tomography after MPTP: observations relating to the cause of Parkinson's disease. *Nature (London)*, **317**, 246–8
13. Snow, B.J., Peppard, R.F., Guttman, M., Okada, J., Martin, W.R.W., Steele, J.C., Eisen, A., Carr, J., Schoenberg, B. and Calne, D.B. (1990). PET scanning demonstrates a presynaptic dopaminergic lesion in Lytico-Bodig (the ALS-PD complex of Guam). *Arch. Neurol.*, **47**, 870–4
14. Adam, M.J. and Jivan, S. (1988). Synthesis and purification of L-[^{18}F]6-fluorodopa. *Int. J. Appl. Radiat. Isot.*, **39**, 1203–6
15. Gershanik, O.S. and Nygaard, T.G. (1990). Parkinson's disease beginning before age 40. In Korczyn, A.D., Melamed, E. and Youdim, M.B.H. (eds.) *Advances in Neurology*, Vol. 53, pp. 251–8 (New York: Raven Press)
16. Bernheimer, H., Birkmayer, W., Horneykiewicz, O., Jellinger, K. and Seitleberger, F. (1973). Brain dopamine and the syndromes of Parkinson and Huntington. *J. Neurol. Sci.*, **20**, 415–55

SECTION 8

Role of the subthalamic nucleus in basal ganglia disorders

15

The role of the subthalamic nucleus in parkinsonism: from pathophysiology to novel non-dopaminergic therapeutic approaches

J.M. Brotchie, I.J. Mitchell, T.Z. Aziz, M.A. Sambrook and A.R. Crossman

INTRODUCTION

In 1817 James Parkinson first described 'shaking palsy' in six patients. In subsequent years parkinsonism became a well-recognized syndrome characterized by paucity of voluntary movements (hypokinesia), rigidity and resting tremor. Parkinsonism still presents a major problem in contemporary neurology clinics, the prevalence in Europe being 1.5 per 1000 of the general population. The prevalence increases with age after the fourth decade of life and parkinsonism affects about 1 per 100 of the population over 60.

In idiopathic parkinsonism, the primary pathological change was first described by Tretakioff in 1919 as being degeneration of the neurons of the substantia nigra pars compacta. These dopaminergic cells project to the striatum. Later is was found that dopamine levels were severely reduced in the striatum of parkinsonian subjects[1]. It is now well established that a deficiency in dopaminergic transmission in the striatum leads to the clinical manifestations of parkinsonism. However, until recently the neural mechanisms mediating these symptoms remained obscure.

NEURAL MECHANISMS UNDERLYING PARKINSONISM: THE CRITICAL ROLE OF THE SUBTHALAMIC NUCLEUS

We have conducted experiments to define the neural mechanisms that accompany parkinsonism in the methyl phenyl tetrahydropyridine (MPTP)-treated primate[2]. We employed the 2-deoxyglucose (2DG) metabolic tracing technique developed by Sokoloff and colleagues[3] to study neural activity in the parkinsonian brain. Metabolic tracing with 2DG provides a means of assessing terminal activity within anatomically discrete brain regions and has also been extremely useful in defining the role of the subthalamic nucleus in a wide variety of dyskinesias[4,5]. Alongside studies using complimentary electrophysiological[6], neurochemical[7] and behavioral techniques[8], 2DG tracing studies have helped to develop a simple model of the alterations in basal ganglia activity that follow lesion of the dopaminergic cells of the substantia nigra and accompany parkinsonian symptoms.

The main points of this model are:

(1) Dopaminergic denervation of the striatum leads to overactivity of the gamma-aminobutyric acid (GABA)ergic striatal outputs to the lateral segment of the globus pallidus.

(2) Lateral pallidal segment neurons are therefore rendered abnormally underactive in the parkinsonian state. The corollary of this abnormal activity is underactivity in the inhibitory pallidosubthalamic connection.

(3) Pallidosubthalamic underactivity leads to disinhibition of the subthalamic nucleus. The subthalamic nucleus is therefore overactive in parkinsonism and there is increased activity in the subthalamic efferents to the medial segment of the globus pallidus.

(4) The outputs of the medial pallidal segment to the thalamus and midbrain tegmentum are also suggested as being overactive in the parkinsonian state.

From this model it was proposed that the subthalamic nucleus was excitatory and provided the driving force behind overactivity of the medial pallidal segment. This model contrasts with the mechanisms thought to underlie the hyperkinetic dyskinesias which represent the antithesis of parkinsonism such as chorea or hemiballism. In these conditions the subthalamic nucleus is known to be underactive or lesioned. The subthalamic nucleus output pathways had traditionally been considered to be inhibitory and to use GABA as their transmitter[9,10]. It has previously been suggested that hemiballism following lesion of the subthalamic nucleus was due to overactivity in basal ganglia outputs from the medial pallidal segment resulting from loss of subthalamic inhibition[11].

We addressed the issue of the nature of subthalamic nucleus outputs in a series of neurochemical studies. In these studies we have presumed the presence of presynaptic uptake mechanisms to be a specific marker for the neurotransmitter released by terminals of a specific neuronal connection. Presynaptic uptake sites for both GABA and excitatory amino-acid (EAA) transmitters were assayed concurrently in regions of the basal ganglia receiving input from the subthalamic nucleus, that is, the globus pallidus and substantia nigra.

Crude synaptosomal membrane preparations were obtained from the brain regions of interest. The membranes were incubated in [^{3}H]-D-aspartate (100 nmol/l) and [^{14}C]-GABA (1 μmol/l) for 30 min (30°C, pH 7.8). The incubation conditions were optimized to allow maximal accumulation of radiolabel by presynaptic uptake mechanisms for EAAs and GABA respectively. Following incubation, unaccumulated radiolabel was removed by cell harvester-mediated filtration. The amount of accumulated radiolabel was measured using dual labelling liquid scintillation counting. The pharmacological profile of the uptake of both radioligands was as expected for uptake of EAA and GABA by their specific uptake sites[12].

Following lesion of the subthalamic nucleus there was a marked decrease in EAA uptake by presynaptic mechanisms in both the globus pallidus (89%) and substantia nigra (90%) (Figure 1). There were, however, no alterations in presynaptic GABA uptake. No changes in either uptake system were seen following lesions of the subthalamic region that did not include the subthalamic nucleus.

These experiments demonstrated that the transmitter used by subthalamic nucleus efferents is not GABA, and is in fact excitatory, using an EAA. Indeed, electrophysiological studies in the rat also identify an excitatory influence of the subthalamic nucleus on the medial pallidal segment[13,14]. These findings are consistent with the report that blockade of EAA transmission in the medial pallidal segment of an otherwise normal monkey

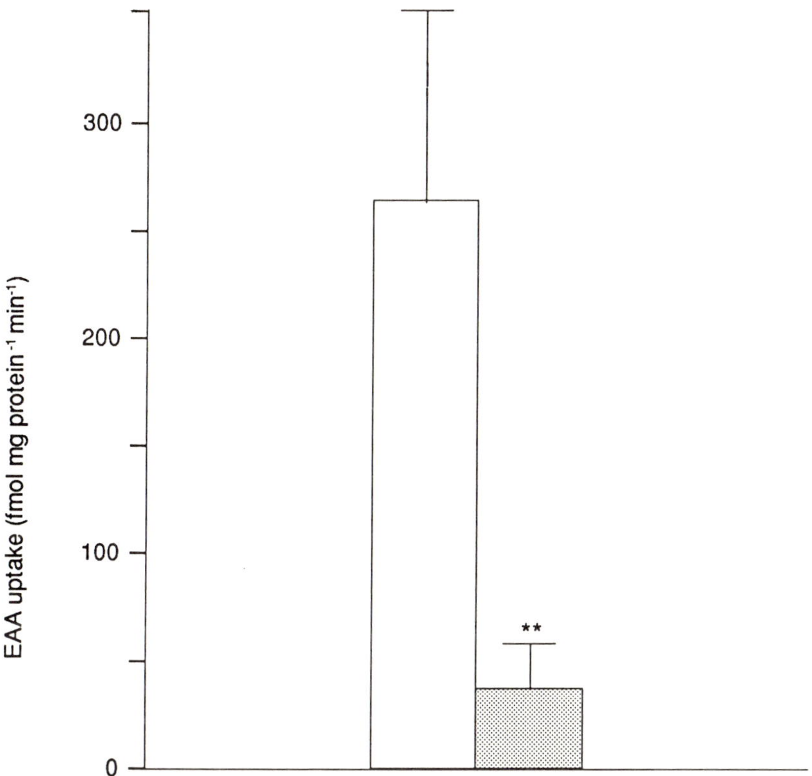

Figure 1 Levels of presynaptic excitatory amino-acid (EAA) uptake, assayed by [^{3}H]-D-aspartate, in the globus pallidus of the rat. Following lesion of the subthalamic nucleus a marked reduction in the level of EAA uptake (shaded bar) is seen in the globus pallidus, compared with control (unlesioned, clear bar); $^{**}p < 0.01$

leads to choreiform or hemiballistic movements[15]. These dyskinesias are very similar to those known to involve lesion of subthalamic nucleus outputs[16–18].

DOPAMINE AGONIST THERAPIES IN PARKINSONISM

In mice, catecholamine depletion following treatment with reserpine causes a severe parkinsonian syndrome. However, in such parkinsonian animals normal motor function can be restored by increasing brain dopamine levels[19]. These studies paved the way for the use of dopamine agonists in the treatment of Parkinson disease. The dopamine precursor, levodopa (L-dopa) was found to be effective in diminishing symptoms when given orally[20]. For over two decades parkinsonian patients worldwide have benefited greatly from the use of dopamine agonist therapies.

Unfortunately, many problems are encountered with dopamine agonist therapy. These can become as incapacitating as the original disease. With time, the control of the patients' response to treatment becomes more unpredictable. This progression culminates in the appearance of dyskinesias[21]. The most debilitating of these include dystonia (this can appear when not on treatment, at peak dose or during the wearing-off of a dose) and chorea (associated with onset and wearing-off of therapeutic effect). Iatrogenic dystonia and chorea cannot be avoided by novel administration protocols, such as chronic intravenous or duodenal infusion[22,23], or slow-release preparations of levodopa. Dyskinesias still appear and may even be more severe[24]. However, there have been proposals that selective D_1 receptor agonists can have antiparkinsonian effects without the appearance of dyskinesias[25].

At present, the levodopa-induced dyskinesias remain a major limitation of the use of dopamine agonist therapy in parkinsonism. Little can be done in terms of dosage regimens to alleviate the dyskinesia without provoking an unacceptable return of akinetic symptoms.

NEURAL MECHANISMS UNDERLYING LEVODOPA-INDUCED DYSTONIA AND DYSKINESIA: A CENTRAL ROLE OF THE SUBTHALAMIC NUCLEUS

Animal studies on levodopa-induced dystonia and chorea have been very few and little is known concerning their pathophysiology. Recently, studies have been conducted in primate models of both levodopa-induced dystonia and chorea to investigate the mechanisms underlying these dyskinesias. In these studies monkeys rendered parkinsonian by the neurotoxin MPTP have received chronic dopamine agonist treatment to alleviate their symptoms. In the parkinsonian primate, as in the patient, dyskinesias appear to be unavoidable sequelae of dopamine agonist therapy[25,26]. We have conducted experiments in the MPTP-treated macaque to investigate the roles of different basal ganglia regions in the production of levodopa-induced dyskinesias. We have employed 2DG metabolic tracing to define the changes in terminal activity that accompany these dyskinesias.

In these experiments cynomolgus monkeys were rendered parkinsonian by MPTP administration (4–22 mg i.v., cumulative doses). A group of parkinsonian animals received regular treatment with dopamine agonists (levodopa plus carbidopa or apomorphine). Such treatment led to the appearance of severe dyskinesias at peak dose which were characterized by either chorea or dystonia. During a period of levodopa-induced dyskinesia, a single bolus injection of [^{3}H]-2DG was given (2–3 mCi/kg, 30 Ci/mmol, i.v.). After 45 min an intravenous overdose of pentobarbitone was given. The brains were frozen rapidly to -45°C. Sections of the brain were cut and exposed to tritium-sensitive film. Autoradiographs were analyzed, optical density measurements being taken in basal ganglia and related regions. Autoradiographs prepared from dystonic and choreic animals were compared with those from MPTP-treated animals treated with levodopa that had not developed dyskinetic side-effects.

The uptake of 2DG, and hence terminal activity, was found to be increased in the subthalamic nucleus of those animals displaying dyskinetic side-effects to dopamine agonist therapy compared to non-dyskinetic animals. However, terminal activity in the medial segment of the globus pallidus and in the basal ganglia-related thalamus was found to be decreased in the dyskinetic animals. The magnitude of these changes in neural activity was greater in dystonic than in choreic animals (Figure 2).

These findings indicate possible neural mechanisms underlying levodopa-induced dystonia and chorea as follows:

(1) Increased terminal activity in the inhibitory pallidosubthalamic pathway leads to underactivity of subthalamic nucleus output neurons.

(2) Decreased activity in the excitatory input from the subthalamic nucleus to the medial pallidal segment causes underactivity in pallidal neurons.

(3) Decreased activity in GABAergic pallidothalamic connections leads to overactivity of thalamic neurons.

These proposed neural mechanisms are interesting as they are very similar to those proposed in other forms of dyskinesia such as hemiballism and chorea due to lateral pallidal manipulations, in that they are characterized by underactive subthalamic nucleus outputs. Also of interest with respect to this model are the recent reports indicating that in the MPTP-treated primate, lesion of the basal ganglia-related thalamus can alleviate levodopa-induced chorea. However, lesion of these areas appears to be incapable of alleviating levodopa-induced dystonia[27]. It is possible that additional, as yet undiscovered, mechanisms are involved in the production of levodopa-induced dystonia.

In summary, it appears that despite attempts of both clinical and basic scientists, dystonia in parkinsonian patients treated with dopamine agonists will remain an intractable and debilitating side-effect. We have therefore, in recent years begun to search for novel therapeutic strategies that would lead

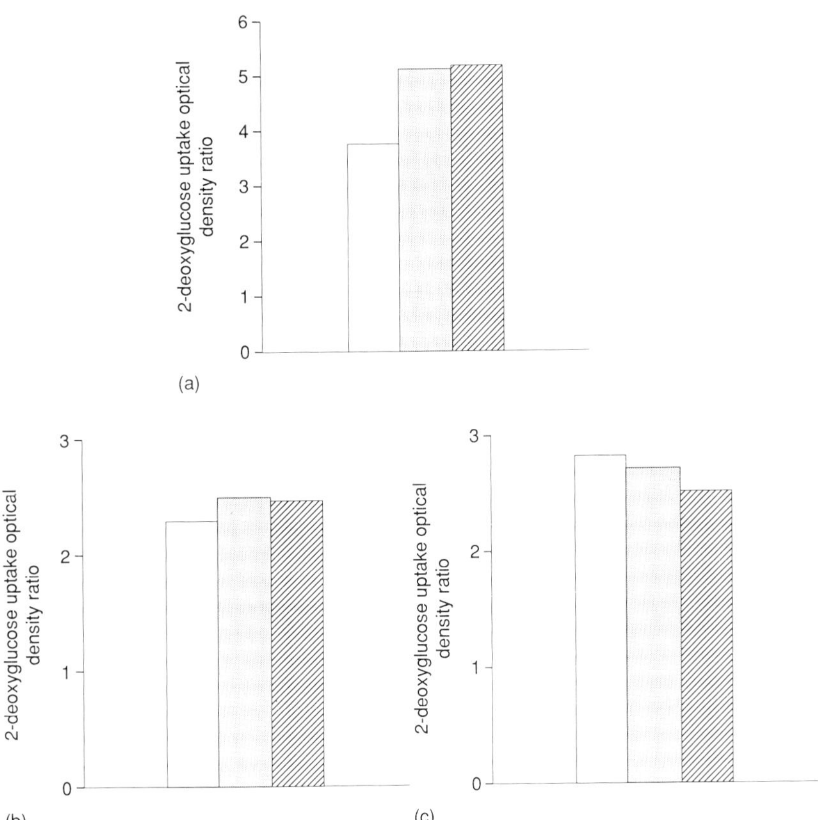

Figure 2 Levels of terminal activity demonstrated by 2-deoxyglucose autoradiography in (a) the subthalamic nucleus; (b) the medial segment of the globus pallidus, and (c) the ventro-anterior/ventro-lateral (VA/VL) thalamus. Uptake of 2-deoxyglucose is shown in parkinsonian animals, treated with levodopa, that were non-dyskinetic (clear bars), showing signs of levodopa-induced chorea (shaded) and dystonia (hatched). The vertical axis, in each graph, is the ratio of the optical density of the region of study to that of the corpus callosum

to a reduction in the reliance on dopamine agonist therapy and might avoid the appearance of dyskinetic side-effects.

ALTERNATIVE APPROACHES TO THE TREATMENT OF PARKINSONISM

The computational processes underlying the control of movement by the basal ganglia remain elusive. However, most schemes suggest a processing of information in a sequential manner taking input from the cortex and sending output to the thalamus[28–30]. In such schemes, the striatum serves as the major input region, whilst the medial segment of the globus pallidus and the substantia nigra pars reticulata serve as the major output centres by virtue of their connections with the thalamus and midbrain tegmentum. Loops within this sequential processing involve both the substantia nigra pars compacta and the subthalamic nucleus.

Dopamine agonist therapy in parkinsonism is generally held to alleviate symptoms by increasing dopamine levels in the input regions of the basal ganglia, mainly the striatum. As such treatment is accompanied by dystonic side-effects we have attempted to define possible therapeutic approaches to parkinsonism that act by manipulating neurotransmission in the output regions of the basal ganglia. Our work has concentrated specifically on the outputs from the medial segment of the globus pallidus.

The subthalamo–pallidal axis: a site of action for novel treatments of parkinsonism?

The realization that parkinsonism was characterized by overactivity of subthalamic nucleus efferents to the medial segment of the globus pallidus, and that these connections use an EAA as transmitter has led to novel approaches for the treatment of parkinsonism. In animal models of parkinsonism we have investigated means by which manipulation of the subthalamic nucleus control of pallidal output might alleviate parkinsonian symptoms.

A neurosurgical approach

It was proposed that lesion of the overactive subthalamic nucleus would reduce subthalamic excitation of the medial pallidal segment and reverse parkinsonian symptoms. Bilateral lesions of the subthalamic nucleus with the excitotoxin ibotenate reverse all the cardinal symptoms in MPTP-treated monkeys[31]. We have taken these important findings as the basis of experiments to assess the possible clinical relevance of subthalamotomy as a treatment for parkinsonism. Our approach has been to employ standard neurosurgical equipment and techniques in MPTP-treated monkeys.

Cynomolgus monkeys were treated with MPTP (2–3 mg/kg i.v., cumulative dose) until a severe, but stable parkinsonian condition equivalent to grade III–IV on the Hoehn and Yahr scale was seen. The clinical state of the animals was assessed using a clinical rating scale (maximum score +16 represented severe parkinsonism, minimum score −8 representing extreme hyperactivity or dyskinesia, a score of zero represented normal behaviour). The clinical rating scale was assessed at 10 min intervals for 50 min on three occasions and summed. Additionally, locomotor activity was monitored by cage-mounted photo-electric activity counters for a 50 min period. Parkinsonism was assessed both pre- and postoperatively. Stereotaxic surgery was performed under general anesthesia using ventriculography-guided stereotaxic procedures. The subthalamic nucleus was lesioned unilaterally

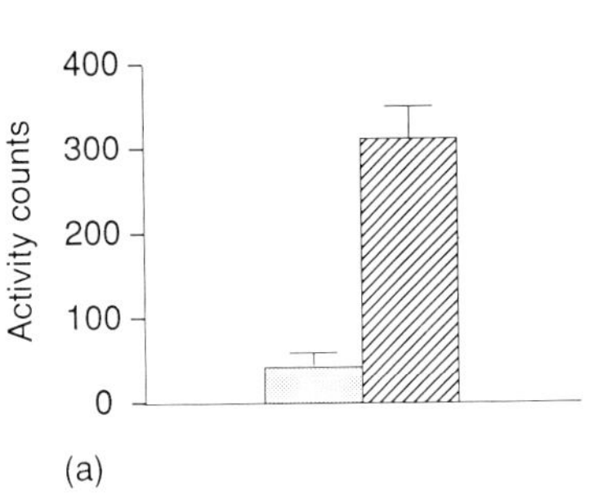

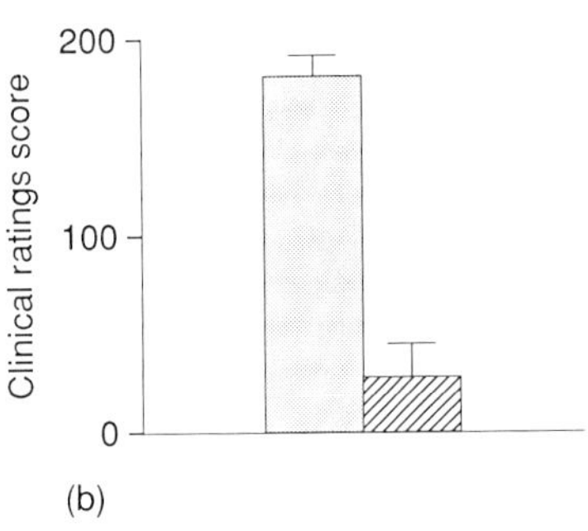

Figure 3 The potent antiparkinsonian effects of unilateral subthalamotomy in the MPTP-treated macaque (shaded bars, MPTP-treated; hatched bars, MPTP treatment followed by lesion of subthalamic nucleus). In (a), activity counts in a 50 min period of assessment are shown. In (b), the total clinical rating score of assessment at 10 min intervals over 3 separate 50 min periods is shown. In both cases data obtained following unilateral subthalamotomy were significantly different to those seen in the untreated parkinsonian state ($p < 0.01$, $n = 6$)

with a standard Radionics radiofrequency lesion generator. The electrode had tip dimensions 2.5 mm × 0.5 mm and the lesioning parameters were 70°C for 2 min. The incision was closed in layers.

Prior to subthalamotomy, all animals were severely parkinsonian. The mean ± SE clinical rating was 181 (± 12.6) per 150 min and mean activity was 46.8 (± 15) counts per 50 min. Following unilateral radiofrequency lesion of the subthalamic nucleus, a marked bilateral improvement of clinical state was seen within 20 h postoperatively. There was a very marked alleviation of akinesia and tremor was abolished. In addition there was a return of facial expression, increased vocalization and the resumption of an erect posture. Parkinsonism as measured by the clinical rating scale was significantly reduced (to 30 ± 19) compared to the preoperative states. Similarly there was a significant increase in locomotor activity measured by the activity counter, mean activity counts being 310 ± 43 ($p < 0.05$) (Figure 3). These potent antiparkinsonian effects of subthalamotomy remained until the animals were killed (up to 6 months postoperatively). A variable degree of contralateral hemiballism was associated with these subthalamic lesions. However, this gradually subsided over a period of a few weeks or months. It is also of interest that in one animal, levodopa-induced dystonia was abolished by unilateral subthalamotomy.

A remarkable finding of this study is that unilateral subthalamic nucleus lesion can cause bilateral reversal of akinesia and tremor.

A pharmacological approach

It was proposed that pharmacological blockade of the overactive EAA-utilizing subthalamic input to the medial pallidal segment would alleviate parkinsonism. This hypothesis was tested in both rat and primate models of parkinsonism by intracerebral microinjection of EAA antagonists directly into the medial pallidal segment.

There are known to be several types of EAA receptor[32]. The most widely accepted classification divides EAA receptors into subtypes selectively activated by and named after the specific agonists N-methyl-D-aspartate (NMDA), α-amino-3-hydroxy-5-methyl-4-isoxazolepropionic acid (AMPA), kainate and trans-1-amino-1,3-cyclopentanedicarboxylic acid (ACPD). The NMDA receptor-operated channels are characterized by having a wide number of regulatory sites, such as the strychnine-insensitive glycine site. In these studies the broad spectrum EAA antagonist kynurenate and a range of subtype-selective antagonists have been used.

Experiments were performed in marmosets and in male Sprague–Dawley rats. Stainless steel cannulae were implanted using standard stereotaxic procedures, under general anesthesia, so as to lie directly above the pallidal complex. Following recovery from this surgery, parkinsonism was induced in the marmosets by administration of MPTP (6 mg/kg i.p.) and by reserpine (5 mg/kg s.c.) in the rats. Following induction of parkinsonism, injection needles were inserted down the cannulae to allow injections of EAA antagonists directly into the medial pallidal segment without the need for anesthetizing the animals. Injections were made bilaterally in the marmosets and unilaterally in the rats. All injection volumes were 0.5 μl. In the MPTP-treated primates, parkinsonism was assessed using a clinical rating scale. On this scale, a score of zero represented a total immobility and very severe parkinsonism, whilst a score of 7 represented clinically normal behavior. In rats, the hypokinesia was assessed by obtaining a locomotor score that was a measure, in arbitrary locomotor units (ALU), of the distance moved by the animal.

In the rat, reserpine administration produced a severe parkinsonian syndrome characterized by paucity of voluntary movements, catalepsy and rigidity. The mean locomotor score for these animals was 4 ± 1 ALU per 15 min. MPTP-treated marmosets exhibited hypokinesia, bradykinesia and rigidity.

In the reserpinized rat and the MPTP-treated marmoset models of parkinsonism, injections of the broad spectrum EAA antagonist kynurenic acid into the medial pallidal segment had a dramatic effect on parkinsonian symptoms. Kynurenate alleviated parkinsonian symptoms reversibly in a dose-dependent manner in both rat and primate models[33] (Figure 4). Following injection of 210 mmol/l kynurenate in the rodent study, the parkinsonian symptoms were alleviated and well-coordinated spontaneous locomotion was observed (locomotor score 206 ALU per 15 min) (Figure 4). Similarly, in the MPTP-treated marmoset, injections of 210 mmol/l kynurenate produced a return to normal behavior. The animals climbed off the floor of the cage and spent much of the time running and jumping from the walls and ceiling of the cage. These antiparkinsonian effects of EAA antagonism were specific to the medial pallidal segment, no antiparkinsonian effects being seen at injection sites in other regions of the basal ganglia or surrounding structures[33].

To delineate the EAA subtype involved in these antiparkinsonian effects of EAA antagonism, injections of subtype-selective antagonists were made. In both the rodent and primate models of parkinsonism, symptoms were

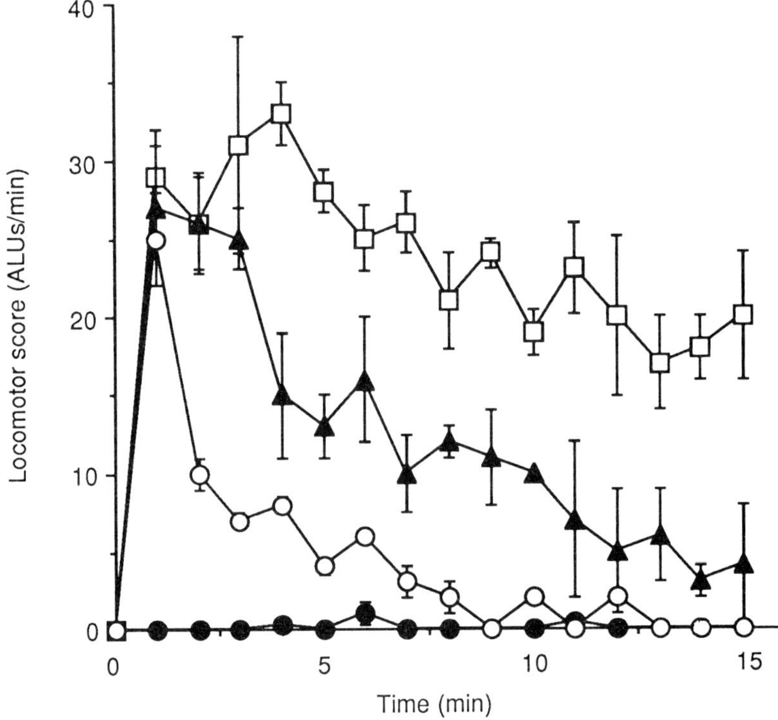

Figure 4 Antiparkinsonian effects of the broad spectrum excitatory amino-acid (EAA) antagonist injected into the medial pallidal segment of the reserpinized rat. The locomotion of reserpinized rats is shown, measured in arbitrary locomotor units per minute (ALUs/min), in each minute following unilateral injection of a variety of kynurenate doses[33]; 210 mmol/l, □; 105 mmol/l, ▲; 53 mmol/l, ○; vehicle, ●

alleviated by both the NMDA receptor-specific antagonist 3-(carboxypiperazin-4-yl)-propyl-1-phosphonic acid (CPP) and the AMPA receptor-selective antagonist 6-cyano-7-nitroquinoxaline-2,3-dione (CNQX). In addition, 7-chlorokynurenate, an antagonist at the NMDA receptor-associated glycine site was a potent and highly effective antiparkinsonian agent in the medial pallidal segment of both rat and primate. The dose–response curves for these antiparkinsonian effects in the MPTP-treated marmoset are shown in Figure 5a.

However, despite its high potency, CPP had a lower efficacy than either 7-chlorokynurenate, CNQX or kynurenate in alleviating parkinsonian symptoms in the MPTP-treated marmoset. At all doses tested, CPP resulted in the appearance of 'anesthetic-like' side-effects (Figure 5b). Anesthetic effects are well known to occur as a result of NMDA antagonism, for example, with ketamine[34]. Such effects probably explain the limited antiparkinsonian actions of CPP in this instance. No anesthetic-like side-effects were seen with either the glycine or AMPA receptor antagonists, and only at the highest doses of the broad spectrum antagonist kynurenate (Figure 5b).

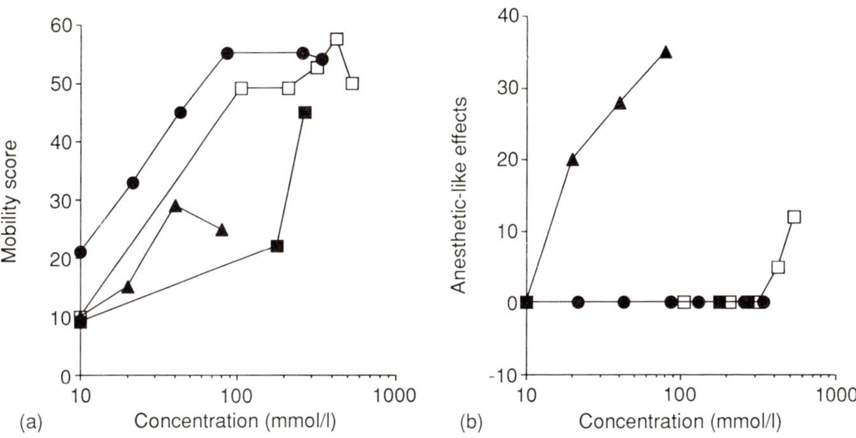

Figure 5 Dose–response curves for (a) the antiparkinsonian, and (b) anesthetic-like effects of excitatory amino-acid (EAA) antagonists in the medial pallidal segment are shown. The compounds tested were: kynurenate (KYN), □; 3-(carboxypiperazin-4-yl)-propyl-1-phosphonic acid (CPP), ▲; 6-cyano-7-nitroquinoxaline-2,3-dione (CNQX), ●; and 7-chlorokynurenate (7-Cl KYN), ■. Values taken are median scores

It therefore appears that blockade of pallidal EAA transmission at either the NMDA receptor-associated glycine site or at the AMPA receptor is an effective means of alleviating parkinsonian symptoms in primate and rat models. The effects of the glycine site antagonist are interesting in that they show that it is possible to block transmission at the NMDA-receptor operated channel without inducing anesthetic side-effects. This finding may be suggestive of two subtypes of NMDA receptor-channel complex, one of which is responsible for the antiparkinsonian effects of NMDA antagonism and is more tightly regulated by the glycine site. Indeed, subtypes of NMDA receptors have recently been described.

In conclusion, these studies show that reversal of overactive subthalamic nucleus inputs to the medial pallidal segment either by subthalamic lesion or by blockade of EAA transmission in the medial pallidal segment can alleviate parkinsonian symptoms. Such approaches may lead to non-dopaminergic treatments for parkinsonism, based on manipulation of basal ganglia outputs. Novel therapies for Parkinson disease would help to reduce our reliance on current dopamine agonist therapies and decrease the incidence of the debilitating side-effects that at present appear unavoidable.

REFERENCES

1. Hornykiewicz, O. (1966). Dopamine and brain function. *Pharmacol. Rev.*, **18**, 925–64
2. Mitchell, I.J., Clarke, C.E., Boyce, S., Robertson, R.G., Peggs, D., Sambrook, M.A. and Crossman, A.R. (1989). Neural mechanisms underlying parkinsonian symptoms based upon regional uptake of 2-deoxyglucose in monkeys exposed to 1-methyl-4-phenyl-1,2,3,6-tetrahydropyridine (MPTP). *Neuroscience*, **32**, 213–26

3. Sokoloff, L., Reivich, M., Kennedy, C., Des Rosiers, M.H., Patlack, C.S., Pettigrew, K.D., Sakurada, O. and Shinohara, M. (1977). The [^{14}C] deoxyglucose method for the measurement of local cerebral glucose utilization: theory, procedure, and normal values in the conscious and anesthetized albino rat. *J. Neurochem.*, **28**, 897–916
4. Mitchell, I.J., Jackson, A., Sambrook, M.A. and Crossman, A.R. (1989). The role of the subthalamic nucleus in experimental chorea: evidence from 2-deoxyglucose metabolic studies and horseradish peroxidase tracing studies. *Brain*, **112**, 1533–48
5. Mitchell, I.J., Jackson, A., Sambrook, M.A. and Crossman, A.R. (1985). Common neural mechanisms in experimental chorea and hemiballismus in the monkey. Evidence from 2-deoxyglucose autoradiography. *Brain Res.*, **339**, 346–50
6. Filion, M., Tremblay, L. and Bedard, P.J. (1988). Abnormal influences of passive limb movement on the activity of globus pallidus neurons in parkinsonian monkeys. *Brain Res.*, **444**, 165–76
7. Pan, H.S., Penney, J.B. and Young, A.B. (1985). γ-amino acid and benzodiazepine receptor changes induced by unilateral 6-hydroxydopamine lesions of the medial forebrain bundle. *J. Neurochem.*, **45**, 1396–404
8. Turski, L., Klockgether, T., Turski, W.A., Schwarz, M. and Sontag, K.-H. (1990). Blockade of excitatory transmission in the globus pallidus induces rigidity and akinesia in the rat: implications for excitatory neurotransmission in the pathogenesis of Parkinson's disease. *Brain Res.*, **512**, 125–31
9. Nauta, H.J.W. and Cuenod, M. (1982). Perikaryal labelling in the subthalamic nucleus following injection of [^{3}H]-gamma amino butyric acid into the pallidal complex: an autoradiographic study in the cat. *Neuroscience*, **7**, 2725–34
10. Shibazaki, T., Hammond, C., Rouzaire-Dubois, B. and Feger, J. (1980). Subthalamic inhibition of identified entopeduncular output neurons in intact and lesioned rats. *Neuroscience Lett.* (Suppl. 5), 538
11. Martin, J.P. and Mccaul, I.R. (1959). Acute hemiballismus treated by ventrolateral thalamolysis. *Brain*, 104–8
12. Brotchie, J.M. and Crossman, A.R. (1991). D-[^{3}H]-aspartate and [^{14}C]-GABA uptake in the basal ganglia of rats following lesions of the subthalamic region suggest a role for excitatory amino-acid but not GABA-mediated transmission in subthalamic nucleus efferents. *Exp. Neurol.*, **113**, 171–81
13. Robledo, P. and Feger, J. (1990). Excitatory influence of rat subthalamic nucleus to substantia nigra pars reticulata and the pallidal complex: electrophysiological data. *Brain Res.*, **518**, 47–54
14. Nakanishi, H., Kita, H. and Kitai, S.T. (1987). Intracellular study of rat substantia nigra pars reticulata neurons in an *in vitro* preparation: electrical membrane properties and response characteristics to subthalamic stimulation. *Brain Res.*, **437**, 45–55
15. Robertson, R.G., Farmery, S.M., Sambrook, M.A. and Crossman, A.R. (1989). Dyskinesia in the primate following injection of an excitatory amino acid antagonist into the medial pallidal segment of the globus pallidus. *Brain Res.*, **476**, 317–22
16. Hammond, C., Feger, J., Biolac, B. and Souteyrend, J.P. (1979). Experimental hemiballismus produced by unilateral kainic acid lesion in the corpus Luysii. *Brain Res.*, **171**, 577–80
17. Whittier, J.R. and Mettler, F.A. (1949). Studies on the subthalamus of the rhesus monkey. II. Hyperkinesia and other physiologic effects of subthalamic lesions, with special reference to the subthalamic nucleus of Luys. *J. Comp. Neurol.*, **90**, 319–72
18. Martin, J.P. (1927). Hemichorea resulting from a local lesion of the brain (syndrome of body of Luys). *Brain*, **50**, 637–51
19. Carlsson, A., Lindquist, M. and Magnusson, T. (1957). 3,4-dihydroxyphenylalanine and 5-hydroxytryptophan as reserpine antagonists. *Nature*, **180**, 1200
20. Cotzias, G.C., Van Woert, M.H. and Schiffer, L.M. (1967). Aromatic amino-acids and modification of parkinsonism. *N. Engl. J. Med.*, **276**, 374–9
21. Nutt, J.G. (1990). Levodopa-induced dyskinesia: Review, observations and speculations. *Neurology*, **40**, 340–45
22. Quinn, N.P., Parkes, J.D. and Marsden, C.D. (1984). Control of on/off phenomenon by continuous intravenous infusion of levodopa. *Neurology*, **34**, 1131–6
23. Lees, A.J. (1989). The on–off phenomenon. *J. Neurol. Neurosurg. Psych.* (Special Suppl.) 29–37

24. Cedarbaum, J.M., Kutt, H. and McDowell, F.H. (1989). A pharmacokinetic and pharmacodynamic comparison of Sinemet CR (50/200) and standard Sinemet (25/100). *Neurology*, **39** (Suppl. 2), 38–44
25. Bedard, P.J., Di Paolo, T., Falardeau, P. and Boucher, R. (1986). Chronic treatment with L-dopa but not bromocriptine induces dyskinesia in MPTP-parkinsonian monkeys. Correlation with [^{3}H]spiperone binding. *Brain Res.*, **379**, 294–9
26. Clarke, C.E., Botce, S., Robertson, R.G., Sambrook, M.A. and Crossman, A.R. (1989). Drug-induced dyskinesia in primates rendered parkinsonian by the ontracarotid administration of MPTP. *J. Neurol. Sci.*, **90**, 307–14
27. Page, R.D. (1990). Thalamotomy to alleviate levodopa induced dyskinesia. *Thesis*, University of London
28. Mitchell, I.J., Brotchie, J.M., Brown, G.D.A. and Crossman, A.R. (1991). Modeling the functional organisation of the basal ganglia: a parallel distributed processing approach. *Movement Disord.*, **6**, 189–204
29. Alexander, G.E. and Crutcher, M.D. (1990). Functional architecture of basal ganglia circuits: neural substrates of parallel processing. *Trends Neurosci.*, **13**, 266–71
30. Alexander, G.E., Delong, M.R. and Strick, P.L. (1986). Parallel organisation of functionally segregated circuits linking basal ganglia and cortex. *Ann. Rev. Neurosci.*, **9**, 357–81
31. Bergman, H., Wichmann, T. and Delong, M.R. (1990). Reversal of experimental parkinsonism by lesions of the subthalamic nucleus. *Science*, **249**, 1436–8
32. Collingridge, G.L. and Lester, R.A.J. (1990). Excitatory amino-acid receptors in the vertebrate central nervous system. *Pharmacol. Rev.*, **40**, 143–210
33. Brotchie, J.M., Mitchell, I.J., Sambrook, M.A. and Crossman, A.R. (1991). Alleviation of parkinsonism by antagonism of excitatory amino-acid transmission in the medial segment of the globus pallidus in rat and primate. *Movement Disord.*, **6**, 133–8
34. Thomson, A.M., West, D.C. and Lodge, D. (1985). An NMDA receptor mediated synapse in rat cerebral cortex: a site of action of ketamine. *Nature*, **313**, 479–81

SECTION 9

General discussion

16

Juvenile parkinsonism with pallidal posture and spastic paraplegia

N. Yanagisawa

INTRODUCTION

The term 'juvenile parkinsonism' has been used to describe a wide variety of motor disorders characterized by akinesia, rigidity and/or dystonia, with relatively young onset[1]. In the effort to delineate disease entities from this vaguely defined syndrome, which may be composed of heterogeneous conditions, a type of young onset dopa-responsive dystonia was proposed as an entity by Segawa and co-workers under the name of 'hereditary progressive dystonia with marked diurnal fluctuation'[2]. Recently, on the other hand, a wider concept of dopa-responsive dystonia was proposed[3] (see also Chapter 7).

As the variety of clinical pictures of parkinsonism and dystonia of young onset is so great, and heterogeneity is assumed, delineation of subtypes of dystonia/parkinsonism of young onset, from various aspects, is needed.

In a neurology meeting in 1968, we described two siblings exhibiting unique extrapyramidal symptoms by the name of 'familial dystonia with rigidity'[4]. Later in 1974 in a Japanese article[5], we described these two cases, and an additional sporadic case, as a syndrome of juvenile parkinsonism with pallidal posture and spastic paraplegia. All of them showed uniform clinical pictures hitherto not reported. Recently, one of these cases came to autopsy and unique changes in the substantia nigra with abnormally less pigmentation of neurons in the compact zone were reported[6,7] (see also Chapter 18).

In this chapter essential parts of the previous descriptions of these cases will be detailed and the nosological position will be discussed from the present knowledge of the related disorders.

CASE RECORDS

Case 1, Ts.O., male

The pedigree of this patient and patient Tk.O. is presented in Figure 1. The youngest brother showed hyperreflexia with ankle clonus on examination in 1967.

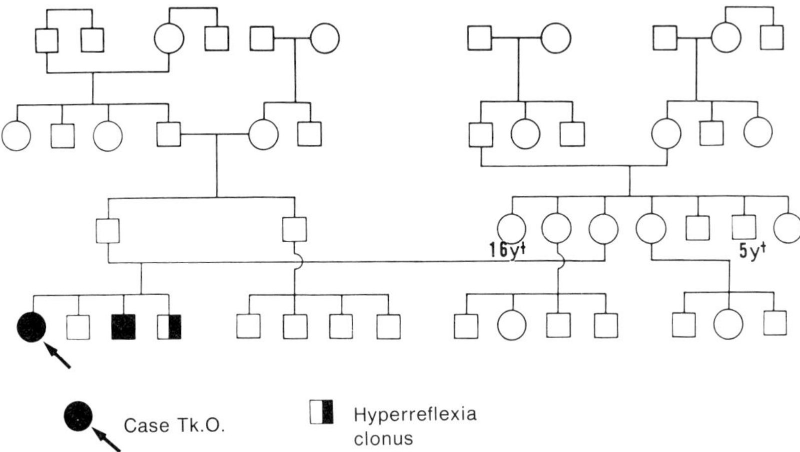

Figure 1 Pedigree of O family

Delivery and development were normal. At 6 years of age, he tended to stumble on running. At 7 years, inversion and plantar extension of the foot developed on walking, and he fell easily with extreme inversion of the foot. These symptoms were worse on fatigue. At 8 years, writing difficulty developed; the arm became stiff while continuing writing. Extension and pronation of the arm developed on psychic tension or with the effort of skilful motion. Around this age, forward bending of the trunk developed and upright standing became impossible.

These symptoms progressed gradually until around 17 years of age, and became stationary thereafter. Marked deterioration was observed in the afternoon or with fatigue. At the age of 18, the patient stood on tiptoe. Thoracic kyphosis, and semiflexion at the elbow and pronation of the hand was a predominant posture. Neurological examination at age 20 showed the following:

(1) Thoracic kyphosis and slight scoliosis convex to left.

(2) Hypertrophy of right sternomastoid, shoulder girdle and arm muscles; diffuse atrophy of lower extremity muscles.

(3) Rigidospasticity in four limbs; pes equinovarus and contracture at the ankle.

(4) Marked hyperreflexia at the knee and ankle. Babinski sign was equivocal.

(5) Tremor with high frequency on voluntary muscular contraction or under postural tension.

(6) Freezing phenomenon on alternating hand movement.

(7) Blephalospasm.

The patient was able to walk a few steps with flexed knees and hips and 'X'

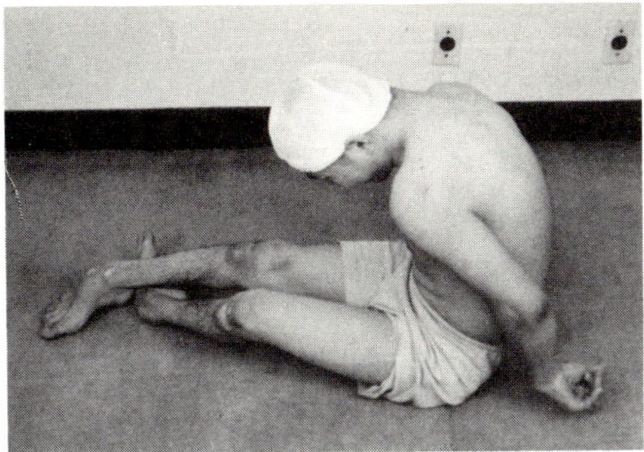
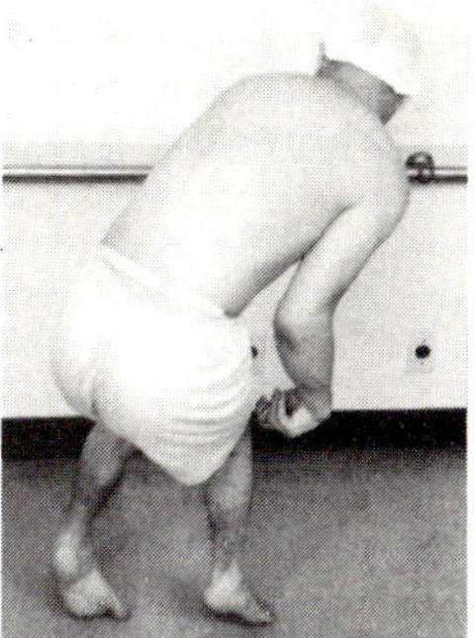

Figure 2 Patient Ts.O. at 20 years of age. Postures when sitting on the floor and standing holding a bar[5]

legs. The postures when sitting on the floor, and standing by holding a bar are shown in Figure 2.

Electromyography at this time disclosed unique characteristics of motor disorders. At rest, small tonic discharges appeared in all extremity muscles tested. In response to muscle stretch, tonic reflex corresponding to rigidity appeared (Figure 3a). Reciprocal innervation was disturbed in rigid muscles (Figure 3b). A unique pattern shown was a high frequency grouping of action potentials at a constant rate of 13 Hz in stretch reflexes and in voluntary contraction, which is apparent in both isometric as well as in isotonic contractions (Figure 4).

Case 2, Tk.O., female

This patient was the elder sister of Ts.O. (Figure 1). Delivery and development were uneventful. At 6 years of age, she stumbled and got tired easily on walking. She was noted to drag her feet. At the age of 7–8, the right lower extremity became stiff and she had difficulty in flexing or extending the foot around the ankle joint. Subsequently the right upper extremity became stiff and difficult to move. She was liable to adopt a posture with extension at the elbow and flexion at the wrist. Around the age of 14, she noticed episodes of generalized hypotonia and loss of power, which recovered after sleep. No relation to medication was noticed, nor was any possible causative factor for these hypotonic episodes noted. From the age of 21, attacks of dizziness with the feeling of an empty stomach appeared which lasted for 1–2 hours. Such attacks of dizziness appeared once or twice a year.

These symptoms progressed gradually. Hypertonia was more marked in the afternoon or with fatigue.

At 26 years of age (1967), we made a neurological examination. The patient developed generalized hypertonia on the effort of purposive movement or of standing. She could stand on tiptoe with a unique posture: head and trunk bent forward, and the arms extended at the elbow and pronated and flexed at the wrist. Flexion at the hip and knee and pes equinovarus was observed.

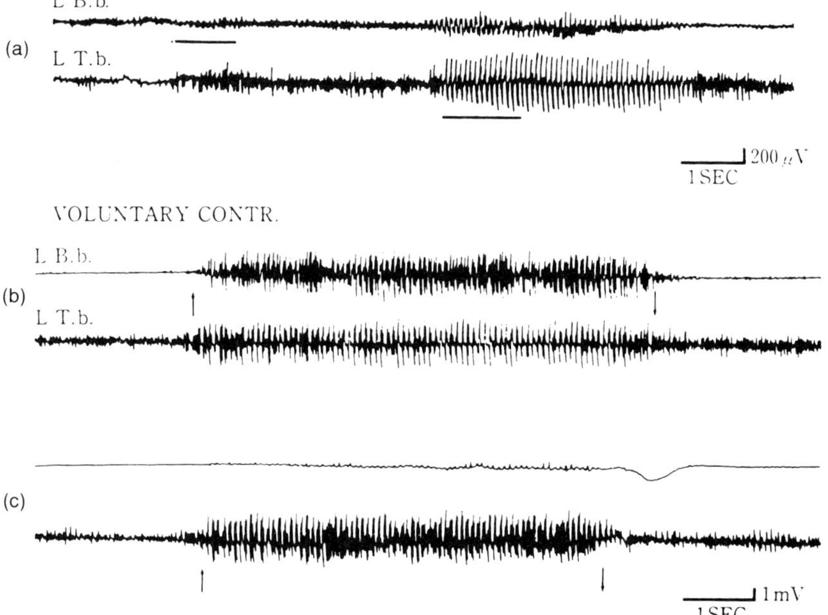

Figure 3 Electromyograph of left arm of patient Ts.O. Simultaneous recording of biceps brachii (B.b.) and triceps brachii (T.b.) muscles. (a) Responses to muscle stretch indicated by a bar under record. Tonic stretch reflex (rigidity) was observed in T.b. (b) and (c). Isometric voluntary contraction during the period indicated by arrows under records. Reciprocal inhibition of antagonist muscle was disturbed in T.b., which was a rigid muscle, but it was maintained well in B.b without rigidity (c). Regular grouping at 13 Hz developed in both reflex and voluntary contractions[5]

This posture was similar to her brother's, Ts.O., but of a milder degree. On standing, fine trembling of the body was observed. Slight atrophy of the lower extremities, and rigidospasticity of both upper and lower extremities was noted. The deep tendon reflex was markedly hyperactive and ankle clonus was present. The big toe was extended at rest, but further extension on stimulation of the sole was not observed (the striatal toe sign). The face was expressionless with half-opened mouth.

Routine laboratory examinations revealed no abnormality. The electroencephalogram was normal with predominant 10 Hz alpha activity. The cerebrospinal fluid was normal in pressure, cell counts and protein content. Pneumoencephalography disclosed no ventricular dilatation. Electromyography showed similar findings to those of the patient's brother, including tonic non-reciprocal discharges in flexors and extensors in the arm and leg. Tonic stretch reflexes in the arm flexors and extensors and voluntary contraction showed high frequency grouping at 12–15 Hz.

I had no chance to follow these siblings after 1967 and both of them were said to have shown a remarkably favorable response to levodopa. The elder

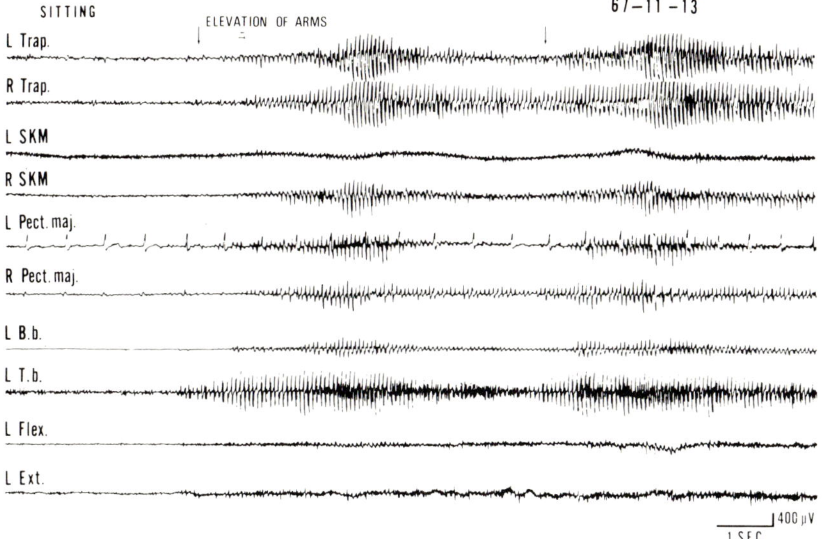

Figure 4 Electromyograph of patient Ts.O. Simultaneous recording of trapezius, sternomastoid, pectoralis major, biceps brachii, triceps brachii, forearm flexor and extensor muscles. With the effort of elevation of arms, regular grouping at 13 Hz developed in shoulder and arm muscles[5]

sister died and was autopsied and the pathology was reported[6]. The younger brother is healthy with minimal motor signs under levodopa treatment and in a normal professional career (Yokochi, personal communication).

Case 3, H.K., male

The family history was non-contributory and there was no consanguinity between the parents. There were no neuropsychiatric disorders in relatives, including two siblings, so far examined.

There was asphyxia for ten minutes on delivery. Physical and mental development were normal.

At the age of 8, this patient felt pain and spasm on the dorsal left foot and showed adduction of the left leg on running. Gradually he dragged the left leg on walking. When I examined the patient 6 months after onset, he noticed stiffness and trembling of the left arm when holding a cup with water.

The patient showed flexed posture on standing with the legs adducted. He walked on tiptoe and could run. The facial expression was normal and Myerson's sign was negative. His speech was normal. Muscle atrophy was noted in the lower legs. Cogwheel rigidity was observed in the flexors and extensors of the upper extremity, and rigidospasticity in the thigh flexors and extensors. The deep tendon reflex was slightly hyperactive in both upper and lower limbs and Babinski sign was positive on both sides. The ankle joint showed contracture with pes equinus. Voluntary movement was generally slow and there was no sign of ataxia. Rigidity and gait disturbance were exaggerated by fatigue and in the late afternoon.

Laboratory tests including ceruloplasmin levels were normal. Electro- and pneumoencephalograms were normal. On cerebrospinal fluid examination, the initial pressure was 320 mmH_2O by lumbar puncture, but cell counts and chemistry were normal.

Levodopa and trihexyphenidyl were only slightly effective at the beginning of administration but the effects did not last. In 1970, he was referred to the Department of Neurology, Tokyo University Hospital. On examination, motor disorders were principally the same as those of 2 years before. Thoracic hyphosis, rigidity in extremities, pes equinovarus and diurnal fluctuation of symptoms were marked, and he could walk with his heels on the floor in the early morning but he could not even stand by himself, due to marked pes equinus, in the afternoon.

He received operations for adductor spasm and Achilles tendon elongation, on both sides, in November 1970 in an orthopaedic clinic, without obvious improvement.

He was referred to the Neurological Clinic in 1973 at the age of 13, and examined. Regarding neurological status, there was no intellectual impairment or psychic symptoms. The face was slightly expressionless and dull with narrow eyelids. On sitting, thoracic kyphosis was marked with head and trunk bent forward (Figure 5). The abdominal muscles showed marked hypertonia. The usual postures showed slight flexion at the elbow, adduction at the wrist and flexion of fingers, flexion at the hip and knee and marked adduction resulting in the knees pressing each other and equinovarus foot (Figure 5).

In the cranial nerve areas, ocular movements were normal but blephalospasm and positive Myerson's sign were noted. Protrusion of the tongue was restricted, and alternating movement of the tongue was limited in range but was regular and fast. Speech was monotonous and fast and articulation was unclear in all sounds. Moderate rigidity was noted in the neck. There was diffuse muscular atrophy in the lower legs. Cogwheel rigidity was generalized in all extremities, but more marked in the upper extremities. Deep tendon

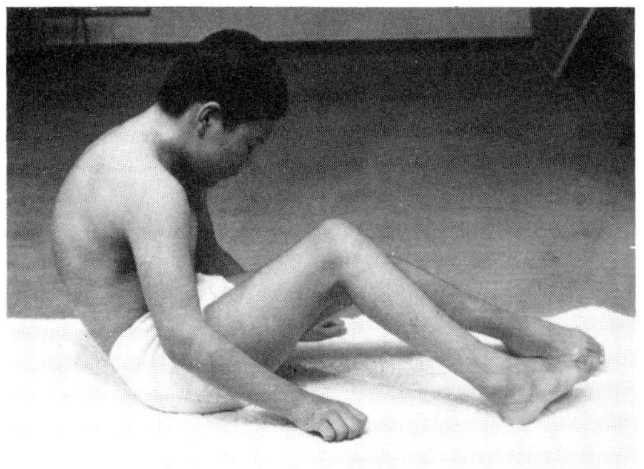

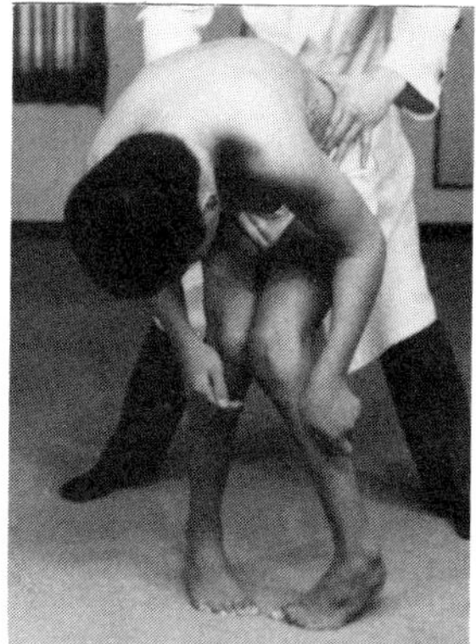

Figure 5 Case H.K. at 13 years of age. Postures when sitting on the floor and standing supported[5]

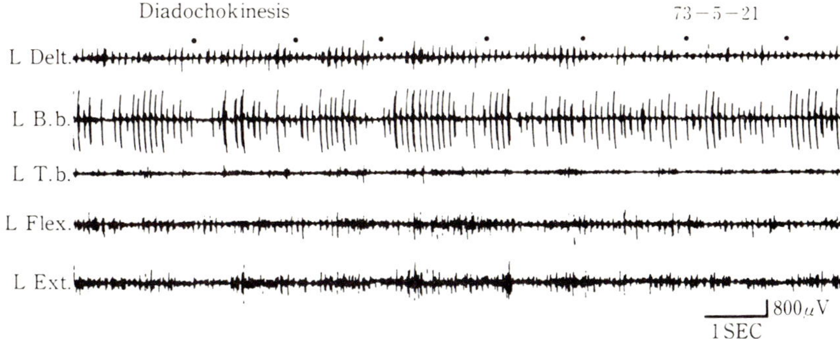

Figure 6 Electromyograph of patient H.K. Simultaneous recording of deltoid, biceps brachii, triceps brachii, forearm flexors and extensors of the left side. The effort of alternating pronation and supination, indicated by dots, developed slow freezing motion with regular grouping of action potentials at 11 Hz[5]

reflex was normal in the arm and the quadriceps and hyperactive at the thigh adductor. Muscle strength with isometric contraction was fair to normal in all limbs. On and off of quick contractions were delayed, and bradykinesia in alternating pronation and supination was marked. Fine tremor was noted in all voluntary contractions. There were no signs of ataxia or sensory disturbance. Electromyography showed distinctive features similar to cases 1 and 2: tonic involuntary contractions, rigidospastic stretch reflexes and regular groupings at 10–12 Hz were observed in both upper and lower extremities (Figure 6).

SUMMARY OF CLINICAL PICTURES

The characteristics of the clinical pictures of the three cases are summarized in Table 1. Parkinsonian features such as masked face, positive Myerson's sign and the freezing phenomenon in arm movement (alternating pronation and supination) were also common findings. However, parkinsonian resting tremor was absent. Muscle atrophy was observed in the lower legs in all three cases, but it was considered as disuse atrophy.

Table 1 Summary of the clinical features of the three cases

Onset at 6–8 years of age and progressive course
Marked bending of head and trunk (pallidal posture), pes equinovarus
Bradykinesia, akinesia
Rigidospasticity in extremities
Hyperreflexia
High frequency (11–15 Hz) grouping of electromyograph on voluntary or reflexive muscular contraction
Diurnal fluctuation of symptoms, marked increase in severity of motor disorders in the afternoon or after physical tasks
No intellectual or psychic impairment

Babinski sign was positive in two patients but in the remaining one (Tk.O.), constant extension of the big toe was observed and it did not respond further to stimuli to the sole, so it was considered as the striatal toe sign. Hyperreflexia was pathological and it was considered as the pyramidal tract sign because ankle clonus was present in patient Tk.O. and the hyperactive adductor reflex was present in patient H.K.

DISCUSSION

The nosological position of the three cases in 1974

In the article of 1974, the common clinical picture of the three cases, hitherto not reported, characterized particularly by marked pallidal posture, as described by Denny-Brown[8], or somersault posture as described by Martin[9], was stressed. This resembles that of animals with bilateral lesions in the globus pallidus, caused either by carbon disulphide intoxication[10] or by electrolysis[11].

Juvenile paralysis agitans[12], progressive pallidal atrophy[13], idiopathic torsion dystonia, Wilson disease, the rigid form of Huntington disease, Hallervorden–Spatz disease and lipidosis were all excluded on the grounds of the clinical features and examinations.

Hereditary dystonia with marked diurnal fluctuation (HPD), as described by Segawa, was indicated by the diurnal fluctuation of symptoms common to the cases under consideration, but our cases did not show the characteristic lumbar lordosis and much lower severity of motor disorders of HPD.

The present nosological position of the three cases, especially patient Tk.O.

Patient Tk.O. came to autopsy, and abnormality of pigmented cells in the compact zone of the substantia nigra was disclosed[7] (see also Chapter 18). There was a decrease in cell population, but a unique, hitherto unreported, finding was uniform depigmentation of the remaining nigral cells.

The unique pathology of patient Tk.O. and the distinctive clinical picture tempt us to consider these cases as a new disease entity.

At this point the relationship between these cases and other parkinsonism or dystonias should be discussed, using our present knowledge. In 1974, juvenile Parkinson disease (paralysis agitans) of the Ramsey Hunt type was differentiated, and the points of differentiation, based on the clinical picture still seem valid. Idiopathic torsion dystonia shows dystonic posture or dystonic movements, including action dystonia, but does not feature rigidity in principle or symmetrical flexion postures as shown in the cases under discussion.

The difference from adult-onset Parkinson disease is obvious. However, variations in the clinical picture of the same disease depending on age should be considered particularly in the basal ganglia disorders. Age-dependent differing characteristics of phenotype of basal ganglia disorders are well-known. This is clearly demonstrated by the young onset rigid form of Huntington's disease and the differing effects of dopa-receptor blocking agents: young subjects show dystonia while elder subjects show chorea/dyskinesia as side-effects of medication for psychiatric disorders.

Yokochi was eager to differentiate clinical types of juvenile parkinsonism[1]. He divided them into three groups, but Yokochi's Type III, which is characterized by dystonia, still shows a wide variety of clinical pictures, and one may infer that it is composed of heterogeneous conditions. The clinical type similar to the present three cases was not included in Yokochi's Type III.

The relation of these three cases to HPD needs further discussion. Segawa has described HPD in this volume based on his observation of 18 patients, of whom 12 were familial from 6 families. The onset of disorders was at 6.0 ± 2.8 years of age, with initial symptoms of fatigability or gait disturbance due to leg dystonia and/or pes equinovarus. Dystonia expanded to all limbs in 5–6 years. The clinical characteristics of HPD at the full-blown stage are as follows:

(1) Postural dystonia, developing from legs to arms. Lumbar lordosis on standing is common, but the patient may adopt a flexed posture on sitting. Retrocollis may exist, but no torsion of the body or neck.

(2) Muscular rigidity, reducing on repetitive muscle stretch.

(3) Postural tremor with frequency at 8–10 Hz, becoming marked after 30 years of age.

(4) Gait disturbance.

(5) Bradykinesia.

(6) Hyperreflexia; no Babinski sign.

(7) Laterality of symptoms, preferring the left side of the body.

The course is progressive for the first two decades, then stationary.

The three cases in the present discussion have some clinical features in common with HPD. However, differences exist between the two conditions regarding the severity of motor disorders, posture and rhythm of tremor. The problem is whether such differences are sufficient to separate these two conditions as different entities. As patient Tk.O. showed a unique pathology which may constitute a disease entity, the relation between the two conditions is crucial. A definite answer cannot be obtained from the information so far available and we should await further researches, especially on gene abnormalities.

For the moment, it seems important to describe the clinical features of Tk.O. and the other two cases in further detail, in order to understand this condition. No case of Segawa's HPD ever developed the severity of generalized rigidity, with atrophy of leg muscles and contracture at the knee and ankle, to the extent of these three cases. Patient Ts.O., the brother of Tk.O., has improved markedly with levodopa and is now engaging in business activity, but he still shows a definite dystonia to an extent which no HPD patients show when under medication (Segawa, personal communication).

The high frequency grouping of the electromyogram of tremor in voluntary, postural or reflex contraction, at a rate of 11–15 Hz is also different from the postural tremor of HPD which may be seen beyond the age of 30. The postural tremor of HPD is in the range 8–10 Hz (see Chapter 1) which is the same range as that of Parkinson disease; the 11–15 Hz grouping does not overlap the parkinsonian tremor. Rather, such high frequency tremor may be observed in young subjects with other basal ganglia disorders, including Hallervorden–Spatz disease[14].

Whether these differences are the expression of different diseases or a matter of degree in the same disease remains to be shown. At present, the record of patient Tk.O. who had loss and depigmentation of nigral cells in the compact zone, and developed unique disorders with a favourable response to levodopa, is valuable for the purpose of clarification of syndromes of dystonia or parkinsonism of young onset.

REFERENCES

1. Yokochi, M. (1979). Juvenile Parkinson's disease – Part I. clinical aspects. *Adv. Neurol. Sci. (Tokyo)*, **23**, 1048–59
2. Segawa, M., Hosaka, A., Miyagawa, F., Nomura, Y. and Imai, H. (1976). Hereditary progressive dystonia with marked diurnal fluctuation. In Eldridge, R. and Fahn, S. (eds.) *Adv. Neurol., Vol. 14: Dystonia*, pp. 215–33. (New York: Raven Press)
3. Nygaard, T.G. and Duvoisin, R.C. (1986). Hereditary dystonia parkinsonism syndrome of juvenile onset. *Neurology*, **36**, 1424–8
4. Toyokura, Y. and Yanagisawa, N. (1968). Familial dystonia with rigidity. Presented at *4th Conference on Neurological Medicine*, Nagoya, January
5. Yanagisawa, N. (1974). Equilibrium, postural mechanisms and the extrapyramidal system. *Adv. Neurol. Sci. (Tokyo)*, **18**, 767–78
6. Narabayashi, H., Yokochi, M., Iizuka, R. and Nagatsu, T. (1986). Juvenile parkinsonism. In Vinken, P.J., Bruyn, G.W. and Klawans, H.L. (eds.) *Handbook of Clinical Neurology*, Vol. 5 (49), pp. 153–65. (Amsterdam: Elsevier Science Publishers)
7. Gibb, W.R.G., Narabayashi, H., Yokochi, M., Iizuka, R. and Lees, A.J. (1991). New pathologic observations in juvenile onset parkinsonism with dystonia. *Neurology*, **41**, 820–2
8. Denny-Brown, D. (1962). *The Basal Ganglia and Their Relation to Disorders of Movement.* (London: Oxford University Press)
9. Martin, J.P. (1967). *The Basal Ganglia and Posture.* (London: Pitman Medical)
10. Richter, R. (1945). Degeneration of the basal ganglia in monkeys from chronic carbon disulfide poisoning. *J. Neuropath. Exp. Neurol.*, **4**, 324–53
11. Denny-Brown, D. and Yanagisawa, N. (1976). The role of the basal ganglia in the initiation of movement. In Yahr, M.D. (ed.) *The Basal Ganglia*, pp. 115–49. (New York: Raven Press)
12. Hunt, R. (1917). Progressive atrophy of the globus pallidus (primary atrophy of the pallidal system). *Brain*, **40**, 58–148
13. Jellinger, K. (1968). Progressive Pallidumatrophie. *J. Neurol. Sci.*, **6**, 19–44
14. Yanagisawa, N., Shiraki, H., Minakawa, M. and Narabayashi, H. (1966). Clinico-pathological and histochemical studies of Hallervorden–Spatz disease with torsion dystonia with special reference to diagnostic criteria of the disease from the clinico-pathological viewpoint. In Tokizane, T. and Schadé, J.P. (eds.) *Progress in Brain Research*, Vol. 21B, *Correlative Neurosciences part B: Clinical Studies*, pp. 373–425. (Amsterdam: Elsevier)

17

The distinction between early onset idiopathic parkinsonism (juvenile Parkinson disease) and dopa-responsive dystonia (hereditary progressive dystonia, Segawa dystonia)

D.B. Calne, T.G. Nygaard and B.J. Snow

In previous papers[1,2] evidence has been presented unifying the nosology of dopa-responsive dystonia and hereditary progressive dystonia.

THE PROBLEM

In recent years it has become recognized that a number of children present with any or all of the following clinical features:

(1) dystonia
(2) rigidity
(3) bradykinesia
(4) diurnal variation of symptoms
(5) dominant family history
(6) therapeutic response to levodopa.

The accumulated evidence indicates that this constellation of findings can generally be resolved into two diagnostic categories, with quite different prognostic implications.

TWO DISORDERS

The two diagnostic options are:

(1) dopa-responsive dystonia (DRD), also termed hereditary progressive dystonia, or Segawa dystonia, and

(2) early onset idiopathic parkinsonism, juvenile Parkinson disease, idiopathic dystonia-parkinsonism, hereafter referred to as EOIP.

The problem is most evident in the first decade of life. Thereafter, the possibility of unusually old cases of DRD or exceptionally young patients with idiopathic parkinsonism is often easier to resolve.

There is no firm evidence to separate EOIP from the general spectrum of idiopathic parkinsonism (Parkinson disease). It is well established that various features of a neurological disorder will vary with the age of onset. This heterogeneity is exemplified by the young-onset, rigid form of Huntington disease (the Westphal variant). By analogy, EOIP is characterized by a number of differences from late-onset disease. The most distinctive, that has contributed to much previous confusion, is the greater frequency and prominence of dystonia in untreated cases of young versus elderly patients with idiopathic parkinsonism.

DIFFERENTIAL DIAGNOSIS

Much of the previous confusion has derived from some rather surprising overlap between DRD and EOIP. Features that are often considered a hallmark for DRD, such as diurnal variation, are also seen in EOIP, and vice versa.

The classical studies delineating DRD were undertaken by Segawa and colleagues[3–6], while those for EOIP were documented by Narabayashi, Yokochi, Yoshimura and colleagues[7–9]. Much of the recent evidence that contributes to a resolution of the complexity derives from the work of Nygaard and colleagues[1] and Snow and colleagues[2]. In the light of the knowledge gained from these and other studies, it is now possible to discern the relative diagnostic importance of the various features of each condition. It is equally significant that we can identify features hitherto regarded as carrying substantial diagnostic weight, which may now be regarded as having rather limited value.

The present situation is conveniently summarized in tabular form. Table 1 shows the diagnostic features that have considerable significance. The weaker discriminants include dystonia, diurnal variation, family history and hyperreflexia.

Table 1 Diagnostic discriminants

Dopa-responsive dystonia	*Early onset idiopathic parkinsonism*
Onset first decade	onset 1st–4th decade
Progressive 1st–2nd decade	progressive through life
Increasing doses of dopa not required	increasing doses of dopa are required
Stable response to dopa	fluctuating response to dopa
Negligible dopa dyskinesia	prominent dopa dyskinesia
Normal flurodopa-PET	reduced fluorodopa-PET
Predominantly female	predominantly male
Seldom resting tremor	often resting tremor

DIFFERENCES IN PROGNOSIS AND THEIR IMPLICATIONS

DRD responds extremely well to low doses of dopaminomimetics over long periods of time. EOIP is an inexorably progressive illness, although the rate of advance is slower in young versus elderly patients[10,11]. EOIP becomes difficult to manage because major therapeutic problems develop, in particular, dyskinesia, severe fluctuations in response, and psychiatric reactions to medications. The natural history and fluorodopa positron-emission tomography (PET) suggest that DRD is associated with dopaminergic dysfunction in the nigrostriatal pathway, involving either reduced synthesis of dopamine or altered receptor numbers or affinity, without any great depletion of dopaminergic neurons[2]. In contrast, EOIP seems to have all the findings expected of a progressive, inexorable loss of neurons from the dopaminergic nigrostriatal pathway[2]. Unfortunately, pathological observations are limited.

THE FUTURE

Further information is needed to confirm or refute these proposals. In particular, we can expect the answers to come from new observations in the fields of molecular biology, pathology (morphometric, neurochemical, and immunocytochemical), and positron emission tomography (with dopamine receptor ligands and, if possible, a marker for tyrosine hydroxylase).

REFERENCES

1. Nygaard, T.G., Snow, B.J., Fahn, S. and Calne, D.B. (1990). Dopa-responsive dystonia: clinical characteristics and definition. Presented at the *Symposium of Hereditary Progressive Dystonia*, November, Tokyo
2. Snow, B.J., Okada, A., Martin, W.R.W., Duvoisin, R.C. and Calne, D.B. (1990). PET scanning in dopa-responsive dystonia, parkinsonism-dystonia, and young-onset parkinsonism. Presented at the *Symposium of Hereditary Progressive Dystonia*, November, Tokyo
3. Segawa, M., Nomura, Y., Yamashita, S., Kase, M., Nishiyama, N., Yukishita, S., Ohta, H., Nagata, K. and Hosaka, A. (1990). Long-term effects of L-dopa on hereditary progressive dystonia with marked diurnal fluctuation. In Berardelli, A., Benecke, R., Manfredi, M. and Marsden, C.D. (eds.) *Motor Disturbances II*, pp. 306–18. (London: Academic Press)
4. Segawa, M., Nomura, Y., Tanaka, S., Hakamada, S., Nagata, E., Soda, M. and Kase, M. (1988). Hereditary progressive dystonia with marked diurnal fluctuation – Consideration on its pathophysiology based on the characteristics of clinical and polysomnographical findings. In Fahn, S., Marsden, C.D. and Calne, D.B. (eds.) *Advances in Neurology*, Vol. 50, pp. 367–76. (New York: Raven Press)
5. Segawa, M., Nomura, Y. and Kase, M. (1986). Hereditary progressive dystonia with marked diurnal fluctuation: Clinicopathophysiological identification in reference to juvenile Parkinson's disease. In Yahr, M.D. and Bergmann, K.J. (eds.) *Advances in Neurology*, Vol. 45, pp. 227–33. (New York: Raven Press)
6. Segawa, M., Hosaka, A., Miyagawa, F., Nomura, Y. and Imai, H. (1976). Hereditary progressive dystonia with marked diurnal fluctuation. In Eldridge, R. and Fahn, S. (eds.) *Advances in Neurology*, Vol. 14, pp. 215–33. (New York: Raven Press)
7. Yokochi, M., Narabayashi, H., Iizuka, R. and Nagatsu, T. (1984). Juvenile parkinsonism – some clinical, pharmacological, and neuropathological aspects. In Hassler, R.G. and Christ, J.F. (eds.) *Advances in Neurology*, Vol. 40, pp. 407–13. (New York: Raven Press)

8. Yoshimura, N., Yoshimura, I., Asada, M., Hayashi, S., Fukushima, Y., Sato, T. and Kudo, H. (1988). Juvenile Parkinson's disease with widespread Lewy bodies in the brain. *Acta Neuropathol.*, **77**, 213–18
9. Narabayashi, H., Yokochi, M., Iizuka, R. and Nagatsu, T. (1986). Juvenile parkinsonism. In Vinken, P.J., Bruyn, G.W. and Klawans, H.L. (eds.) *Handbook of Clinical Neurology*, Vol. 49, pp. 153–65. (Amsterdam: Elsevier Science)
10. DeJong, D., and Delisle Burns, J. (1967). Parkinson's disease – a random process. *Can. Med. Assoc. J.*, **97**, 49–56
11. Diamond, S.G., Markham, M.D., Hoehn, M.M., McDowell, F.H. and Muenter, M.D. (1989). Effect of age at onset on progression and mortality in Parkinson's disease. *Neurology*, **39**, 1187–90

18

A case of nigrostriatal dopamine deficiency of juvenile onset

H. Narabayashi

INTRODUCTION

Parkinson disease is defined today as a condition, idiopathic and slowly progressive in nature, presenting a mixture of various grades of rigidity, tremor and akinesia, and showing levodopa responsiveness. All these criteria indicate the slowly progressive deterioration of the nigrostriatal dopaminergic system.

The term juvenile parkinsonism has been used by Yokochi[1,2] and Narabayashi[3] to describe the cases with parkinsonian symptoms starting before the age of 40, where onset is much earlier than that of classical Parkinson disease, in which the symptoms first start after around the age of 50. Although 'juvenile' has customarily been used for cases of various diseases occurring in the first and second decades of life, this term applied to parkinsonism seems not so narrow in usage.

'Early starting' parkinsonism is another term used to describe the cases starting earlier than Parkinson disease. The border between the earlier starting cases and juvenile parkinsonism is also not strictly defined. Some authors[4–13] propose use of the term 'juvenile' for the cases starting below the age of 20 and 'early starting' for the cases starting after 20, although the borderline between the two groups cannot be clearly defined.

The important point is whether differences can definitely be seen in the clinical pictures, course of the disease and also in neuropathology between these two groups of cases. Some authors have described differences between the two, but others have reported difficulty in differentiating between them.

Obviously we should be extremely careful about the possible heterogeneity in etiology of earlier starting cases, especially in cases with very early onset. Progressive pallidal atrophy of Hunt[6] might be one example. These days, response to levodopa can be used to differentiate whether the condition is due to nigrostriatal dopamine deficiency and to exclude pathology in the striatal or the pallidal neurons. Dopa-responsiveness is taken as one of the essential conditions to define Parkinson disease and also juvenile parkinsonism.

The following is a case of juvenile onset that fits the criteria of Parkinson disease, as described at the beginning of this paper and seems important to help us understand the various manifestations of the nigrostriatal dopamine deficiency.

CASE T.O.

This patient was a woman, who died when 39 years old. In her case the disease started around the age of 6 years. The initial symptom was slight foot-dystonia with difficulty in walking, more on the right, which spread very slowly to the other side of the body and trunk. The difficulty was relatively slight in the morning after sleep and worse in the afternoon. The patient was first seen by the author at the age of 24, when she could neither stand nor walk and was almost bedridden in the afternoon, although she was a little better in the morning. In the supine position, the main feature was severe rigidity, which was diffuse in the four extremities and trunk and was accompanied by slight dystonic posture of the trunk and inversion of the feet, more on the right side than on the left. In the sitting position the patient's posture was abnormal, with her trunk bent forward, head drooped, and the right arm externally rotated at the shoulder.

At that time only anticholinergics were available, and they produced no noticeable change. Left-sided stereotaxic thalamotomy, performed at the age of 24, markedly reduced rigidity on the right side of the body; and this positive effect lasted for thirteen years. However, with unilateral surgery, improvement of activity in daily life was not marked. Her response to levodopa, when it became commercially available in Japan in early 1970, was remarkable, as the drug had an almost normalizing effect. However, within 1 year very severe dopa-induced dyskinesia appeared, with choreo-ballistic-type movement of extremities and trunk, which was observed only on the unoperated side and was induced by only 0.3 g of levodopa alone. As a result, continuation of medication became almost impossible. Application of a high dose of bromocriptine produced no change.

With the aim of abolishing dyskinesia on the left side of the body, right-sided microthalamotomy was performed at the age of 37. After the surgery, rigidity and drug-induced dyskinesia totally disappeared on both sides, and the medication of small doses of levodopa and bromocriptine was enough to produce smooth improvement and almost normalized activity in daily life. Thereafter, she spent the remainder of her life in the coutryside, being almost normal physically and mentally, using about 1.0 g of levodopa alone, and enjoyed life writing Japanese traditional poems, until her death at the age of 39 due to paralytic ileus and peritonitis.

Neuropathological findings can be summarized as follows: macroscopically, pigmentation of the nigral area was not seen, similarly to Parkinson disease. However, as judged from light microscopy, neuronal loss of the compact zone of the substantia nigra was slight, especially when the long duration (32 years) of the disease is considered. The remaining neurons there contained almost no melanin pigment but did have some Lewy bodies; and the shape of the neurons was round, resembling those of a child's brain.

These findings were described elsewhere by the author and his colleagues.

Although these pigmentless neurons within the substantia nigra compact zone were relatively well preserved, the grade of neuronal degeneration was different between the ventrolateral part and the medial part of the compact zone[14]. More severe glial fiber proliferation was evident by glial fibrillary acidic protein staining within the former area than in the latter. Such regional difference in pathology within the substantia nigra compact zone is quite interesting and will be discussed below.

DISCUSSION

Today, Parkinson disease is defined as a disorder due to a dopamine deficiency within the striatum, that is caused by nigral degeneration and occurs mostly in the elderly. The triad of rigidity, tremor and akinesia, are symptoms interpreted on the basis of this pathology. Progressive worsening of the clinical picture is also interpreted as the result of nigral neuronal loss becoming more severe. This specific case of T.O. is interesting and important for elucidating in more detail the pattern of degeneration within the substantia nigra as well as for explaining the reason for the progressive worsening of clinical symptoms.

The clinical picture of the case was quite characteristic: juvenile onset, starting with dystonic signs of the feet, and very slow progression, finally reaching the almost bedridden state. Rigidity in the later stage, that is, during admission for the second-side surgery, was accompanied by cogwheeling. Difficulty of voluntary movement was due to diffuse rigidity. Tremor was almost absent unless the patient was trying to perform difficult and delicate purposeful movements. Improvement by levodopa therapy was quite marked and even dramatic, but was soon followed by the severest grade of dyskinesia, which finally could be controlled by microelectrode thalamotomy[15]. All these clinical features strongly indicate that the condition was due to nigrostriatal dopamine deficiency as in Parkinson disease and that such biochemical changes could start at a much earlier age than in Parkinson disease.

Pathology was also similar to that of Parkinson disease: neuropathological findings, decoloration of the nigral area and loss, or non-existence, of melanin pigment were similar to those seen in Parkinson disease. There were a few Lewy bodies, and the population of substantia nigra compact zone neurons was abnormally low, although not severely depleted. Relative cell loss was more severe in the ventrolateral part of the substantia nigra compact zone, from where the projection goes mainly to the putamen, and less in the medial part, which mainly sends projections to the caudate nucleus. Such a regional difference in pathology within the substantia nigra compact zone is characteristic in Parkinson disease brains, as described by several authors[16,17], and may again indicate that a similar pathological process could possibly occur in the substantia nigra compact zone of the juvenile onset case.

From these clinical and neuropathological findings, the patient was interpreted as a case of nigrostriatal dopamine deficiency syndrome similar to Parkinson's disease, but of juvenile-onset.

Akinesia in this case was interpreted as mostly secondary akinesia due to rigidity, and primary akinesia was minimally involved[18,19]. Bilateral surgical intervention, with a 13-year interval between the two procedures, alleviated the rigidity and secondary akinesia almost completely, as well as the drug-induced dyskinesia on both sides. Postoperatively the patient could manage to stand and to walk slowly alone without medicine. The dose of levodopa necessary to improve the remaining difficulty, which was interpreted as the primary akinesia and different from the secondary one, became almost half of the preoperative dose. This suggests that the main reason of motor difficulty in this case was rigidity or dystonic-rigid state of the muscles. The role of the primary akinesia was judged to be minimal.

Rigidity and primary akinesia may have a different anatomical basis, as discussed in the following paragraphs.

As already described by several authors, microelectrode stereotaxic surgery on the ventrolateral nucleus of the thalamus alleviates almost completely the rigidity and secondary akinesia in parkinsonism by lesioning the pallido-thalamic projection at its end-point, but not the primary akinesia. Thus rigidity and primary akinesia are considered to be two different symptoms depending on different anatomical substrates, although both may belong to the nigrostriatal dopamine deficiency syndrome. Since the cell loss and the glial reaction in this case were prominent in the ventrolateral part of the substantia nigra compact zone and much less so in the dorsomedial part, rigidity, which was alleviated by surgery, might mainly be the consequence of pathology of the former part projecting to the putamen.

The role of primary akinesia in this case was taken to be small, and this akinesia is suspected to have been related to involvement of the nigrocaudal projection, where the pathology was less severe.

It is well established that the pallido-thalamic projection is the main exit of the extrapyramidal impulses, mostly originating in the putamen, subthalamic nucleus and pallidum. The projection for primary akinesia is still not clearly explained, but the caudate nucleus is assumed to be most responsible for this symptom.

Figure 1 illustrates the schema of the neuronal network underlying the nigrostriatum, proposed by the author as a kind of working hypothesis. Nigroputaminal and nigrocaudal projections are differently represented. Intensive anatomical, physiological and pharmacological studies are currently being carried out on these two divisions of the nigrostriatal projections.

Long-term (3–8 years postoperative) follow-up of 162 patients with unilateral or bilateral operation was reported by the author[20]. Of these, 10 (6%) became drug-free postoperatively for 4–8 years. Seven of them were hemiparkinsonism cases, two were of earlier onset with bilateral operation, and one was a tremor-type case. All of the other patients still require, and take, levodopa by the same or a little lower dose than preoperatively. From a review of these postoperative drug-free cases, the common feature, except in the one case of tremor as the dominant symptom, is that most of the cases were still in a relatively early stage of the disease, that is, stage I or II of the Hoehn-Yahr classification, at the time of the operation, or were cases of

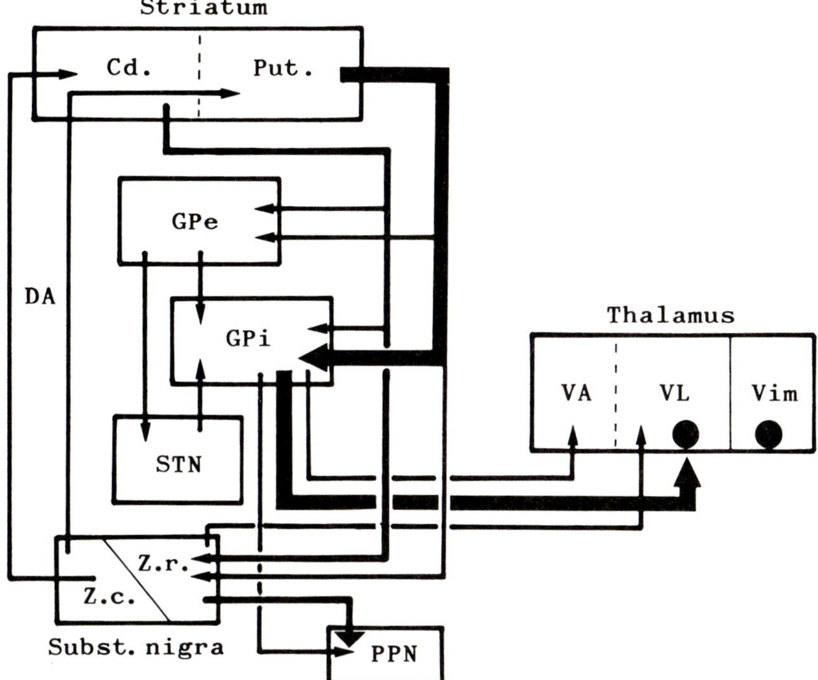

Figure 1 Diagram of the outflow from the nigrostriatum, proposed by the author. Cd., caudate nucleus; Put., putamen; Gpe, external segment of globus pallidus; GPi, internal segment of globus pallidus; STN, subthalamic nucleus; Z.r., reticular zone of the substantia nigra; Z.c., compact zone of the substantia nigra; VA, ventral anterior nucleus; VL, ventrolateral nucleus; Vim, ventral intermediate nucleus; PPN, pedunculopontine nucleus

younger onset. In these cases difficulty of movement can be ascribed as more due to rigidity. After exact surgical intervention, which was enough to eliminate rigidity, tremor and akinesia, the need for levodopa became absent or much less, as seen in patient T.O. in whom pathological changes were more prominent in the nigroputaminal tract, with less involvement of the nigrocaudal tract.

These findings and analyses seem to be important to understand the progression and worsening of the clinical picture in Parkinson disease patients[21]. It is always observed in parkinsonian patients that the first sign of the disease starts from one extremity on one side of the body and then slowly progresses to the other side. In the first step of the disease, pathology may be limited to the nigroputaminal projection, presenting mostly as rigidity, tremor and the secondary akinesia. Surgical treatment would be enough to alleviate all motor symptoms, and patients in this stage often become drug-free postoperatively.

When the clinical picture involves bilateral extremities and trunk and more akinesia with slight difficulty of postural control, the nigrocaudal pathology may have begun. In this stage, a certain dose of levodopa becomes necessary, even after improvement by surgical treatment. Most of the cases of surgical treatment with the aim of alleviating rigidity and tremor belong to this stage. Hughes and colleagues[22] clearly stated that akinesia is not changed for better or worse by ventrolateral thalamic surgery, and that the levodopa effect is similar on both operated and non-operated sides.

Furthermore, the locus ceruleus, the norepinephrine system, will also be added to the pathology with related clinical symptoms in the more advanced stage. This has been described elsewhere in detail[23–5] and will not be discussed further.

It is noteworthy that the speed of progression seems to differ according to the age of patients. In the younger-starting cases, progression in clinical symptoms seems to be slower, suggesting pathology remaining within the dopamine system. In the present case, the patient could remain in an almost normal condition under treatment with a small dose of medicine after bilateral surgical procedure. Many of the younger patients can stay in the highly improved state or become almost normalized when pharmacological therapy, by levodopa and dopamine agonists, and/or surgical therapy is carefully and successfully applied. In contrast, elderly patients tend to deteriorate continuously even after similar improvement by these therapeutic efforts.

In conclusion, careful observation of clinical pictures and responses to either pharmacological or surgical treatment over the long term is important for an understanding of the progressive worsening of the clinical picture and spread of the pathological process in Parkinson disease.

REFERENCES

1. Yokochi, M. (1979). Juvenile Parkinson's disease. 1. Clinical aspects. *Adv. Neurol. Sci. (Tokyo)*, **23**, 1048–59
2. Yokochi, M. (1979). Juvenile Parkinson's disease. 2. Pharmaco-kinetic study. *Adv. Neurol. Sci. (Tokyo)*, **23**, 1060–73
3. Narabayashi, H., Yokochi, M., Iizuka, R. and Nagatsu, T. (1986). Juvenile parkinsonism. In Vinken, P.J., Bruyn, G.W. and Klawans, H.L. (eds.) *Handbook of Clinical Neurology*, Vol. 5(49), pp. 153–65. (Amsterdam: Elsevier Science)
4. Brett, E.M. (1972). Juvenile parkinsonism. *Dev. Med. Child. Neurol.*, **14**, 391–402
5. Giovanniini, P., Piccolo, I., Genitrini, S., Soliveri, P., Girotti, F., Geminiani, G., Scigliano, G. and Caraceni, T. (1991). Early-onset Parkinson's disease. *Movement Disorders*, **6**, 36–42
6. Hunt, R. (1917). Progressive atrophy of the globus pallidus. *Brain*, **40**, 58–147
7. Martin, W.E., Resch, J.A. and Baker, A.B. (1971). Juvenile parkinsonism. *Arch. Neurol.*, **25**, 494–500
8. Mayer, J.M., Mikol, J., Haguenau, M., Dellanave, J. and Pépin, B. (1986). Familial juvenile parkinsonism with multiple systems degeneration. A clinicopathological study. *J. Neurol. Sci.*, **72**, 91–101
9. Nygaard, T.G. and Duvoisin, R.C. (1986). Hereditary dystonia-parkinsonism syndrome of juvenile onset. *Neurology*, **36**, 1424–8
10. Quinn, N., Critchley, P. and Marsden, C.D. (1987). Young onset Parkinson's disease. *Movement Disorders*, **2**, 73–91
11. Scott, R.M. and Brody, J.A. (1971). Benign early onset of Parkinson's disease: A syndrome distinct from classic postencephalitic parkinsonism. *Neurology*, **21**, 366–8
12. Yokochi, M. and Narabayashi, H. (1981). Clinical characteristics of juvenile parkinsonism. In Rose, F.C. and Capildeo, R. (eds.) *Research Progress in Parkinson's Disease*, pp. 35–9. (Kent, UK: Pitman Medical)

13. Yokochi, M., Narabayashi, H., Iizuka, R. and Nagatsu, T. (1984). Juvenile parkinsonism – Some clinical, pharmacological, and neuropathological aspects. In Hassler, R.G. and Christ, J.F. (eds.) *Advances in Neurology, Vol.* 40, pp. 407–13. (New York: Raven Press)
14. Gibb, W.R.G., Narabayashi, H., Yokochi, M., Iizuka, R. and Lees, A.J. (1991). New pathological observations in juvenile onset parkinsonism with dystonia. *Neurology*, **41**, 820–2
15. Narabayashi, H., Yokochi, F. and Nakajima, Y. (1984). Levodopa-induced dyskinesia and thalamotomy. *J. Neurol. Neurosurg. Psychiatr.*, **47**, 831–9
16. Gibb, W.R.G. and Lees, A.J. (1991). Anatomy, pigmentation, ventral and dorsal subpopulations of the substantia nigra, and differential cell death in Parkinson's disease. *J. Neurol. Neurosurg. Psychiatr.*, **54**, 388–96
17. Goto, S., Hirano, A., Matsumoto, S. (1989). Subdivisional involvement of nigrostriatal loop in idiopathic Parkinson's disease and striatonigral degeneration. *Ann. Neurol.*, **26**, 766–70
18. Narabayashi, H. (1980). Clinical analysis of akinesia. *J. Neural Transm.*, Suppl. 16, 129–36
19. Narabayashi, H. (1983). Pharmacological basis of akinesia in Parkinson's disease. *J. Neural Transm.*, Suppl. 19, 143–51
20. Narabayashi, H. (1990). Surgical treatment in the levodopa era. In Stern, G. (ed.) *Parkinson's Disease*, pp. 597–646. (London: Chapman and Hall)
21. Narabayashi, H. (1990). Clinical analysis of juvenile and classical parkinsonism and underlying pathophysiological mechanisms. Presented at the *XIth International Congress of Neuropathology*, September, Kyoto
22. Hughes, R.C., Polgar, J.G., Weightman, D. and Walton, J.N. (1971). L-dopa in parkinsonism and the influence of previous thalamotomy. *Br. Med. J.*, **1**, 7–13
23. Narabayashi, H., Kondo, T., Hayashi, A., Suzuki, T. and Nagatsu, T. (1981). L-threo-3,4-dihydroxyphenylserine treatment for akinesia and freezing of parkinsonism. *Proc. Japan Acad.*, (Ser.B), **57**, 351–4
24. Narabayashi, H., Kondo, T., Yokochi, F. and Nagatsu, T. (1986). Clinical effects of L-threo-3,4-dihydroxyphenyl serine in cases of parkinsonism and pure akinesia. In Yahr, M.D. and Bergmann, K.J. (eds.) *Advances in Neurology, Vol.* 45, pp. 593–602. (New York: Raven Press)
25. Narabayashi, H. and Kondo, T. (1987). Results of a double-blind study of L-threo-DOPS in parkinsonism. In Fahn, S., Marsden, C.D., Calne, D. and Goldstein, M. (eds.) *Recent Developments in Parkinson's Disease, Vol.* 2, pp. 279–91. (New Jersey: Macmillan Healthcare Information)

Index

age at onset
 childhood-onset parkinsonism 28
 childhood-onset torsion dystonia 28
 dopa-responsive dystonia 24, 28, 98, 183, 216
 early-onset parkinsonism 22, 53, 56, 68, 70, 183, 216
 hereditary progressive dystonia 3, 13, 46, 74–79, 81–84, 125
 juvenile-onset dopamine deficiency 221–227
 juvenile parkinsonism 12, 22, 38, 40, 46, 211
 Parkinsonism disease 22, 38, 68, 183
 parkinsonism-dystonia 46
 primary dystonia 65, 66
amantadine 52, 53
anticholinergic drugs
 action dystonia 8, 9
 childhood-onset parkinsonism 27
 childhood-onset torsion dystonia 27, 28
 dopa-responsive dystonia 26, 28, 62
 hereditary progressive dystonia 8, 88
 primary dystonia 117

Babinski sign 91, 165, 206, 213
biopterin
 dopa-responsive dystonia 24, 26
 hereditary progressive dystonia 11, 58, 111, 119, 126
 juvenile parkinsonism 133, 138
 parkinsonism, early onset 58
 primary dystonia 11, 118
bromocriptine
 dopa-responsive dystonia 26, 31
 dystonia–parkinsonism 61
 early-onset parkinsonism 52
 hereditary progressive dystonia 8, 89
 Parkinson disease 134, 136

carbamazine 26
carbidopa 25, 62
cerebral palsy 8
cerebrospinal fluid (CSF) profiles 117–123
 childhood-onset parkinsonism 31
 dopa-responsive dystonia 24, 26, 31
 hereditary progressive dystonia 5, 126
 juvenile parkinsonism 138
 Parkinson disease 118
 primary dystonia 117
 torsion dystonia 31

childhood-onset parkinsonism 21, 23, 27–31
childhood-onset torsion dystonia 27, 28
computerized tomography (CT) scanning
 early-onset parkinsonism 51, 57
 hereditary progressive dystonia 6, 9
 torsion dystonia 9, 144

decarboxylase inhibitors 6, 25
diurnal fluctuations
 dopa-responsive dystonia 10, 24, 25, 183
 dystonia–parkinsonism 61–70
 early-onset parkinsonism 51–59, 183
 hereditary progressive dystonia 3, 10, 13, 22, 73–79, 87, 143, 155
 juvenile parkinsonism 11, 12, 44, 139, 211
 parkinsonism–dystonia 183
dopa-responsive dystonia 21–35
 age of onset 25, 28, 98, 183, 218
 cases
  Japanese 24
  North American 23, 97–104
  others 24
 classification and history 21–23
 clinical observations 24–26

differential diagnosis 10, 27–31
drugs
anticholinergics 26, 28
bromocriptine 26, 31
carbabamazine 26
levodopa 22, 28
trihexyphenidyl 22, 25
inheritance 26, 97–103, 110
laboratory studies
biopterin metabolites 26
cerebrospinal metabolites 26
positron-emission tomography (PET) 24, 26, 31, 181–186, 217
sex hormones 102
drugs
amantadine 52, 53
anticholinergic 8, 9, 26–28
bromocriptine 8, 26, 31, 52, 89
carbamazine 26
carbidopa 25, 62
decarboxylase inhibitors 6, 25, 62
5-hydroxytryptophan 125–132
levodopa, *see under* levodopa
tetrahydrobiopterin 8
trihexyphenidyl 22, 25, 61
Duchenne muscular dystrophy 8
dystonia
bromocriptine 61
differential diagnosis 8
levodopa induced 192–194
neurochemistry 117–123
tetrahydrobiopterin 118
dystonia–parkinsonism
carbidopa 62
classification 68–70
clinical features 65
differential diagnosis 69
follow-up study 61–64
inheritance 65, 70
levodopa 62, 70
magnetic resonance imaging (MRI) 65–67

early-onset parkinsonism, *see under* parkinsonism of early onset

familial association, *see under* inheritance

gamma-aminobutyric acid (GABA) 175, 190

Hallervorden–Spatz disease 8, 212
hereditary progressive dystonia with marked diurnal fluctuation 3–19
age of onset 3, 13, 46, 74–79, 81–84, 125
associated diseases 89
bromocriptine 8, 89
cases 5, 89–91
cerebrospinal fluid profile 5, 126
clinical characteristics 3–5, 12, 13
clinical course 87–88
comparison to juvenile parkinsonism 37, 44
computerized tomography (CT) 6
differential diagnosis 8–12, 215–218
diurnal fluctuation 3, 5, 10, 13, 22, 73–79, 87, 143, 155
drugs
anticholinergic 8, 62
bromocriptine 8, 89
5-hydroxytryptophan 89, 125–132
levodopa 6, 13, 17, 73, 88, 155, 166
tetrahydrobiopterin 8, 88, 125–132
familial variation 73–96
inheritance 8, 15, 73–96, 107–113
Japanese study 73–96
magnetic resonance imaging (MRI) 6, 9, 144
neurological symptoms 86, 87
pathophysiology 13–15
polysomnography 5, 9, 143–146
positron-emission tomography (PET) 5, 6
saccadic deficits 159–177
sex ratio 81
sleep abnormalities 155
symptoms at onset 84–86
treatment 6–8, 88, 89
tyrosine hydroxylase 13, 107–113
hereditary spastic paraplegia 8
homovanillic acid (HVA)
dopa-responsive dystonia 24, 26
hereditary progressive dystonia 119, 126
juvenile parkinsonism 138
primary dystonia 117
Huntington disease 146, 148, 153, 154
5-hydroxyindolacetic acid (5HIAA)
dopa-responsive dystonia 26
hereditary progressive dystonia 5, 89, 119, 126

juvenile parkinsonism 139

inheritance
dopa-responsive dystonia 97–103, 110
dystonia-parkinsonism 61, 70
early-onset parkinsonism 56
hereditary progressive dystonia 8, 15, 73–96, 107–113
Japanese familial study 73–96
juvenile Parkinson disease 40
North American study 97–103
Parkinson disease 38, 40, 103
parkinsonism-dystonia 70
torsion dystonia 107

juvenile onset dopamine deficiency 219–225
juvenile parkinsonism 37–48
age of onset 12, 22, 38, 40, 46, 211, 219
cases 205–211
cerebrospinal fluid profile 138
classification 45, 212–214
clinical features 12, 211
comparison with hereditary progressive dystonia 44
definition 38
differential diagnosis 11, 215–218
epidemiology 38–41
incidence 40
inheritance 40
levodopa 12, 38, 41
Lewy bodies 41–43
magnetic resonance imaging (MRI) 65
pallidal posture 205–215
pathobiochemistry 133
pathology 41
subgroups 43
symptoms 12, 41
tetrahydrobiopterin 133, 136–139

levodopa
childhood-onset parkinsonism 28
childhood-onset torsion dystonia 28
dopa-responsive dystonia 22, 28
dystonia-parkinsonism 66
early-onset parkinsonism 52, 56
hereditary progressive dystonia 6, 13, 17, 73, 88, 155, 166
juvenile parkinsonism 12, 38, 41
Parkinson disease 22, 92, 117
primary dystonia 117
saccadic deficits 166
torsion dystonia 9
Lewy bodies 22, 42, 221
linkage analysis 107–113

magnetic resonance imaging (MRI)
early-onset parkinsonism 51
hereditary progressive dystonia 6, 9, 144
juvenile parkinsonism 65
Parkinson disease 143
primary dystonia 65–67
3-methoxy-4-hydroxyphenylglycol (MHPG) 5, 9
1-methyl-4-phenyl-1,2,3,6-tetrahydropyridine (MPTP) 15, 173–175, 192, 195

neopterin
dopa-responsive dystonia 26
hereditary progressive dystonia 119
primary dystonia 118
neuroimaging 181–186
nigrostriatal dopamine deficiency 219–225

Parkinson disease
age of onset 22, 38, 68, 183
bromocriptine 134, 136
cerebrospinal fluid profile 118
definition 221
differential diagnosis 15, 37, 45, 51, 56, 73, 173, 213, 221
dopamine agonists 192
hemi 143, 148
inheritance 38, 40, 103
juvenile 11, 22, 65, 215–218, 220
levodopa 22, 92, 117
Lewy bodies 42
magnetic resonance imaging (MRI) 143
pars compacta 66
polysomnography 146, 148
saccadic deficits 173, 174
tetrahydrobiopterin 136, 139
tyrosine hydroxylase activity 139
voluntary saccade 5
parkinsonism
alternative treatments 194, 195
dopamine agonist therapies 192

neurosurgery 195
pharmacology 196–199
role of subthalamic nucleus 189–201
subthalamic–pallidal axis
tetrahydrobiopterin 134–136
parkinsonism, childhood onset 27
parkinsonism-dystonia 46, 70, 183
parkinsonism, early onset 51–59
bromocriptine 52
characteristics 56–58
comparative study 54–56
computerized tomography (CT) 51, 57
differential diagnosis 51, 57
inheritance 56
levodopa 52, 56
long-term follow-up 52–54
magnetic resonance imaging (MRI) 51
pregnancy and menstruation 58
parkinsonism, juvenile, *see under* juvenile parkinsonism
polysomnography 143–158
hereditary progressive dystonia 5, 9, 143–146
other movement disorders 146–151
pathophysiological considerations 151–155
position-emission tomography (PET) 181–186
dopa-responsive dystonia 24, 26, 31, 181–186, 217
hereditary progressive dystonia 5, 6
parkinsonism-dystonia 183–186
young-onset parkinsonism 183–186

saccadic deficits 159–177
assessment of brain function 167–172
behavioral paradigms 161
calibration 163
clinical observations 165
dopamine 174, 175
eye movement analysis 161
levodopa 166
Parkinson disease 173, 174
quantitative analysis 166
recording procedures 160
visually and memory guided 166
sex hormones 58, 102
Southern blot analysis 108
subthalamic nucleus and parkinsonism 189–201

tetrahydrobiopterin
hereditary progressive dystonia 8, 88, 125–132
juvenile parkinsonism 133, 136–139
Parkinson disease 134–136
primary dystonia 118
trihexyphenidyl
dopa-responsive dystonia 22, 25
dystonia parkinsonism 61
early-onset parkinsonism 61
primary dystonia 81
tyrosine hydroxylase gene 107–113

Westphal phenomenon 4, 15
Wilson disease 8, 212

young-onset parkinsonism, *see under* early-onset